Chair Massage

Kishwaukee College Library
21193 Malta Road
Malta, IL 60150-9699

Chair Massage

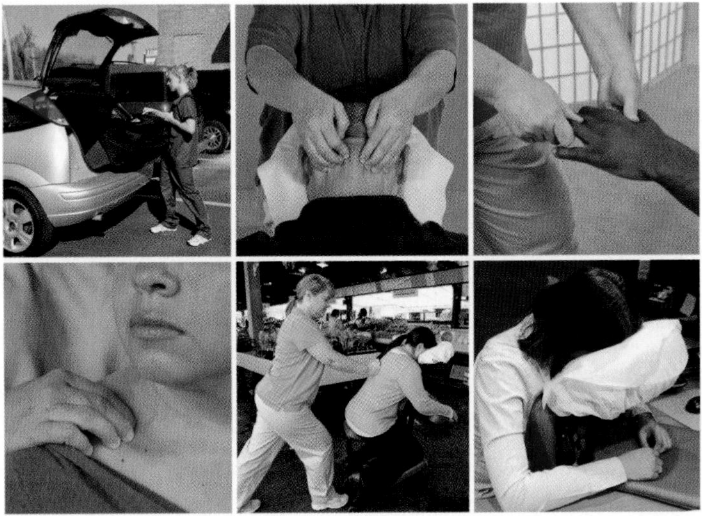

Patricia M. Holland, MC, LMT
Instructor and Dean of Students
Cortiva Institute–Tucson
Owner and Practitioner, Mindful Touch Therapeutic Massage
Tucson, Arizona

Sandra K. Anderson, BA, LMT, ABT, NCTMB
Co-Owner and Practitioner, Tucson Touch Therapies
Treatment Center and Education Center
Tucson, Arizona

MOSBY

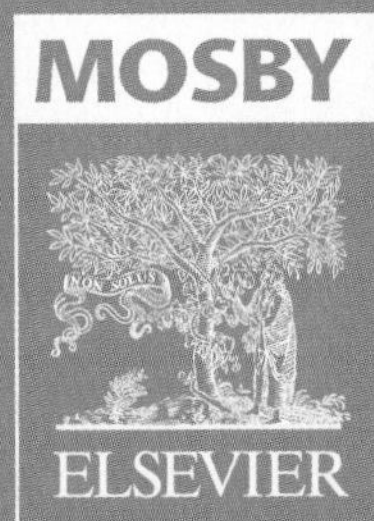

ELSEVIER

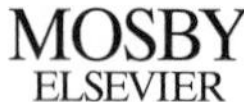

3251 Riverport Lane
St. Louis, Missouri 63043

CHAIR MASSAGE ISBN: 978-0-323-02559-1

Copyright © 2011 by Mosby, Inc., an affiliate of Elsevier Inc.

No part of this publication may be reproduced or transmitted in any form or by any means, electronic or mechanical, including photocopying, recording, or any information storage and retrieval system, without permission in writing from the publisher. Details on how to seek permission, further information about the Publisher's permissions policies and our arrangements with organizations such as the Copyright Clearance Center and the Copyright Licensing Agency, can be found at our website: www.elsevier.com/permissions.

This book and the individual contributions contained in it are protected under copyright by the Publisher, (other than may be noted herein).

Notices

Knowledge and best practice in this field are constantly changing. As new research and experience broaden our understanding, changes in research methods, professional practices, or medical treatment may become necessary.

Practitioners and researchers must always rely on their own experience and knowledge in evaluating and using any information, methods, compounds, or experiments described herein. In using such information or methods they should be mindful of their own safety and the safety of others, including parties for whom they have a professional responsibility.

With respect to any drug or pharmaceutical products identified, readers are advised to check the most current information provided (i) on procedures featured or (ii) by the manufacturer of each product to be administered, to verify the recommended dose or formula, the method and duration of administration, and contraindications. It is the responsibility of practitioners, relying on their own experience and knowledge of their patients, to make diagnoses, to determine dosages and the best treatment for each individual patient, and to take all appropriate safety precautions.

To the fullest extent of the law, neither the Publisher nor the authors, contributors, or editors, assume any liability for any injury and/or damage to persons or property as a matter of products liability, negligence or otherwise, or from any use or operation of any methods, products, instructions, or ideas contained in the material herein.

ISBN: 978-0-323-02559-1

Vice President and Publisher: Linda Duncan
Senior Editor: Kellie White
Senior Developmental Editor: Jennifer Watrous
Publishing Services Manager: Patricia Tannian
Senior Project Manager: Sharon Corell
Design Direction: Kim Denando

Working together to grow libraries in developing countries
www.elsevier.com | www.bookaid.org | www.sabre.org
ELSEVIER BOOK AID International Sabre Foundation

Printed in China
Last digit is the print number: 9 8 7 6 5 4 3 2 1

To my parents, Rosemary and Jerry Holland. I wish you were here.
To Laurie Anne Calland. Gratitude abounds.
Patricia M. Holland

To David Kent Anderson, my husband and my best friend. He started his professional bodywork career doing chair massage.
Sandra K. Anderson

Reviewers

John Combe, LMT, NCTMB
Therapist/Educator, Combe's Wellness Center
The Dalles, Oregon

Matt B. Isolampi, CNMT, LMT, MMT
Massage Therapy Instructor, Westside Tech, OCPS
Winter Garden, Florida

Michaela Johnson, BA, LMT
Practitioner, Massage, Shiatsu, and CranioSacral Therapies
Tucson, Arizona

Scott G. Rayburn, CMT, LMT
D.B.A. Waterock Massage Therapy
Massage Therapy Instructor
Central State Massage Academy
Oklahoma City, Oklahoma

Leslie Rosenthal, NCTMB, BSW, MPH
Owner, Massage Works
Long Beach, California

Joe Smelser, BA, LMP
Instructor, Cortiva Institute–Seattle
Seattle, Washington

Preface

Chair massage is a type of bodywork that is performed in an upright, portable massage chair with the client fully clothed and without using any lotions or oils. The focus of the treatment is usually on the shoulders, neck, upper back, head, and arms, which are typically the areas of the body that hold the most stress and tension. This type of massage is seen as a stress-reliever and is often available in the workplace and in many other public settings, such as conferences, fairs, shops, health food stores, sporting events, and more. These treatments take as little as 15 minutes and can be an excellent source of extra income for the bodywork practitioner. In addition to generating revenue, practitioners can also use chair massage as a method for networking and bringing in clientele for their practices involving bodywork on a massage table or futon (such as shiatsu and Thai massage). Some practitioners even incorporate chair massage with their work on the table or futon. Clients who are extremely sore from injury or have conditions that are more easily addressed in the seated position (such as certain shoulder issues) can benefit greatly from chair massage. From the chair, the practitioner can ease the client onto the massage table or futon to continue the session.

Chair Massage is important to the massage profession because it promotes seated massage as a viable modality that can stand on its own merits. The text provides practical and useful information for bodywork practitioners to design, implement, and maintain a successful chair massage business or to complement an existing practice. *Chair Massage* was written because the authors wanted to pass on the knowledge and skills that have proved to be successful for them in their bodywork practices and educational endeavors. The intention for this book is to present information in a format that will educate, inspire, and prepare readers to integrate seated massage into an existing practice, create a new business exclusively with seated massage, or develop classes to educate practitioners in this modality.

WHO WILL BENEFIT FROM THIS BOOK?

Chair Massage grew out of a need for a concise, comprehensive textbook that can be used for many bodywork programs. It is designed as a teaching aid for massage therapists and other bodywork practitioners who are learning chair massage, either as a continuing education course or within a primary bodywork program. Chair massage is a topic of great interest to students and professionals because of the potential for extra dollars and the networking opportunities it provides.

Chair Massage was designed with the flexibility of the modality of chair massage in mind. The text includes both Western bodywork techniques, such as those from massage therapy, and the channels and points from traditional Chinese medicine. In addition, a section on various other energy modalities is included so that practitioners can see how some or all of these can be incorporated into chair massage treatments. Practitioners of Asian bodywork techniques will find *Chair Massage* as useful as massage therapists will.

The book can be adapted to courses of varying lengths and depths and encompasses all the elements necessary to teach students and professionals to become successful chair massage practitioners. Simple techniques are shown first, and as students master these, additional techniques designed for skill enhancement are presented. Good body mechanics is emphasized throughout. Chapters dealing with the business, communication, and ethics of chair massage are also included. All of this information will serve students and professionals well in their bodywork practices, helping them to prevent injury and ensuring career longevity.

ORGANIZATION

Chair Massage leads the reader, in a logical progression, through the information necessary to effectively perform seated massage for both relaxation and therapeutic purposes, to ways to succeed in adding this modality to his or her practice. The first chapter gives the history of seated massage, differences between seated and table massage, and benefits of seated massage for both the practitioner and the client. This background gives the reader a context for the importance and usefulness of this modality. A chapter on equipment, logistics, and hygiene is designed to give readers an understanding of what is needed to perform seated massage and what they can expect when traveling to various locations. A sequence of photos exhibiting how to properly move the massage chair in and out of a vehicle is shown in this chapter so practitioners do not harm themselves when transporting equipment.

Moving into the practice of chair massage, a chapter with a basic routine with foundational techniques is included. It also has an anatomy and kinesiology review, palpation considerations, ways to adjust pressure to meet each client's needs, proper body mechanics, and cautionary sites. The next chapter covers specific body area routines for shoulders, arms and hands, the low back, and the neck and scalp, including an anatomy and kinesiology review and cautionary sites for each of the regions, and a segment on how to close the treatment session. The detailed section addressing techniques for low back is important because of the high incidence of low-back pain in clients. The segment on closing the session completes the reader's view of the experience of a chair massage session from start to finish.

The next chapter on additional techniques and adaptations gives the reader more tools to work with, such as special considerations for working on clients in wheelchairs. Elderly clients, or those with certain injuries and physical limitations, may be unable to hoist themselves onto a massage table or lie down on a futon, or they may be uncomfortable lying on a massage table or futon. For these clients, chair massage may be most practical. In addition, chair massage techniques can be easily applied to people in wheelchairs or anyone seated in an ordinary chair or bed and propped with pillows. This chapter explains all of these concepts and includes a special photo sequence shot at an assisted-living home that provides real-life examples.

Included in each of the technique chapters is a brief description of traditional Chinese medicine pressure points that practitioners may find useful when working with various client conditions. Knowledge of certain traditional Chinese medicine points along channels gives the therapist more techniques to use during chair massage treatments, thus increasing the ability to create client-centered treatments. Practitioners who are unfamiliar with traditional Chinese medicine can still locate and press points along channels to help alleviate certain client conditions. Practitioners who are familiar with traditional Chinese medicine will find it unnecessary to refer to another text immediately before and during sessions. The reader can simply flip to the appendix for a refresher, rather than searching for the pertinent information in various Asian bodywork and acupuncture texts, where chair massage is either not briefly synthesized or not included.

The book ends with two important chapters dealing with business aspects of seated massage, communications, and ethics. The business chapter provides marketing methods and practical considerations, such as setting fees and drawing up contracts. The ethics chapter explains the importance of boundaries and ethical presentation of self as a professional massage therapist and bodyworker and communicating effectively with clients.

Appendixes on traditional Chinese medicine, including information about one of the foundations of chair massage, and more kinesiology and anatomy review provide brief, yet thorough, additional resources in the book itself, making separate books on those topics unnecessary for students studying chair massage.

DISTINCTIVE FEATURES

Because chair massage is essentially learned by doing, it is important that students have relevant, readily applicable learning material. These features include the following:

- More than 450 full-color illustrations, most of them photos, clearly showing techniques, concepts, traditional Chinese medicine channels, and points
- Brief descriptions of tsubos (points on traditional Chinese medicine channels) that practitioners may find useful to press for various client conditions
- Special boxes called Perspectives, which contain interviews with practitioners who offer chair massage and can give practical advice from a business standpoint
- Sample dialogues for use during sessions
- Sample business forms and templates
- A brief anatomy and kinesiology review in each of the technique chapters
- An appendix dedicated to anatomy and kinesiology
- An appendix dedicated to a review of traditional Chinese medicine channels
- Resources for chair massage supplies and information

LEARNING AIDS

The following enhance student understanding and retention of the material:

- Outlines and Objectives at the beginning of each chapter help students organize their study material.
- Key Terms are identified and defined at the beginning of each chapter.
- Boxes with tips are provided in each of the technique protocols.
- Study questions at the end of each chapter encourage critical thinking through multiple choice, fill-in-the-blank, and short-answer questions.
- Activities at the end of each chapter assist students in deepening their understanding of the material and help them prepare for practicing professional chair massage.
- Glossary of terms in the back of the book provides a quick reference for the terms that appear throughout the text.

ANCILLARIES

An Evolve website for instructors accompanies this book and includes the following:

- A test bank of multiple choice and fill-in-the-blank questions in ExamView format
- An image collection of all images in the book in PowerPoint and JPG formats
- An instructor's resource manual with lesson plans, teaching objectives, and answers to short-answer questions from the book

NOTE TO THE STUDENT

Students will find the practical and comprehensive nature of this book to be beneficial in their process of learning a new skill or fine-tuning an existing skill. They are encouraged to be curious, creative, and courageous as they explore this modality and while finding a place for it in their work. Students are also encouraged to pay attention to their body mechanics, their palpation skills, and the therapeutic relationship with their clients. All of these are part of developing a meaningful chair massage practice.

About the Authors

Patricia M. Holland, MC, LMT

Patricia has two certifications from the prestigious Desert Institute of the Healing Arts (now Cortiva Institute–Tucson) in Tucson, Arizona: 1000-hour massage therapy certification (1993), and 100-hour Thai massage certification (2004). She also holds an MC in counseling and a BS in speech communications. Patricia has been teaching since 1993, including 13 years as the instructor of the Onsite Chair Massage elective at the Desert Institute of the Healing Arts. Currently, in addition to her duties as dean of students at Cortiva Institute–Tucson, she teaches Foundations of Massage and Introduction to Clinic, and coordinates the school's Community Service Outreach Program. Both Introduction to Clinic and the Outreach Program involve teaching students chair massage, and the Outreach Program involves supervision of students as they provide chair massage to the public. Patricia also owns a private massage therapy practice–Mindful Touch Therapeutic Massage–in Tucson.

Sandra K. Anderson, BA, LMT, ABT, NCTMB

Most of Sandra's professional career has been as a bodyworker and a bodywork educator. After graduating with a BA in biology from Ithaca College in Ithaca, New York, she worked in various settings until she moved to Tucson, Arizona, and discovered massage therapy. She graduated from the Desert Institute of the Healing Arts in Tucson (now Cortiva Institute–Tucson) with certification in massage therapy, 1991; in shiatsu, 1999; and in Thai massage, 2002. During this time she also built her private practice and taught at the Desert Institute. For 12 years she instructed students, primarily in the areas of anatomy, physiology, kinesiology, pathology, and shiatsu techniques, and supervised massage and shiatsu student clinics. She was chair of the anatomy and physiology department for 5 years, during which time she developed curriculum and teaching training courses. For 5 years she served as chair of the Examination Committee for the National Certification Board for Therapeutic Massage and Bodywork. She is author of *The Practice of Shiatsu* from Elsevier, and co-author, with Ann Mihina, of *Natural Spa and Hydrotherapy* from Pearson Prentice Hall. Sandra and her husband, David, own Tucson Touch Therapies, a bodywork treatment center in Tucson. In addition to seeing clients, Sandra creates and conducts continuing education workshops.

Acknowledgments

Sandra Anderson, friend, co-author, and taskmaster. Her trust in Patricia's wisdom and process means the world to her.

Patricia Holland, friend, co-author, and listener. Her willingness to go on this book journey with Sandra means everything to her.

Margaret Avery Moon, Jill Bielawski, and Jeff Schadel, Patricia's mentors and instructors at the Desert Institute of the Healing Arts, who introduced Patricia to chair massage and taught her its value and potential.

Norma Ray, networker extraordinaire and friend, who taught Patricia the ropes of coordinating and supervising community service events.

Jan Schwartz, for her generosity in loaning Patricia her beautiful purple Oakworks Portal Pro when she started her chair massage practice.

David Lovitt and his amazing staff at D.M. Lovitt Insurance Agency, for their years of supporting Patricia's business as well as teaching her the fine art of client retention.

Sue Kauffman, a great sister of Sandra's and a great friend.

Michaela Johnson, a good consultant and friend of Sandra's. Her discerning gift for words helped move the chapters in the right direction.

Carol Davis and **Annie Gordon**, great friends who keep Sandra grounded and sane.

The practitioners and staff at Tucson Touch Therapies, all of whom are dedicated professionals who make coming to work wonderful for Sandra.

All the students whom we've taught through the years—the classroom is our greatest teacher.

Jim Visser, for his excellent photography. He made us look good!

All of the businesses where our location shots were taken—we enjoyed visiting each of these places.

Kaldi's Coffee House, in Kirkwood, Missouri.

Kirkwood Farmer's Market, in Kirkwood, Missouri.

Pudd'nhead Books, in Webster Groves, Missouri. A special thank you to **Nikki Furrer**.

St. Agnes Home, in Kirkwood, Missouri. A special thank you to **Diane Strutynski**.

All the models in the photographs, who did an excellent job.

Allison Leonard, who graciously lifted a massage chair in and out of a car approximately 1000 times on an icy cold morning.

Valerie Gibson, Scott Gravagna, and Kate Meyer, massage therapists who gave us a bit of a break during the photo shoot and performed some of the techniques and exercises.

Models **Samantha Bryan, Julia Dummitt, Ochuko Ekpere, April Falast, Sheetal Gattani, Dottie Gray, Kim Levy, Brendan Sullivan**, and **Jennifer Whitmer**.

Kellie White, an extraordinary editor who is a joy to work with.

Jennifer Watrous, an incredible developmental editor. Her attention to detail and affable style make the creation of a book a lot of fun.

Contents

What Is Chair Massage?

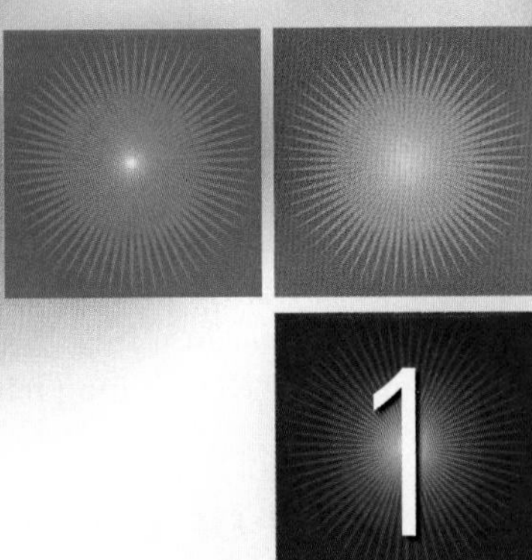

OBJECTIVES

Upon completion of this chapter, the reader will have the information necessary to do the following:

1. Discuss why practitioners and clients would find chair massage appealing.
2. Briefly describe the equipment and techniques used in chair massage.
3. Explain the commonalities and differences between chair and table massage.
4. Delineate the history of chair massage.
5. List and explain the benefits of chair massage from both a Western and an Asian point of view.
6. Outline the advantages chair massage gives the practitioner.
7. List optimal locations for performing chair massage.

KEY TERMS

Anma (amma)	Medical gymnastics
Anmo	Polarity
An wu	Onsite massage
Aura	Qi
Ayurveda	Reiki
Chair massage	Seated massage
Chakras	Sen
Channels (meridians)	Shiatsu
Do-in (tao-yinn)	Swedish Movement Cure (Treatment)
Healing Touch	Thai massage
Jin Shin Jyutsu	Tuina
Ling system	
Marmas	

WHY CHOOSE CHAIR MASSAGE?

Seated massage, also known as **chair massage** and **onsite massage**, is a versatile modality. It is called chair massage because it is most often performed on clients who are seated on specially designed portable massage chairs, although regular sitting chairs can also be used. Because the clients are sitting, chair massage is sometimes called seated massage. The term *onsite massage* is used because part of the versatility of these treatments is that they can be brought to a wide variety of client locations instead of clients traveling to one location to receive massage. The terms *chair massage, seated massage,* and *onsite massage* will all be used interchangeably in this text.

The versatility of chair massage is also demonstrated by the multitude of professional and personal opportunities it creates for practitioners. It can enhance a menu of services, increase clientele, provide a framework for marketing, stimulate creativity and diversity in treatments to help prevent burnout, offer a chance to work in a variety of settings, and present ways to meet and experience many different types of clients.

Chair massage can be appealing to clients and prospective clients for a range of reasons. People who have never experienced massage may feel more comfortable receiving chair massage because they would not need to disrobe; the treatments are performed through the recipient's clothing. Modesty is preserved while the client is still able to receive a therapeutic treatment. Because of this benefit, chair massage can also be an introduction to safe touch for survivors of trauma.

Because chair massage treatments usually last 10 to 30 minutes, those who do not have a lot of free time or a lot of disposable income can still reap the benefits of receiving bodywork. The practitioner usually travels to client locations, such as a workplace, athletic event, or street fair, so clients do not need to take extra time to travel to the massage location; it is already where they are. For those on limited incomes, chair massage can be an excellent way to receive bodywork without much expense. Because treatment times are usually shorter than they are for table massage treatments, fees are less.

Massage chairs are useful for working with clients who are more comfortable sitting upright such as a woman who is pregnant or clients who find it difficult to get on and off a massage table. For example, people who are elderly or those with physical limitations may find sitting on a massage chair much more appealing. Techniques can even be adapted to clients who are in wheelchairs or just sitting at their desks or sitting on kitchen chairs.

As with other types of massage, chair massage is a nice complement to other health practices because the benefits of massage dovetail nicely with the benefits of such practices as exercise, yoga, meditation, and proper nutrition. Receiving chair massage can inspire clients to receive longer treatments on a massage table, thus giving them increased opportunities to experience health and well-being. Even if clients choose not to do this but decide to continue receiving chair massage, an initial chair massage can still be the beginning of the client's long relationship with bodywork.

OVERVIEW OF CHAIR MASSAGE

Equipment and Techniques

Whereas chair massage can be considered simply massage therapy that is performed with the client sitting on a chair, it can also be thought of as a distinct bodywork modality. Although it is true that most techniques used in performing table massage can be easily adapted to performing chair massage, there are other factors that make chair massage unique.

As previously discussed, the equipment used for chair massage is a specially designed massage chair (Figure 1-1). A straight-backed sitting chair can also be used. The client sits on the chair backward and leans forward on the chair back while propped by pillows or other support bolsters (Figure 1-2). Yet another option is a specially designed tabletop massage support (Figure 1-3).

For hygiene purposes, a single use cover is placed on the face cradle (face rest) of massage chairs and tabletop massage supports. Coverings on pillows or other supports are used for only one client; the practitioner needs to have enough for each client scheduled during the treatment times. Also, the practitioner needs to have hand cleaner and paper towels readily available for use in between each client.

The client remains fully clothed while receiving chair massage. If certain articles of clothing or other items the client is wearing would hamper the effects of the massage, they should be removed. For example, jackets, ties, large rings, bracelets, watches, bulky necklaces, dangling earrings, and, sometimes, shoes should all be removed before

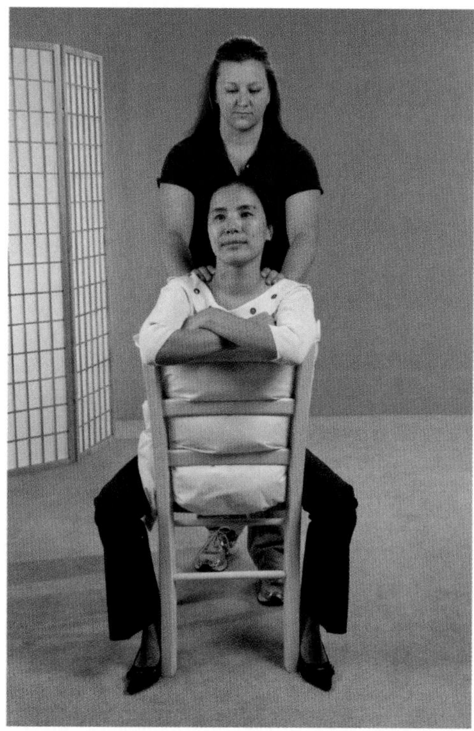

FIGURE 1-2 Client on a straight-backed chair, leaning forward.

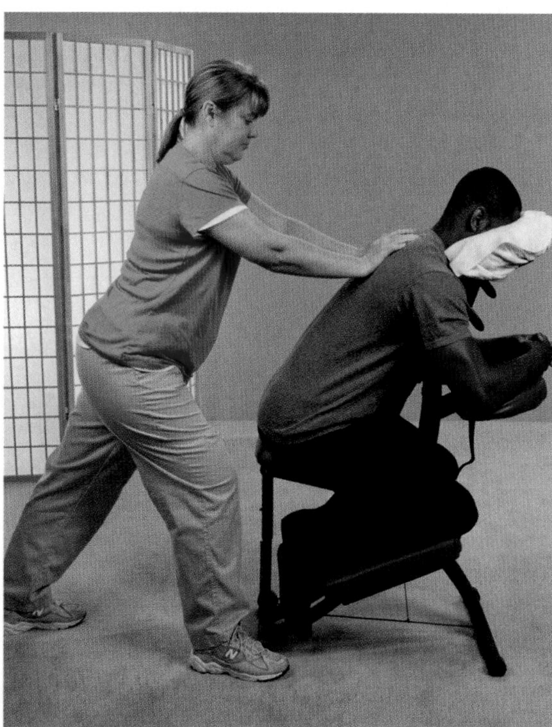

FIGURE 1-1 Client on a massage chair.

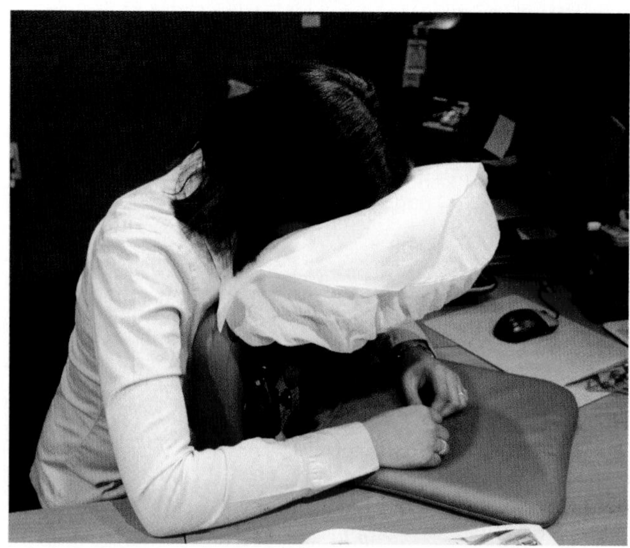

FIGURE 1-3 Client using a tabletop massage support.

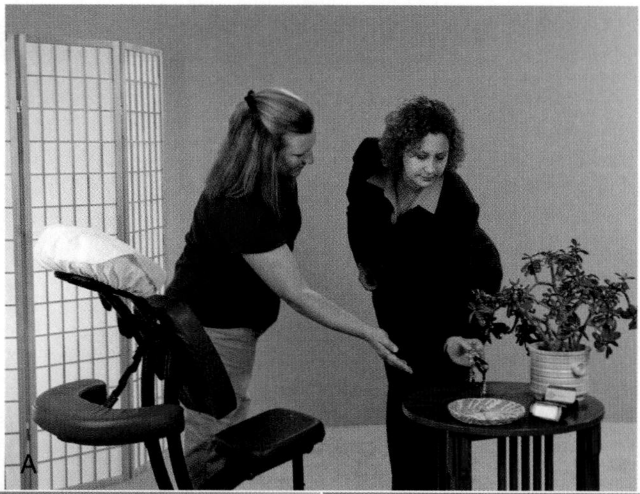

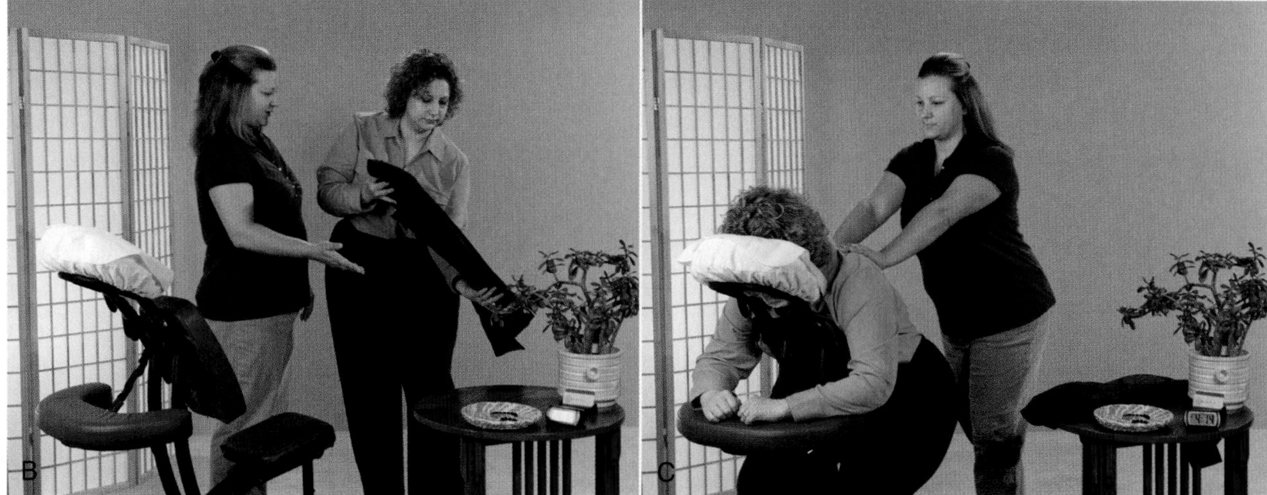

FIGURE 1-4 **A,** Client removes jewelry. **B,** Client removes jacket. **C,** Client receives chair massage with jacket and large jewelry placed nearby.

the start of the treatment (Figures 1-4 A, B, and C). This ensures the comfort of the client and enables the practitioner to effectively perform the treatment.

Because the client remains fully clothed, no lubricant is usually used during the performance of chair massage techniques. However, some practitioners may choose to massage the client's arms, hands, upper back, and possibly the legs using lubricant during certain treatments. When applied skillfully, the following techniques are just as therapeutically beneficial to clients receiving chair massage as they are to those receiving table massage:

- Palm pressure
- Finger and thumb pressure
- Deep gliding
- Kneading
- Compressions
- Elbow and forearm pressure
- Friction
- Range-of-motion techniques
- Stretches
- Percussion

Other modalities lend themselves to being performed on sitting clients as well. For example, **Healing Touch**, **polarity**, **reiki**, **Jin Shin Jyutsu**, and other energy balancing therapies can be carried out as complete treatments, or aspects of them can be incorporated along with massage techniques during the session (Box 1-1). The same is true for Asian bodywork modalities such as **shiatsu**, **Thai massage**, and **tuina**. In fact, as is discussed in the section titled "History of Chair Massage," Asian bodywork techniques form part of the foundation of chair massage techniques.

Even though a typical chair massage treatment can last anywhere from 10 to 30 minutes, shorter and longer treatments can also be performed. Almost the entire body can be addressed by chair massage: the head and scalp; neck and shoulders; upper, middle, and lower back; forearms; wrists and hands; and the upper and lower legs. The upper chest and abdomen can even be addressed by having the client turn around and sit backward on the massage chair. In the case of a straight-backed chair, the client would turn and face forward, or if the client were leaning forward onto a table or desk, the client would simply sit up.

BOX 1-1 Other Modalities

Healing Touch

Healing Touch is energy therapy, endorsed by the American Holistic Nurses Association, which supports healing on physical, emotional, mental, and spiritual levels. The practitioner assesses for energetic disturbances and selects appropriate techniques to clear, integrate, and energize the human energy field, also referred to as the person's **aura**, and balance the person's energy centers, or **chakras**. Chakras refer to wheel-like vortices, which, according to the traditional medicine of India, **Ayurveda**, are areas of the body that receive the energy of the universe then assimilate and express it as the person's life force. Healing Touch is performed on a massage table with the client fully clothed and shoes removed. The practitioner uses light touch on the client's body and the surrounding human energy field. Healing Touch facilitates overall wellness including pain management, relaxation, stress reduction, assisting the client in healing relationships with self and others, and relief from depression, anxiety, and grief. Clients are also offered suggestions for creating and maintaining balance in their energy field.

More information can be found at the website for Healing Touch International, Inc., www.healingtouchinternational.org.

Polarity

Polarity therapy is based on the concept of the human energy field and was developed by Dr. Randolph Stone in the 1940s. It is derived from Ayurveda, and it incorporates cranial osteopathic manipulation techniques and work on pressure points along channels of energy flow (see shiatsu). The theory of polarity includes that the universal source of life energy is in constant motion, but it is polarized into positive and negative movements around a neutral core; this is also how the energy occurs in the human body. Health occurs when the energy flows smoothly and in an uninterrupted fashion. Practitioners palpate and release energy blockages through the application of touch in varying depths of pressure, specifically on **marmas**, which are energetic points located near the surface of the body. There are about 100 marmas, and they are concentrated at the junctions of muscles and tendons, in the joints, and along blood vessels. Polarity is performed on a massage table with the client fully clothed and shoes removed. The practitioner's right hand is considered to be polarized positive and sends energy to the client, and the left hand is considered to be polarized negative and receives energy from the client. By placing both hands on the client at the same time, in various places on the client's body, the practitioner seeks to balance the client's energy. Practitioners also educate clients on how to perform specific exercises, positive thinking, and proper nutrition to balance their energetic flows.

More information can be found at the website for the American Polarity Therapy Association, www.polaritytherapy.org.

Reiki

Reiki was developed in 1922 by Mikao Usui in Japan. It involves channeling a powerful healing energy that unlocks the inner flow of vital energy within the client. Reiki restores, normalizes, balances, and aligns the energy centers (chakras) and channels (see shiatsu) of the body. This can result in the physical, mental, emotional, and spiritual transformation of the client. The client remains fully clothed on a massage table, and the practitioner either places the hands lightly on the client's body or a few inches above. The hands are usually kept still for three to five minutes before moving to the next position. Overall, the hand positions usually give a general coverage of the head, the front and back of the torso, the knees, and the feet. Some practitioners use a determined set of between 12 and 20 hand positions; other practitioners use their intuition as a guide for their hand placement.

More information can be found at the website for the International Center for Reiki Training, www.reiki.org.

Jin Shin Jyutsu

Jin Shin Jyutsu is an ancient Asian healing art that focuses on balancing the life energy of the body. It was passed down from generation to generation for thousands of years and, by the early 1900s, had fallen into disuse until Master Jiro Murai of Japan developed an interest in it. He passed his information onto Mary Burmeister, who brought it the United States in the 1950s. The principles of Jin Shin Jyutsu involve 26 safety energy locks along energy pathways of the body. When the pathways become blocked, there is local disruption of the energy flow, which can lead, eventually, to an imbalance in the entire pathway. The client lies on a massage table fully clothed, except for shoes. The practitioner holds the client's energy locks in various combinations by placing the fingertips on the client. The result is harmonization and restoration of the client's energy flows.

More information can be found at the website for Jin Shin Jyutsu, Inc., www.jsjinc.net.

Shiatsu

Shiatsu is a Japanese form of bodywork that came to prominence through the efforts of Tokujiro Namikoshi, who founded the Clinic of Pressure Therapy in Hokkaido, Japan, in 1925. Shiatsu is based on the same principles as acupuncture, which is part of traditional Chinese medicine. These principles include the concept that the body's energy, or **qi**, moves along specific pathways called **meridians** or **channels** through the body. The qi can become blocked or deficient in certain areas, resulting in pain, discomfort, or other problems. The practitioner uses various shiatsu techniques, such as hand and finger pressure, gentle stretches, and joint mobilizations, within the client's tolerance to correct imbalances in qi and increase body and mind awareness. Shiatsu is usually performed on a futon on the floor, without the use of oils or lotions, with the client wearing loose-fitting clothes and no shoes.

More information can be found at the website for the American Organization for Bodywork Therapies of Asia, www.aobta.org.

Thai Massage

Thai massage, also known as yoga massage, Thai yoga, and ancient massage, has its roots in Ayurvedic medicine and yoga from India and has also has been influenced by traditional Chinese medicine. Its principles include an understanding of the flow of energy along lines or **Sen** throughout the body. The practitioner uses pressure, stretches, joint range-of-motion techniques, and specific work along the Sen to stimulate the body's smooth flow of energy, loosen tight areas, and give an overall feeling of well-being. Thai massage is usually performed on a futon on the floor, without the use of oils or lotions, with the client wearing loose-fitting clothes and no shoes.

BOX 1-1 Other Modalities—cont'd

More information can be found at the website for the Ancient Massage Foundation, www.ancientmassage.com.

Tuina

Tuina (also spelled Tui-Na), which means push (tui) and grasp (na), is a Chinese form of bodywork that has been carried down through the ages. It is based on the principles of, and is included as part of the formal training for practitioners of traditional Chinese medicine. Tuina is usually performed on a futon on the floor, without the use of oils or lotions, with the client wearing loose-fitting clothes and no shoes. The practitioner brings balance to the client's body by kneading, pressing, rolling, shaking, and stretching it, as well as by using range-of-motion techniques and pressing points along the channel. These techniques open blocked energy channels and encourage the smooth flow of qi, alleviating various conditions the client is experiencing.

More information can be found at the website for the World Tui-Na Association, www.tui-na.com.

Each treatment is, of course, designed around the client's needs. For example, the client may choose to have an overall, relaxing treatment during which as many areas of the body as possible are addressed during the treatment time frame, or the focus may be on one specific area of the body such as the neck, shoulders, or back. Perhaps the client requests a soothing and relaxing treatment, or a more vigorous, stimulating treatment is needed. Many techniques can be used in seated massage, giving practitioners the ability to create client-centered treatments. These techniques are presented in Chapters 3, 4, and 5.

Chair Massage versus Table Massage

Although chair massage has some similarities to massage performed on a massage table, such as in some of the techniques performed and the therapeutic benefits, there are also some differences. For example, as previously discussed, treatment lengths are usually shorter for chair massage, and the equipment is different. Chair massage can be performed in more locations than can table massage, such as public areas, as clients remain fully clothed.

Practitioners should keep in mind that some potential clients do not like to be so visible to others while receiving a treatment. They may feel like everyone is watching them and therefore will choose not to receive a treatment in a public setting. It is possible to address this issue by investing in structures that can create a sense of privacy such as shoji screens or kiosks. Another option is for the practitioner to make arrangements with the client to perform the treatment in a setting that is comfortable for both of them.

Because treatment lengths are shorter, a chair massage may be less costly than a table massage. To give practitioners an idea of the differences and similarities between chair massage and table massage, Table 1-1 compares the two.

HISTORY OF CHAIR MASSAGE

Early Beginnings

Human beings have a natural need to touch each other. Touch is used as a form of recognition, as a means of communication, as part of play, and to care for and comfort others. Unfortunately, touch is also used as a means to control and harm others. But throughout the ages, when touch comes from a place of sincere desire to help others, it has the ability to help facilitate health and wellness within another person. This is the foundation of all forms of massage therapy and bodywork.

There is no doubt that massage and other types of bodywork were practiced long before written history. As time went on, techniques were invented, modified, and refined so that when history began to be recorded, many systems of bodywork, some simple, some sophisticated, had been in use for quite some time. There are many examples of how bodywork has been represented, and many of these portray people being massaged in seated positions. For example, ancient Egyptian scrolls illustrate different types of massage techniques with recipients who are sitting as shown in Figure 1-5. Statues depicting seated Thai massage positions can be found in the gardens of Wat Pho (also known by the traditional name Phra Chetuphon Temple), the royal temple in Bangkok built in the 1500s (Figure 1-6). An Indian painting dating from the early 1700s shows a maharaja's wife being massaged while sitting on a cushioned footstool.

Additionally, many forms of Asian bodywork, such as **anma** (an early form of Japanese massage), shiatsu, Thai massage, and tuina have portions of treatment protocols with the client seated. Because of this history, it is easy to see how chair massage at least partially developed from Asian bodywork, especially the Japanese modality shiatsu. In fact, seated massage can be thought of a hybrid of shiatsu and Western massage therapy.

Asian Bodywork

Ancient Asian practitioners developed a view of the human body as both a physical and energetic being. Although they had awareness of muscles, bones, blood, and organ functions, an awareness remarkably similar in many respects to current Western science, they also determined that energy, called qi, flows in channels in specific areas of the body and connects with the organs. Each person's qi also connects with, and is nourished by, the qi of the universe.

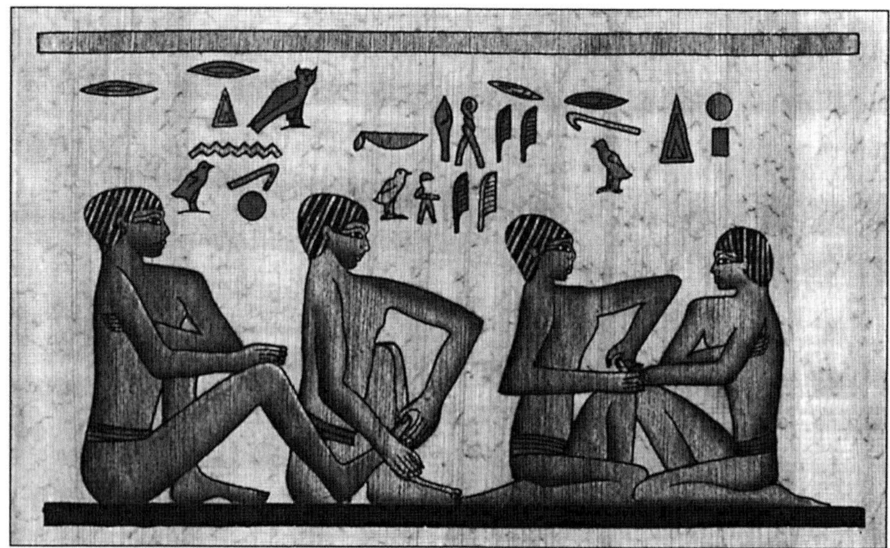

FIGURE 1-5 Modern-day rendering of a circa 2330 BCE wall painting in the tomb of Akhmahor (Ankh-mahor), at Saqqara, known as the physician's tomb, showing massage being given with recipients seated. (From Calvert RN: The history of massage: an illustrated survey from around the world. Rochester, Vt., 2002, Healing Arts Press.)

TABLE 1-1 Chair Massage versus Table Massage

	Chair Massage	Table Massage
Locations	Public area or private treatment space	Private treatment space
Equipment	Specially designed massage chair, straight-backed chair, or tabletop massage support	Massage table, bolsters
Supplies	Face cradle (face rest) covers, hand cleaner, paper towels	Face cradle (face rest) covers, linens, lubricant, hand cleaner
Level of client dress	Fully clothed	Either clothing removed and draped by linens or fully clothed
Techniques used	Palm pressure Finger and thumb pressure Kneading Compression Elbow and forearm pressure Friction Deep gliding strokes Range-of-motion techniques Stretches Percussion Energy techniques Asian bodywork techniques	Palm pressure Finger and thumb pressure Kneading Compression Elbow and forearm pressure Friction Gliding strokes Range-of-motion techniques Stretches Percussion Energy techniques Asian bodywork techniques
Usual treatment length	10-30 minutes	30, 60, or 90 minutes
Cost	$1 per minute*	$60 per hour**

*$1 per minute = $60 per hour; however most chair massage treatments are shorter than table massage treatments so the cost of individual treatments would be lower.
**National average according to the American Massage Therapy Association, 2008, Massage Therapy Industry Fact Sheet. Retrieved October 7, 2008, from http://amtamassage.org/news/MTIndustryFactSheet.html#2.

Arguably, the oldest known forms of bodywork, **an wu** and **do-in** (or **tao-yinn**), developed in China more than 5000 years ago. An wu, a healing and spiritual practice, used techniques similar to Western massage: pressing, gliding, stretching, and percussing the body. The practitioner used his thumbs, fingers, forearms, elbows, knees, and feet on the client's body to release muscle tension and on the points along the channels of qi to stimulate its flow. Do-in (or tao-yinn) was similar to yoga. It is still practiced today as a combination of exercises for channel stretching, breathing, qi flow, and self-massage.

Gradually, an wu came to be known as **anmo**, which began to become a popular medical treatment. By the fifth century CE, anmo had developed into a more sophisticated

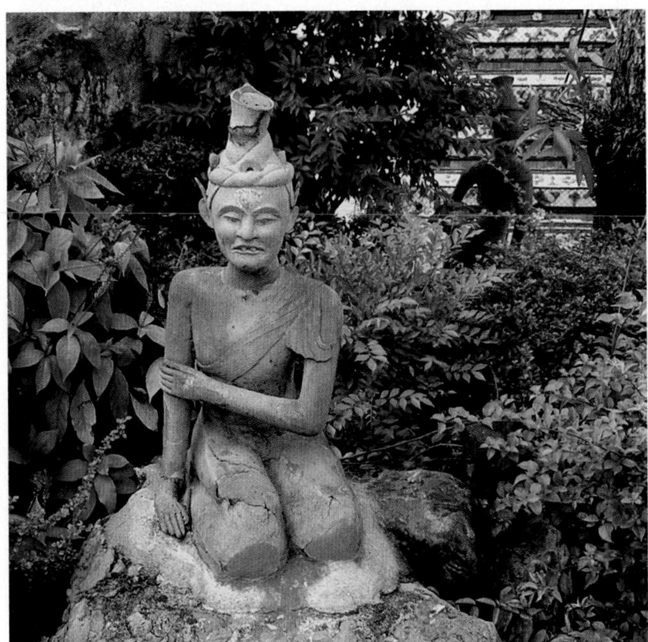

FIGURE 1-6 One of the carved statues in the gardens of Wat Pho, the Royal Monastery in Bangkok, that depict specific techniques of Thai massage. (Photo © John Glines.)

system of theory, diagnosis, and treatment, and, during this time, anmo spread to other Asian countries such as Korea, Japan, and India. By the 1300s, however, anmo had become less popular but did become focused on musculoskeletal disorders and injuries, which laid the foundations for the practice of medical massage called **tuina**.

Acupuncture gradually took over in China as the primary form of medicine. As physicians palpated and massaged patients, they pinpointed the effects of pressing certain locations on qi channels. They also discovered that more specific pressure on these more specific locations had greater effect; these locations were narrowed down into points. Over time, pressure on these points became more and more precise until needles were finally inserted into the points, giving birth to acupuncture. The points were named, numbered, and classified in the system that is still used today and is shown in Figure 1-7. However, palpatory and massage techniques (anmo, tuina, and do-in) remained important foundational techniques that physicians had to master before they were allowed to progress to using needles. Even though acupuncture became the primary form of healing, massaging and pressing along the channels, and points on the channels, remained widespread.

Shiatsu

Because of geographic proximity, Japanese culture and Chinese culture have had a close relationship. During the sixth century CE, acupuncture and anmo were readily infused into Japanese culture. As the years progressed, acupuncture remained relatively the same as when it arrived in Japan. However, anmo was modified and refined and gradually evolved into anma, or amma, a uniquely Japanese bodywork.

During the Edo period (1602-1868), anma reached its height of popularity. New anma techniques and methods were developed, schools were established, and texts were written to teach anma. Also during this time, Japan was closed to the West because European culture was seen as a threat to traditional Japanese culture. All cultural and political contact with the outside world was forbidden. The Dutch were the only people allowed to trade with Japan, and contact was limited to a small island off Nagasaki. The Dutch introduced Western medical information, including anatomy and physiology, to the Japanese; the Japanese taught anma and acupuncture to the Dutch, who took these modalities back to Europe.

Not many professions were open to the visually impaired during this period. Anma was available to them, however, with the reasoning that the blind had greater touch sensitivity. It was also seen as a form of welfare. Soon anma was being practiced mostly by blind practitioners and, because being visually impaired limited the education these practitioners were able to receive throughout this period, their medical knowledge fell below that of the physicians and herbalists. Much technical and clinical wisdom was lost, and anma became known as being useful only for relaxation or as healthcare only used by the poor.

The Meiji period of Japan (1868-1912) saw an overhaul of the Japanese government. It was re-created in a Western framework, and changes were instigated to make Japanese society more like Western society. Western medicine dominated, and the therapeutic value of anma and Asian medicine was rejected. During this time, Western massage therapy was introduced to Japan.

By the beginning of the 1900s, anma had lost so much credibility that it was considered shady employment. The practitioners of true art of anma sought a way to distinguish themselves from less reputable practitioners; a new name for this bodywork was needed. In 1919, Tamai Tempaku published a book called *Shiatsu Ho*, which translates to "finger pressure method." This text united anma with Western anatomy and physiology concepts, and shiatsu practitioners started implementing Western bodywork techniques from Western chiropractic medicine and massage therapy.

In 1925, the Shiatsu Therapists' Association was formed to promote shiatsu as a legitimate profession. In 1955, the Japanese government officially recognized shiatsu as a part of anma; this was the first legal sanction of shiatsu. Shiatsu was officially recognized by Japan as a separate and distinct modality in 1957, the same year the Japan Shiatsu School, opened in 1940 by Tokujiro Namikoshi (1905-2000), was licensed by the minister of Health and Welfare. Because of the influence of renowned Japanese practitioners and teachers such as Namikoshi, his son Toru, and Shizuto Masunaga (1925-1981), shiatsu has spread well beyond Japan's borders.

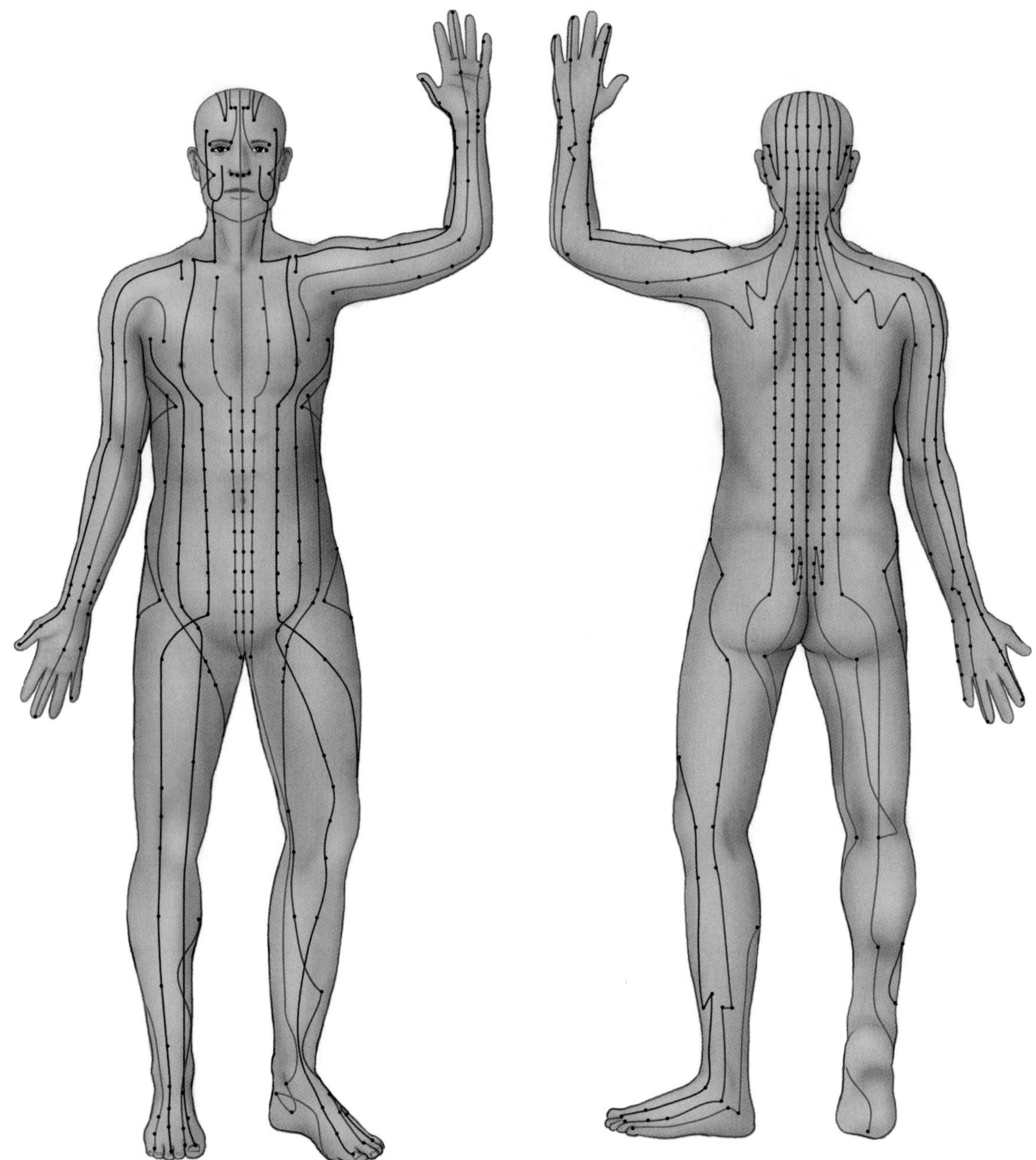

FIGURE 1-7 The major channels and points. (From Anderson S: *The practice of shiatsu.* St. Louis, 2008, Mosby.)

Western Massage Therapy

Modern Western massage therapy has its roots in ancient Greek and Roman culture. The earliest written records about massage include those of the Greek physician Hippocrates (460-377 BCE), who described the use of oils with massage for various healing benefits. Galen (129-199 CE) was a Greek physician who also performed and wrote about massage methods of the time, which included the use of rubbing the body to treat disease and injuries. He eventually traveled to Rome and helped introduce these methods to the Romans.

The Roman Empire lasted approximately 500 years, collapsing around 476 CE, which was the start of the Middle Ages. During this time, the knowledge of ancient healing techniques, including massage, was almost lost entirely. Fortunately, monks in certain monasteries throughout Europe dedicated themselves to collecting, studying, and reproducing classic Greek and Roman texts. Additionally, Islamic physicians in the Middle East kept the knowledge of massage techniques alive. In fact, during the Middle Ages of Europe, Islamic countries became the centers of classical western scientific thought. As a result, the knowledge of

Aristotle, Hippocrates, Galen, and others survives to this day.

In the 16th century, as part of the Renaissance, there was a renovation of medicine. The writings of the ancient Greeks and Romans resurfaced, and their methods of treating injuries and disease generated renewed interest in manual healing techniques, including massage. Massage started to become popular again.

Modern Massage Therapy

Per Henrik Ling (1776-1839) was a prominent figure in the development of modern massage therapy. He did *not* invent what is sometimes called Swedish massage; instead, he can be credited with helping develop it into a more formal treatment process. After learning the massage techniques of the time and adopting other methods once he found them effective, he created a coherent program that used active and passive movements and massage, and he called it **medical gymnastics**. Gymnastics, in this case, meant exercises. They are the basis of today's massage therapies and movement therapies.

Ling was, among other things, a fencing master. As such, he studied movements of the body and came to understand that human body movements were not only for locomotion to perform work but also had the capability of strengthening and healing the body. His system of medical gymnastics included muscle strengthening through active movements and certain techniques applied by the practitioner. The active movements were those the client performed themselves, such as certain types of weight lifting. The practitioner applied techniques to the client's body such as long, compressive motions along muscles, gliding and kneading strokes, friction, percussion, and vibration—in short, what is now widely known as Swedish massage.

In 1813, Ling founded the Royal Institute of Gymnastics in Stockholm, and physicians from Germany, Austria, Russia, and England learned Ling's techniques and spread his teachings throughout their countries. By the late 1800s, people from all over the world, including those from the United States who were interested in natural healing methods, traveled to the institute to learn medical gymnastics, also known by then as the **Ling system**, **Swedish movement cure**, and the **Swedish movement treatment**.

In 1851, Dr. Mathias Roth published the first English-language book on the Swedish movement cure in England, *The Prevention and Cure of Many Chronic Diseases by Movements.* In it, he described the types of equipment that would have been found in a medical gymnast's clinic; all of these were designed for the client to be in proper positions for the active movements and to receive techniques from the practitioner. The equipment included rectangular tables, ladders, rings on which clients would hang from their arms, and chairs and stools. This is the first written record of the modern era showing seated massage. An example can be seen in Figure 1-8.

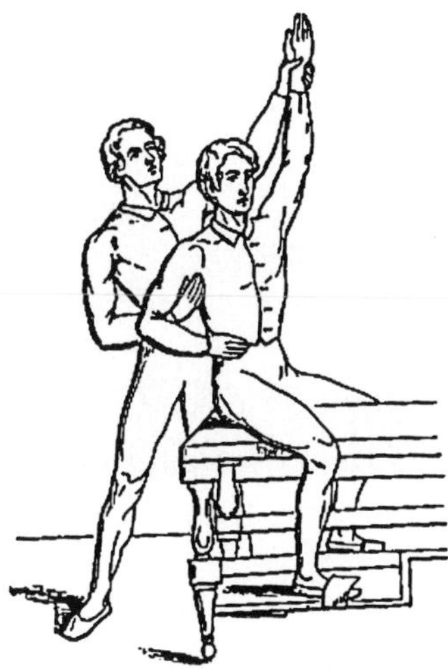

FIGURE 1-8 Practitioner performing a technique of the Swedish movement cure on a seated client. (From Roth M: *The prevention and cure of many chronic diseases by movements.* London, John Churchill, 1851.)

Dr. George H. Taylor, a physician from New York, had developed his own system of therapy using exercises, then learned of institutions in Stockholm, Sweden, that were using similar methods. In 1856, his younger brother, Dr. Charles F. Taylor, went to England to receive training in Ling's techniques from Dr. Roth, with George following in 1858 to learn the techniques for himself. In 1858, both Drs. Taylor brought the Ling system to the United States, and Dr. George H. Taylor wrote the first American text on the Ling system, *Exposition of the Swedish Movement Cure,* in 1860, and founded the Remedial Hygienic Institute in New York, which was devoted to the practice of the Swedish movement cure.

By the late 1800s, recipients of the Swedish movement cure would be placed in any of several different positions such as lying on a table, hanging by their arms from a raised bar, kneeling down, or sitting in a chair, all depending on what part of their bodies they were exercising or receiving massage, as shown in Figures 1-9 and 1-10.

The Swedish movements and massage techniques gradually became more and more accepted as useful treatments. Before long, they were being performed in private offices, rest homes, and sanitariums. Sanitariums, forerunners of today's destination spas, were fashionable in the late 1800s and early 1900s. Possibly the most well known in the United States was the Battle Creek Sanitarium run by Dr. John Harvey Kellogg (1852-1943). Dr. Kellogg coined the term *sanitarium,* and developed the "Battle Creek Idea" that good health and fitness were the result of good diet, exercise, correct posture, fresh air, and proper rest. Wealthy patrons traveled to Battle Creek and stayed for several weeks to restore their bodies to health. While there, they participated in exercise, ate strictly regimented diets, and received hydrotherapy treatments as well as massage. In 1895, Dr. Kellogg wrote *The Art of Massage,* which describes effects of massage,

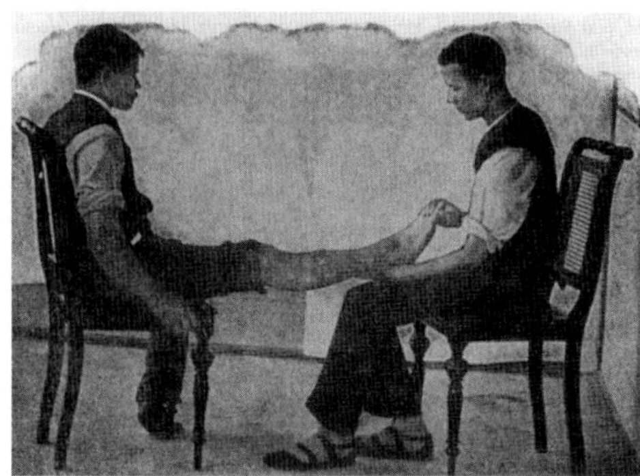

FIGURE 1-9 Seated client receiving passive ankle range of motion. (From Bilz FE: *The natural method of healing.* Leipzeig, FE Bilz, 1898.)

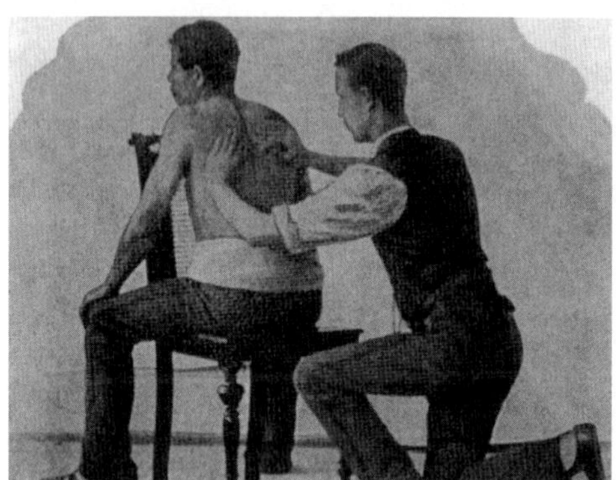

FIGURE 1-10 Client sitting backward on a chair while receiving back massage. (From Bilz FE: *The natural method of healing.* Leipzeig, FE Bilz, 1898.)

techniques and how to perform them, as well as contraindications based on what was known about human anatomy and physiology at the time. This is considered the first actual text on massage therapy.

Massage was also incorporated into nursing. Englishwoman Florence Nightingale (1820-1910) is credited with creating modern nursing practices. She emphasized that fresh air, sunlight, warmth, quietness, hygiene, and proper diet were essential to health and healing. Massage training was included in her school for nurses. By the time of Nightingale's death, nurses routinely received training in and practiced massage therapy on patients.

By World War I (1914-1919), the Swedish movements and massage were integral parts of medical treatment. Injured soldiers received table massage as well as chair massage in special massage units of army hospitals. This practice continued after the war as well. These were the foundations of physical therapy, which began to be a more formalized healthcare profession in the 1920s.

Starting in approximately the 1950s, as Western scientific healing methods, including diagnostic tools, medications, and surgery, were being discovered and developed, natural approaches to healing, including massage therapy, were used less and less in mainstream medicine. Massage for medical reasons was shifted to physical therapy. Physical therapists continued using massage as part of treatment programs up until about the 1960s when more sophisticated physical therapy instruments and equipment started to be developed. Emphasis shifted from hands-on treatment of clients to equipment-based treatment.

Massage therapy was still being practiced throughout this time, but it came to be regarded as only for relaxation and pampering. As such, massages were usually performed on massage tables, with unclothed clients lying under draping, and with the application of lubricant to the client's skin, and clients had to travel to specific locations to receive massage, such as a spa or private office. By the 1980s, massage performed with the client in the seated position had all but disappeared.

David Palmer

Massage Magazine has called David Palmer the father of contemporary chair massage. As was discussed previously, massage has been given to clients who are in the seated position since the beginning of massage and bodywork. David Palmer, then, did not invent chair massage. He did, however, see a unique opportunity to bring the benefits of massage therapy to many groups of people and then created a method to bring it to them. In the process, he fostered a new branch of massage therapy and assisted practitioners and clients in seeing massage therapy in a new way.

Before becoming a bodywork practitioner in 1980, Palmer had worked in the nonprofit sector. He attended the Amma Institute in San Francisco, California, where he learned traditional Japanese massage, and in 1982 he became the director. At this time, massage therapy had not yet become as widely accepted as it is today, and many practitioners could not make a living doing bodywork exclusively. Palmer realized that if massage could be offered to clients in a more affordable and convenient manner, then more people could benefit from its therapeutic effects, and more practitioners would be able to do the work they love.

Palmer recognized that the techniques he had learned and practiced could be adapted to create acupressure-based bodywork for clients in the seated position. He also realized that because these treatments were performed on clothed clients, they could be more appealing to people who might otherwise be reluctant to receive massage, thus blending old techniques with a new perspective. He began offering training in seated massage at the Amma Institute in 1982, and in 1983 he and colleague Stephen Pizzella started a business employing practitioners trained in his seated massage program.

The year 1984 saw the first major endorsement of seated massage when Palmer and Pizzella contracted with Apple Computer in Silicon Valley, California, which eventually led to several practitioners providing more than 300 seated massage treatments each week to its employees. This association generated media exposure about chair massage. Chair massage became so popular, Palmer recognized that a specialized chair that was not only portable but provided support for the client and enabled the practitioner to give a more therapeutic treatment while using good body mechanics was needed. He enlisted the help of cabinetmaker Serge Bouyssou and, also in 1984, the first massage chair was designed. In 1986, Living Earth Crafts made the first production version of Palmer's and Bouyssou's massage chair. It was made mostly of wood and weighed a staggering 28 pounds, but it became the template for the proper way to position clients in almost all subsequent massage chairs.

With the first downturn in the personal computer industry in 1985, Apple was forced to lay off many employees, and Palmer and Pizzella's account ended. Palmer sold his portion of their business to Pizzella in 1986, then founded TouchPro Institute to teach chair massage through continuing education classes, and in 1989 Palmer stepped down as director of the Amma Institute to devote himself fully to the development of the chair massage profession. Since then he has written several books and many articles on the business of chair massage, and he has played a role in the development of current massage therapy marketing methods.

Figure 1-11 is a timeline that shows a brief history of the events that led to the development of modern seated massage.

BENEFITS OF SEATED MASSAGE

Research has shown that just 20 minutes of chair massage can contribute to a client's health and well-being. It is a myth that chair massage is not therapeutic. For example, just the stress relief, or relaxation, alone can help reduce blood pressure, decrease insomnia, and support the immune system. Additionally, clients in massage chairs can be positioned so that deeper, more specific work can be done on tight muscles, such as those in the shoulder, back, and neck. Stretches and joint range-of-motion techniques can help increase flexibility.

Receiving chair massage, as with table massage, has emotional and psychological benefits as well. These benefits include a decrease in anxiety, a feeling of being uplifted, mental clarity, an overall feeling of being more centered and focused, and, perhaps, more body awareness. Some of these effects are immediate, because clients usually feel better right away, and if clients receive chair massage regularly, some of these effects will be quite long lasting.

Benefits of Chair Massage in the Workplace

Human beings are designed to move. Muscles contract and pull on bones, which act as levers to create movement at joints. People who do physical work for a living certainly make use of their muscles and joint movements. Sometimes, though, if they do not use their bodies properly, muscle and joint tightness and injury can occur. Examples of these injuries include muscle strain, herniated disks, generalized low back pain, and repetitive stress injuries, such as carpal tunnel syndrome and tendonitis. Any and all of these conditions can result in lower productivity by the people experiencing them or time off from work to recover, which, in turn, can cost businesses millions of dollars each year.

According to the Bureau of Labor Statistics (BLS), U.S. Department of Labor, "Musculoskeletal disorders (MSDs), often referred to as ergonomic injuries, are injuries or illnesses affecting the connective tissues of the body such as muscles, nerves, tendons, joints, cartilage, or spinal discs. Injuries or disorders caused by slips, trips, falls, motor vehicle accidents, or similar incidents are not MSDs." (A more detailed definition can be found on the BLS website at www.bls.gov/iif/oshdef.htm.)

The BLS also breaks MSDs down into different categories and delineates how many of cases of MSDs result in time away from work. The statistics for 2007 are shown in Table 1-2.

Almost 30% of all workplace injuries requiring time away from work are due to MSDs, and the average number of workdays lost because of these conditions is nine days. Shoulder injuries, half of which are due to overexertion, require up to an average of 18 days for recuperation, whereas injuries from repetitive motion are the conditions resulting in the most required days away from work—up to 20 days.

On the other hand, those who have less labor-intensive jobs such as those involving sitting for long periods of time as happens at a desk in a cubicle, or standing for long periods of time in one small area as happens at a check-out stand in a grocery store, can also experience muscle and joint tightness, and even injury. This can be due to long-term, static positions of muscles (either in shortened or lengthened positions), lack of movement at joints (causing a decrease in flexibility), and an overall decrease in muscle strength. Some examples of conditions people may experience include tight neck and shoulder muscles, tension headaches, tight or painful low backs, and decreased joint range of motion.

Chair massage, then, can be helpful to people in many occupations. Whether one's job is more physical or more mental, there are some overall benefits that everyone can experience:

- Stress reduction
- Increased mental clarity
- Increased blood flow and joint flexibility and decreased muscle tension; this can alleviate the effects of sitting for long periods of time or doing repetitive tasks (such as filing or working on an assembly line)
- Relief from headaches and sore muscles
- Providing a healthy break; people can feel rejuvenated and ready to go back to work
- Improved immune function; provides resistance to colds, flu, and stress-related diseases and disorders

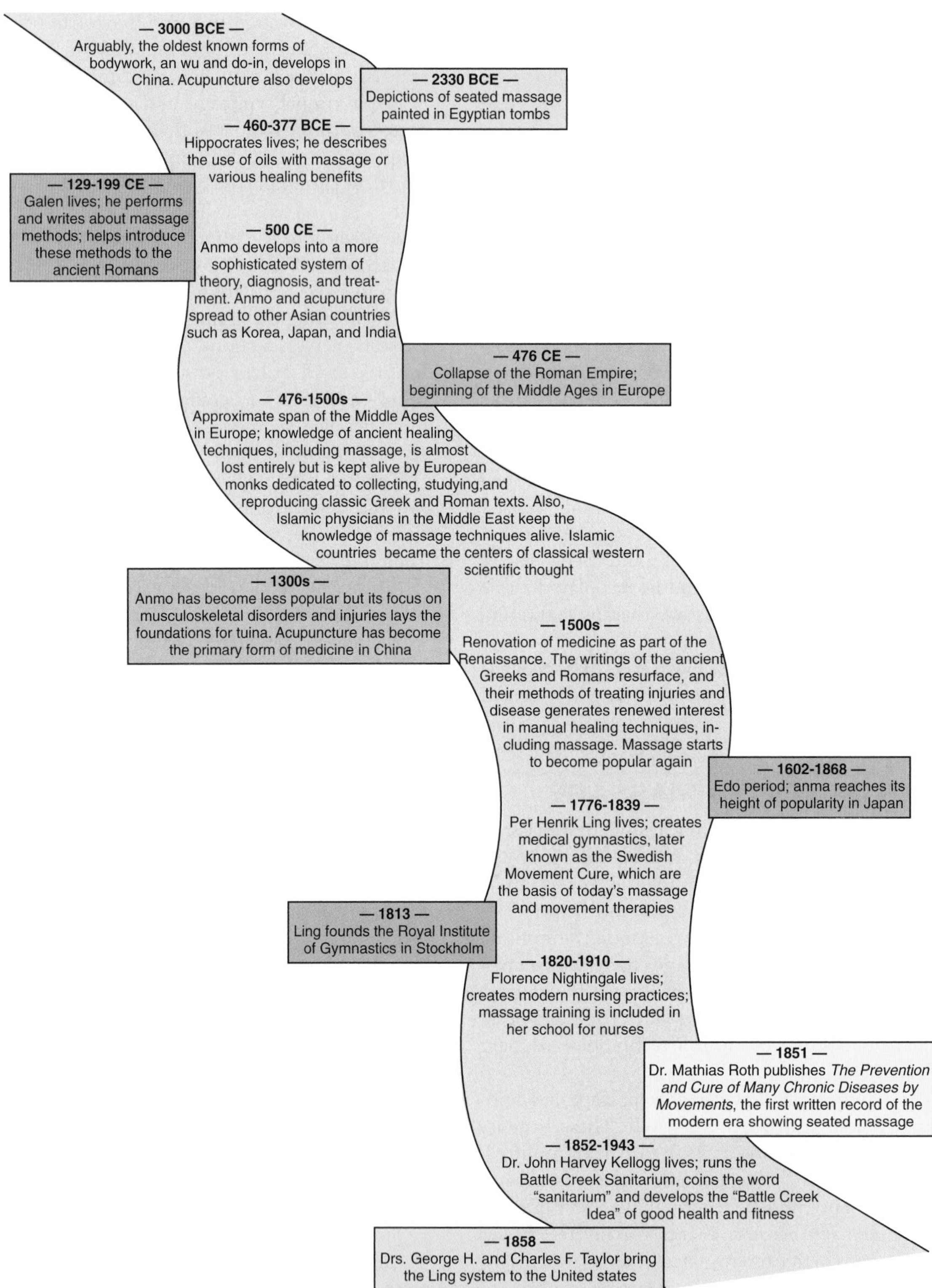

FIGURE 1-11 Timeline of the events that led to the development of modern seated massage.

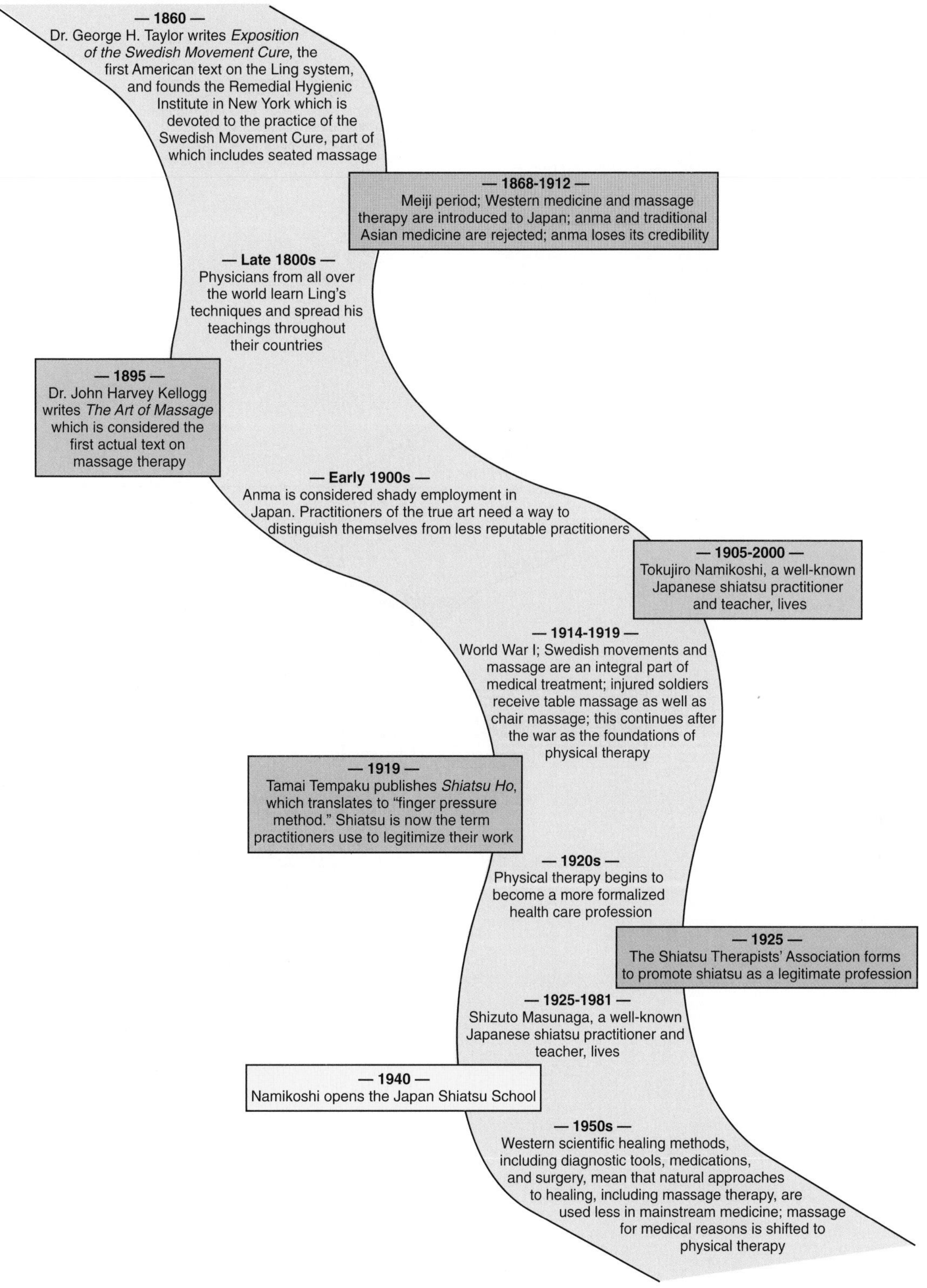

FIGURE 1-11, cont'd.

Continued

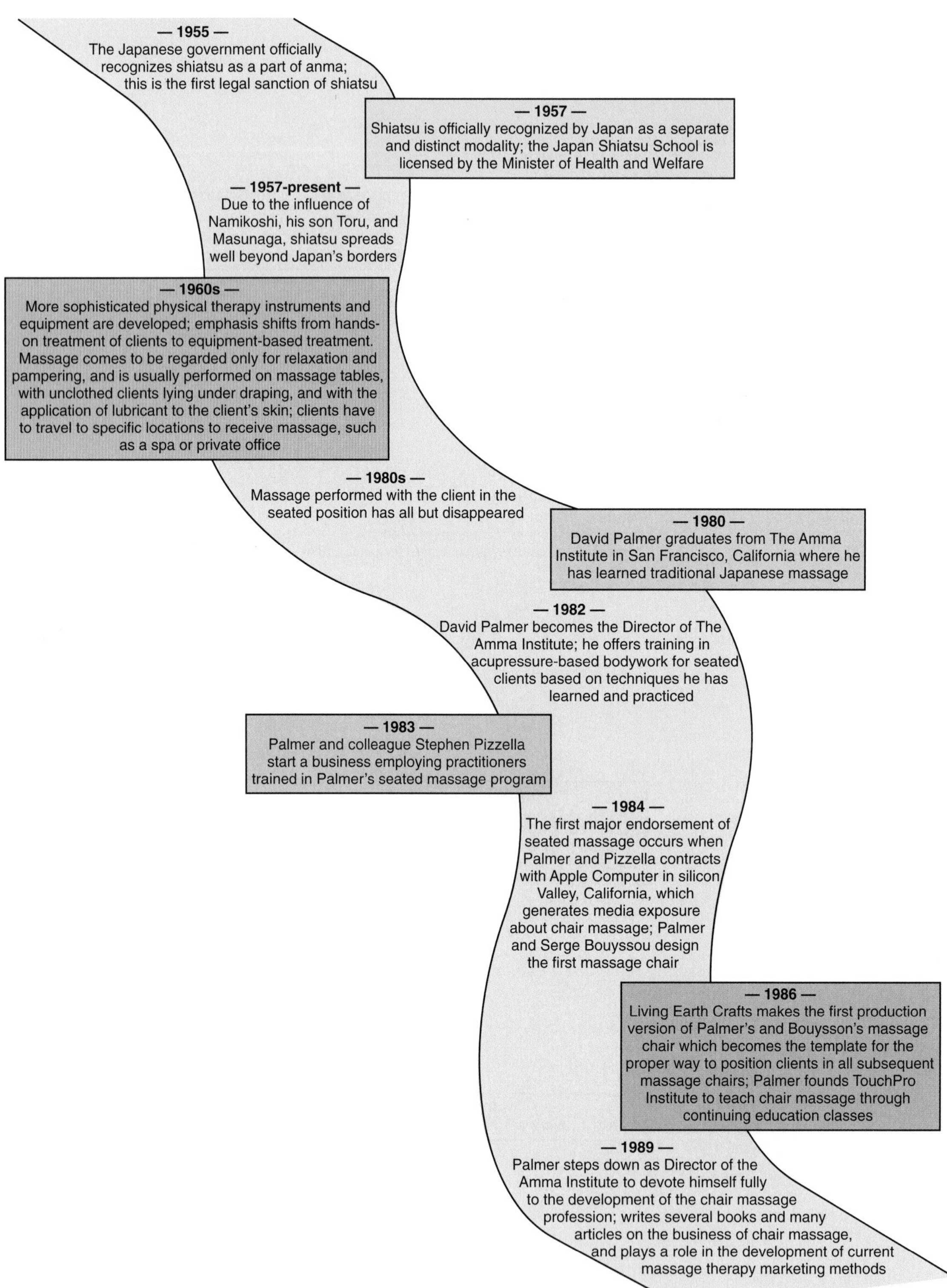

FIGURE 1-11, cont'd.

TABLE 1-2 Cases of Musculoskeletal Disorders Resulting in Time Away from Work for 2007

Musculoskeletal Disorder	Number of Cases Involving Days Away from Work
Sprains, strains, tears	448,380
Repetitive motion	36,700
Carpal tunnel syndrome	11,940
Tendonitis	4,380
Soreness, pain, total	115,540
Back pain	37,130
Overexertion, total	264,930
From lifting	140,330

Data from Bureau of Labor Statistics, U.S. Department of Labor, Survey of Occupational Injuries and Illnesses in cooperation with participating State agencies. Retrieved May 12, 2009, from www.bls.gov/iif/oshwc/osh/case/ostb1973.pdf and www.bls.gov/iif/oshwc/osh/case/ostb1954.txt.

There is no doubt that healthy employees are more productive and lose less time because of illness or injury. Wellness programs in workplaces have been found to reduce workers' compensation claims and absenteeism, as well as assist employees in creating wellness in the workplace. All these reduce costs to businesses. These programs can include methods for employees to exercise, lose weight, stop smoking, and reduce stress. Wellness programs also communicate to the employees that the employer is invested in their health and well-being. It is easy to see that providing seated massage onsite for employees could also be part of programs that contribute to employees' health and wellness. Table 1-3 shows the physical, emotional, and psychological benefits clients may have from receiving chair massage.

Benefits of Chair Massage from the Asian Bodywork View

As noted in "History of Chair Massage," contemporary chair massage has at least partial roots in traditional Asian bodywork, particularly shiatsu. As such, there are benefits of chair massage that can be looked at from the Asian bodywork view, namely, that the body has an energetic component as well as physical ones. Qi, flowing in channels in specific areas of the body, can be accessed and supported by practitioners as they are working on clients. Even if practitioners do not have a background in Asian bodywork, they are still affecting the client's qi simply by placing their hands on the client. Some of the benefits of massage, such as increased mental clarity and focus, can, indeed, be attributed to practitioners interacting with the client's qi.

According to traditional Chinese medicine, upon which shiatsu is based, when a person's qi is out of balance in some way, the result is pain, discomfort, or other disorders. The goal of shiatsu is to help rebalance the client's qi and alleviate discomfort. The channels qi flows through are connected to the organs of the body and, for the most part, share their names. The organs and channels have certain physical, mental, psychological, emotional, and spiritual functions in the body, and the balanced flow of qi in the channels sustains these functions.

TABLE 1-3 Benefits of Chair Massage

Physical	Emotional and Psychological
Muscle tension relief	Decreased anxiety
Increased blood circulation	Increased mental clarity and focus
Decreased blood pressure	Increased body awareness
Increased joint flexibility	
Increased immune function	
Insomnia relief	

Referring back to Figure 1-8, along the channels are points where the qi is accessed easily. When the flow of qi is disrupted for any of many possible reasons, it can be brought back into equilibrium by affecting the qi at the points. As discussed previously, acupuncturists insert needles into the points to balance qi. Shiatsu practitioners, however, use their own qi to support and stabilize their client's qi. They do this through the use of finger, thumb, palm, forearm, elbow, knee and foot pressure, stretches, and range-of-motion techniques. Some types of shiatsu focus on addressing points; other types address the entire channel.

Chapters 3 through 5 are devoted to techniques and sequences that can be used to perform chair massage. Included in Chapters 4 and 5, and Appendix A is information on the location of channels and points in the various regions of the body and how to work them. Also included are benefits of working specific points. For example, certain points can be pressed to alleviate headaches or help with insomnia.

ADVANTAGES CHAIR MASSAGE GIVES THE PRACTITIONER

Offering chair massage gives the practitioner many advantages in the bodywork profession. It makes bodywork more accessible to those who feel constrained by time, money, or modesty issues. It also gives practitioners opportunities to get out into their communities, enhance their communication and marketing skills, and increase their income.

Chair massage enhances a menu of services because it is an option for clients who may not be interested in or able to receive a one-hour table massage. The lower fee can be attractive, and chair massage is accessible to clients of many different body sizes, levels of fitness, and physical abilities and disabilities. In addition, after receiving a chair treatment as an introduction to massage, many clients may then want to experience a longer table treatment. In either case, having chair massage as a modality creates opportunities for practitioners to increase their clientele.

There are several types of work options for seated massage practitioners to choose from. They can become employees for businesses that provide onsite treatments. These businesses can range anywhere from small, local operations to franchises of large, national chains. Instead of employees, certain providers of onsite massage prefer to have independent contractors. Unlike employees, independent contractors set their own treatment schedules, receive payment directly from clients, and use their own equipment. However, they also pay their own taxes and insurance.

Independent contractors usually pay the onsite massage business a set fee, either per treatment performed or length of time spent providing treatments, or sometimes there is a weekly or monthly fee, no matter how many treatments the contractors perform.

Yet another option is for practitioners to be business owners themselves, either solely or in partnership with others. This option can generate the most income for practitioners, but it requires the most work as well. In addition to performing treatments, or hiring others to perform treatments, the practitioner is responsible for all aspects of the business. This includes marketing, scheduling treatments, buying supplies and equipment and keeping them in good working order, maintaining financial records such as for accounting and payroll, and so forth. To assist practitioners in making their best choice, Chapter 6 discusses work options for seated massage practitioners in more detail.

Community Events

Working with a massage chair is a good way for practitioners to get noticed in their communities, providing gateways into bodywork careers. It does not take much time or effort to volunteer at community service events or sports events such as those that raise funds for a particular cause. The practitioner has the opportunity to give back to the community while spreading the word about his or her business. The networking opportunities are almost endless and offer a good way to build a practice.

Chairs are less expensive than massage tables, so there is less of an initial investment in equipment. They can be taken to different locations with minimal effort, which means greater marketing opportunities. Also, chairs take up less room than a massage table, are easier to transport, and it is easier to set up a massage chair and do several hours of treatments at an event than it is to set up a massage table and do brief table treatments.

Practitioners can research upcoming community events and contact the organizers about donating chair massages or offering them at low rates. In addition to performing the actual treatments, practitioners can then pass out their business cards and brochures. During two hours of chair massage, a practitioner could see perhaps 10 to 15 clients, depending on how long each treatment is. Of these, one or two may call to book a full-body table session with the practitioner. Many times practitioners have received calls from new clients who took the practitioner's card when they received a brief treatment at the end of an event. Another option is become a sponsor of the event so that the practitioner's business name, logo, and contact information are on the event's marketing materials.

Diversification

Another avenue practitioners can pursue is business and corporate accounts. These can be quite lucrative, and the income can be steady when sessions are scheduled on a regular basis. Some practitioners, in fact, do chair massage as a stand-alone practice while others do it in conjunction with their private table massage practice or working out of a spa or wellness center or other massage venue. It is a good way to maintain income if other sources decrease for some reason, such as when working for spas that lay off practitioners during their low season.

Staving off boredom is a challenge members of all professions deal with. It is easy to get into a routine where very little changes. Chair massage can be appealing to practitioners because it gets them out of their usual work setting and into different locations. There can be a variety of clients, all with different body types, personalities, and therapeutic needs. Chair massage also offers practitioners a good way to connect with those who work in different professions. Sometimes it is easy for practitioners to become isolated, especially if they have a sole practice. Traveling to different businesses provides glimpses into other walks of life.

Chair massage can stimulate practitioner creativity in treatment options. For example, chair massage can be used in conjunction with table work. Effective chair massage techniques can address problem areas in the upper body that may be awkward to address on a massage table. Intensive shoulder girdle work can be done first on a chair, and then the client can be moved to the table to address the rest of the body. More information about treatment options is presented in Chapters 4 and 5.

It is important to note, however, that not all practitioners have the temperament to perform chair massage in different locations. It will be the most satisfying for outgoing people who like variety and meeting new people. Flexibility is a must as well. Environmental factors can be unpredictable. These factors can include everything from inclement weather during outdoor events, to discovering that promised space to provide treatments is no longer available, to having no clients because the chair massage was not announced to employees before the practitioner's arrival. For those who can keep a cool head and positive attitude while dealing with the unexpected, chair massage can be a rewarding modality.

OPTIMAL LOCATIONS FOR PERFORMING CHAIR MASSAGE

Even though seated massage was designed and marketed for office employees, it has become available in a wide range of settings such as airports, fitness centers, and hotels. Many times it can be found at fundraising walks and runs. It is common for someone's first massage experience to be a five-minute chair massage at a community walk or run. Athletic events are also popular places for chair massage. In fact, at some sporting events people have waited in line for an hour and half just to receive a 10-minute treatment. Having access to the massage at the end of an event may be all that potential clients need to convince them that they could make bodywork a part of their health maintenance plan.

When considering locations where people could benefit from chair massage, and therefore optimal places to market chair massage, practitioners should keep the following in mind:

- High-traffic areas
- Places where people are likely to be stressed
- Events at which people are enjoying themselves and where receiving chair massage could be a continuation of that enjoyment
- Events advocating wellness
- Athletic events
- Places people do their day-to-day activities
- Workplace settings
- Healthcare settings
- Special events
- Places where chair massage could be an oasis from a hectic pace

Box 1-2 shows some examples of places that chair massage can be offered. Practitioners can use this as a guide to generate marketing ideas.

SUMMARY

Seated massage is a versatile modality. It can enhance the practitioner's menu of services and stimulate her or his creativity in providing treatments. Seated massage can be appealing, especially to clients who are modest or more comfortable sitting upright and because it is less expensive and takes less time than table massage. Treatments can be performed using a specially designed massage chair, straight-backed chair, or a tabletop massage support. Even though the client remains fully clothed and no lubricants are used, many of the same techniques performed in table massage can be performed during seated massage and are just as therapeutically effective. Energy modalities and Asian bodywork modalities can also be incorporated into seated massage sessions. A typical chair massage treatment lasts anywhere from 10 to 30 minutes, and chair massage can address almost the entire body.

Chair massage at least partially developed from Asian bodywork, especially the Japanese modality shiatsu, as well as from Western massage therapy. Contributors include Per Henrik Ling, who is credited with the creation of medical gymnastics; Dr. John Harvey Kellogg, who developed the "Battle Creek Idea," which incorporated massage, and wrote the first text on massage therapy; and Florence Nightingale, who incorporated massage training in her school for nurses. Because of these prominent figures and others, massage was a part of medical treatment until the 1950s when Western scientific healing methods began to greatly replace natural approaches to healing. Massage came to be viewed as only for relaxation and pampering, and table massage predominated. In the 1980s, David Palmer, in order to make massage therapy more accessible to potential clients, created acupressure-based bodywork for clients in the seated position. He also helped design the first massage chair, and through his marketing efforts, he brought public attention to the modality of chair massage.

Clients can experience many physical, mental, and psychological benefits from receiving chair massage. Chair massage can be especially helpful to people in many different occupations, whether their jobs require physical effort or require them to sit or stand still for long periods of time. Either case can lead to musculoskeletal disorders such as repetitive motion injuries like carpal tunnel syndrome, sprains, strains, and so forth. Businesses lose a great deal of money each year to workers' compensation claims and absenteeism because of these conditions. Seated massage onsite for employees as part of programs that contribute to employees' health and wellness can reduce money and time lost as a result of injuries.

Chair massage gives the practitioner many advantages. There are several work options from which practitioners can choose, namely, becoming an employee, independent contractor, or business owner. Working with a massage chair at community events is a good way for practitioners to get noticed, and the diversity a chair massage practice provides can stimulate the practitioner's creativity, prevent boredom and burnout, and offer a way for practitioners to connect with those in other professions. Seated massage has become available in a wide range of settings. Optimal places to market chair massage, other than workplace settings, include high traffic areas, places where people are likely to be stressed, athletic events, and special events such as bridal showers and birthday parties.

BOX 1-2 Examples of Chair Massage Locations

Places Where People are Likely to be Stressed
Airports (Figure 1-12)
Hospitals
Conference centers

High-Traffic Areas
Sidewalk cafes
Shopping malls (Figure 1-13 and Figure 1-14)

Places Where People are Enjoying Themselves
Outdoor concerts
Festivals
The beach
Farmer's markets (Figure 1-15)
Parks

Events Advocating Wellness
Health fairs
Walks and runs to raise money for causes such as diabetes and cancer research

Athletic Events (Figure 1-16)
Triathlons
Soccer games
Softball games
Golf tournaments

Places where People Do Their Day-to-Day Activities
Banks
Supermarkets
Schools
Fitness centers
Beauty salons

Workplace Settings
Corporations
Small businesses (Figure 1-17)
Factories

Healthcare Settings
Hospitals
Doctor offices
Dental offices
Nursing homes

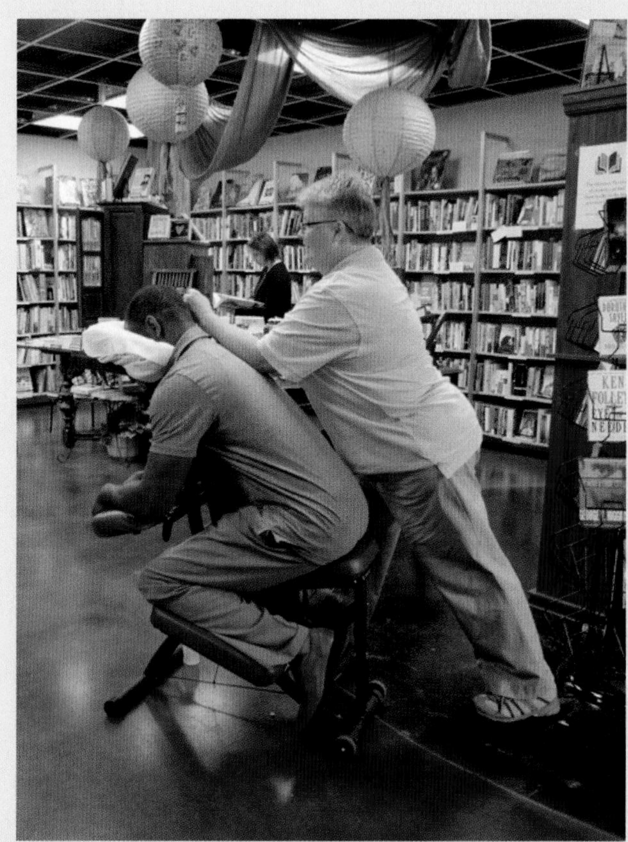

FIGURE 1-13 Chair massage in a bookstore.

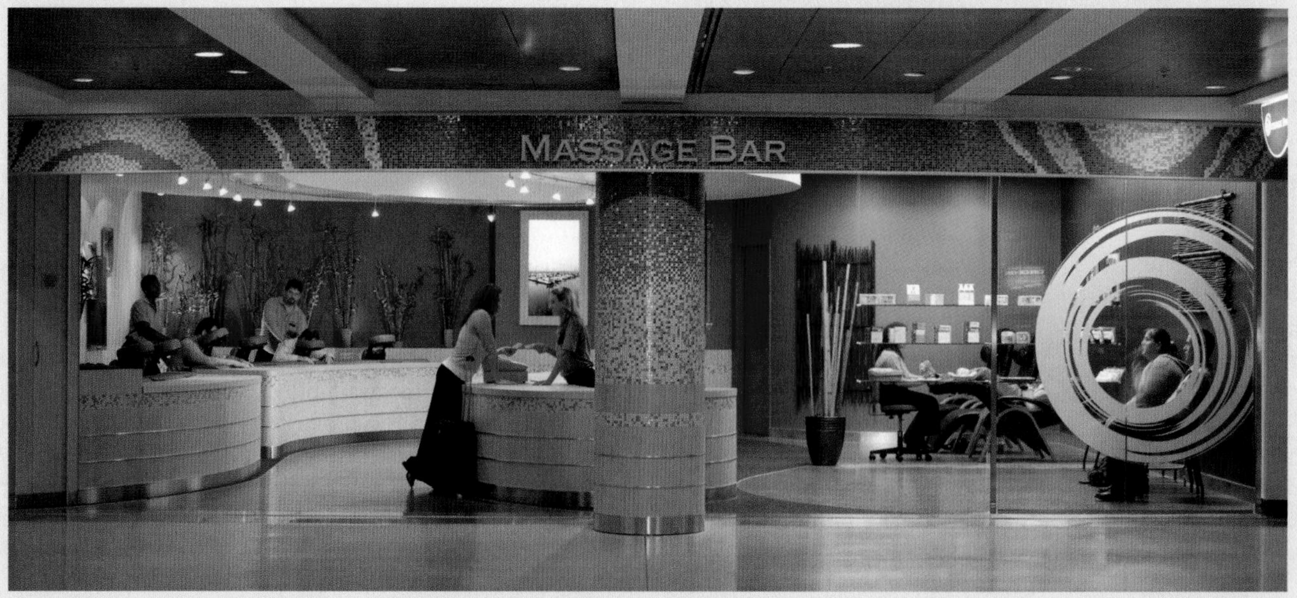

FIGURE 1-12 Massage Bar at the Sacramento, California, airport. (Courtesy Massage Bar.)

BOX 1-2 Examples of Chair Massage Locations—cont'd

Special Events
Birthday parties
Graduation parties
Retirement parties
Bridal showers
Baby showers

Places Where Chair Massage Could Be an Oasis from a Hectic Pace
Conventions
Trade shows

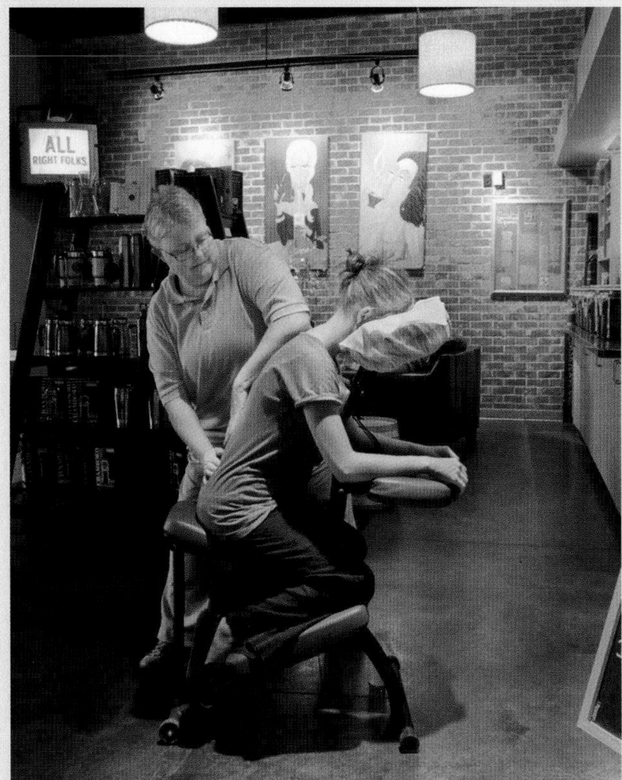

FIGURE 1-14 Chair massage in a coffee shop.

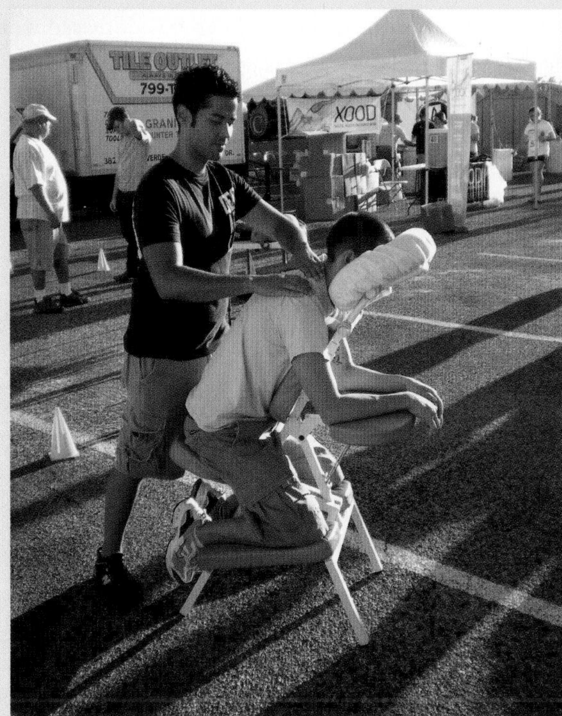

FIGURE 1-16 Chair massage at an athletic event.

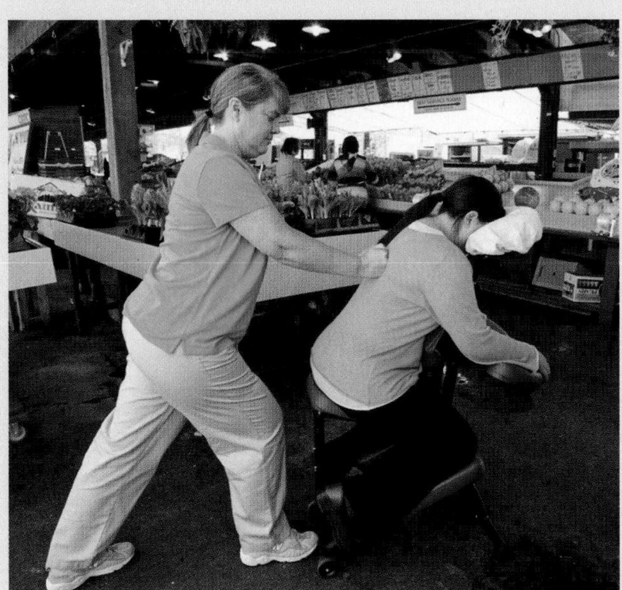
FIGURE 1-15 Chair massage at a farmer's market.

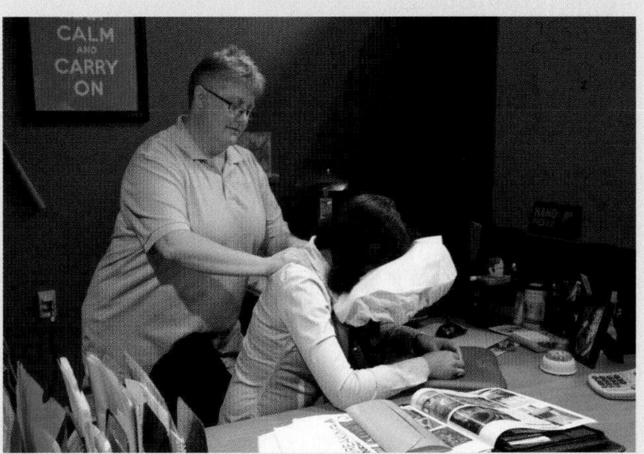

FIGURE 1-17 Chair massage in a business office.

STUDY QUESTIONS

Answers to Study Questions are located on page 227.

Multiple Choice

1. Which of the following techniques is unlikely to be used during the performance of seated massage?
   a. Percussion
   b. Lymphatic massage
   c. Forearm work
   d. Friction
2. What parts of the client's body can be addressed when he or she is seated in a massage chair?
   a. Lower legs
   b. Abdomen
   c. Back
   d. Feet
3. From which of the following did shiatsu most directly develop?
   a. Amma
   b. Tuina
   c. Thai massage
   d. Reiki
4. Who invented the Swedish movement cure?
   a. Hippocrates
   b. John Harvey Kellogg
   c. Dr. George H. Taylor
   d. Per Henrik Ling
5. Which of the following is a benefit of chair massage to people in the workplace?
   a. Stress reduction
   b. Relief from headaches and sore muscles
   c. Improved immune function
   d. All of the above

Fill in the Blank

1. A typical chair massage treatment can last anywhere from ____________________ to ____________________ minutes.
2. The oldest known forms of bodywork, an wu and do-in, developed in China more than ____________________ years ago.
3. In addition to physical benefits, receiving chair massage, as with table massage, has ____________________ and ____________________ benefits.
4. Qi flows in specific streams in the body called ____________________.
5. Chair massage makes bodywork more accessible to those who feel constrained by ____________________, ____________________, or ____________________ issues.

Short Answer

1. Discuss the professional and personal opportunities chair massage creates for practitioners.

   ____
   ____
   ____
   ____
   ____

2. Explain the commonalities and differences between seated and table massage.

   ____
   ____
   ____
   ____
   ____

STUDY QUESTIONS

3. Briefly outline the how Asian bodywork, the ancient Greeks and Romans, and Western massage techniques have all contributed to the development of chair massage.

____

____

____

____

____

4. Explain Per Henrik Ling's contribution to modern massage therapy.

____

____

____

____

____

5. Discuss David Palmer's contribution to the popularity of chair massage.

____

____

____

____

____

ACTIVITIES

1. Receive one or more professional chair massage treatments. In what settings were they performed? How long was each treatment? How did you feel after the treatment as compared to before? What did you like about each treatment? What did you not like?

2. Using your local Yellow Pages and newspapers, make a list of companies and events where you could offer chair massage.

3. Search the Internet for companies that employee chair massage practitioners. Contact these companies to find out the following:
   a. How much practitioners can realistically expect to make doing chair massage—an annual amount as well as an amount per hour/treatment
   b. How their treatments are structured: 10 min, 15 min, 30 min, and so forth
   c. Whether they have employees, independent contractors, or both
   d. What they look for when someone is interviewing to work for them
   e. What types of places (businesses, bridal showers, the mall, and so forth) they send their practitioners to perform chair massage
   f. How they started their business
   g. What the biggest rewards in their business are
   h. What the biggest challenges in their business are

____

____

____

____

____

Essentials of Practice

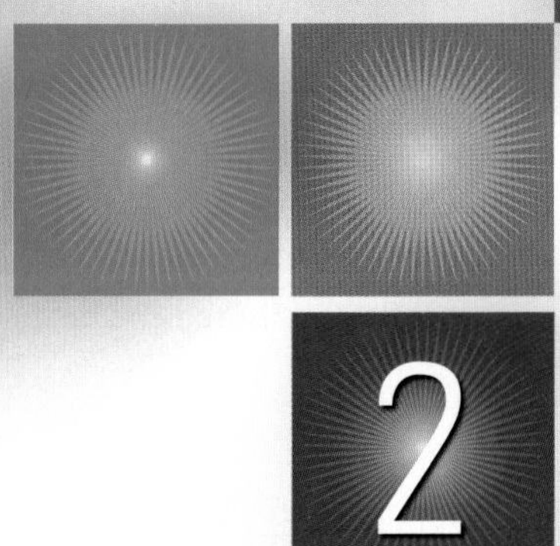

OBJECTIVES

Upon completion of this chapter, the reader will have the information necessary to do the following:

1. Explain ways to provide chair massage without a massage chair.
2. Delineate the factors involved in choosing the right massage chair.
3. Discuss the proper body mechanics involved in handling the massage chair.
4. Explain the proper way to set up, adjust, and take down the massage chair.
5. Explain sanitation and hygiene guidelines for the chair massage practice and practitioner, and explain the importance of proper maintenance of equipment.
6. List and describe all the other supplies necessary for the chair massage practice.
7. Discuss the logistics involved in traveling to locations to perform chair massage.

KEY TERMS

Antiseptics
Body mechanics
Dead lift
Desktop massage support (tabletop system)
Disinfectants
Equipment personality
Hygiene
Microorganisms
Pathogens
Return on investment costs
Sanitation
Universal (standard) precautions

STARTING OFF SIMPLE

Whether practitioners are new to the massage and bodywork profession or have been practitioners for quite some time, the investment in equipment requires careful consideration. These considerations include determining what pieces of equipment are essential, deciding on a price range, choosing the highest-quality equipment available in the price range, and calculating how many treatments need to be performed to make the investment worthwhile. This is also known as **return on investment costs**. Chapter 6, "Essentials of Business," covers the information practitioners need to set up and run their seated massage business. It includes worksheets practitioners may find helpful to calculate their investment costs and return on investment.

Sometimes practitioners are unsure of how they want to build their practice, and they may not want to spend a lot of money on equipment until they are clear on where their path in the massage and bodywork profession lies. This can make providing onsite massage appealing. Compared to the costs of the equipment needed to perform table massage, the initial investment in onsite massage equipment can be low.

The simplest and most inexpensive method of providing seated massage is by using a straight-backed chair with a pillow to support the client (Figure 2-1). Another option is to place pillows on a table, then have the client sit on a stool or chair and lean forward onto the pillows (Figure 2-2). If more propping is required, bolsters made from specially shaped foam rubber or other materials can be purchased and used for client comfort (Figure 2-3). In these cases, the costs involved are relatively minimal and would be for pillows and supporting bolsters, and covers for the pillows and bolsters.

The next step up in onsite massage equipment is the professionally manufactured **desktop massage support** (also called **tabletop systems**). These are designed to be set on a table, desk, or other flat surface. The client places her head in the face cradle (face rest), and a chest (sternum) pad to support the client's torso may be available. Most are adjustable with mechanisms to lock the position of the desktop support in place, ensuring safety of the client. Desktop massage supports can be used for clients who are in wheelchairs (Figure 2-4), in offices with space restrictions or because the company wants as little impact or fuss as possible in the workplace (Figure 2-5), for clients who are unable to kneel on a massage chair for physical reasons (e.g., arthritis in the knees), and for clients who are confined to a bed such as a prenatal client on complete bedrest or a client who is hospitalized. Although access to the client's lower back may be restricted by the chair the client is sitting in, or the bed the client is lying in, the neck, shoulders, and possibly the arms and hands can be massaged easily.

Desktop supports weigh about 10 pounds and so are lighter to carry and easier to store than massage chairs.

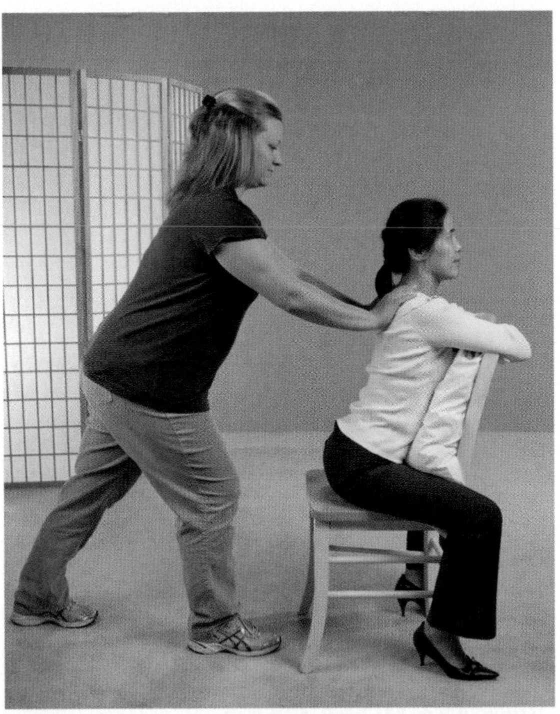

FIGURE 2-1 Client receiving massage in a straight-backed chair.

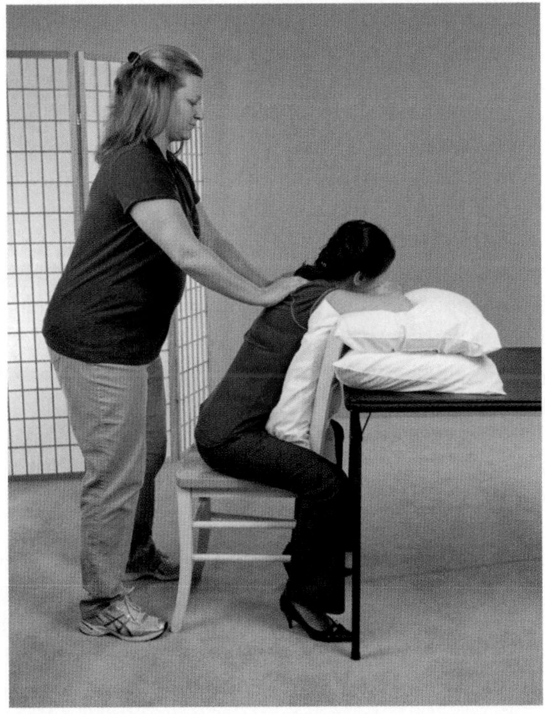

FIGURE 2-2 Client leaning forward onto a table to receive massage.

They usually cost just under $200, which may or may not include a travel bag. Two companies to research for desktop supports are Oakworks (www.oakworks.com), which makes the Desktop Portal portable massage system, and Earthlite (www.earthlite.com), which makes the TravelMate desktop massage support.

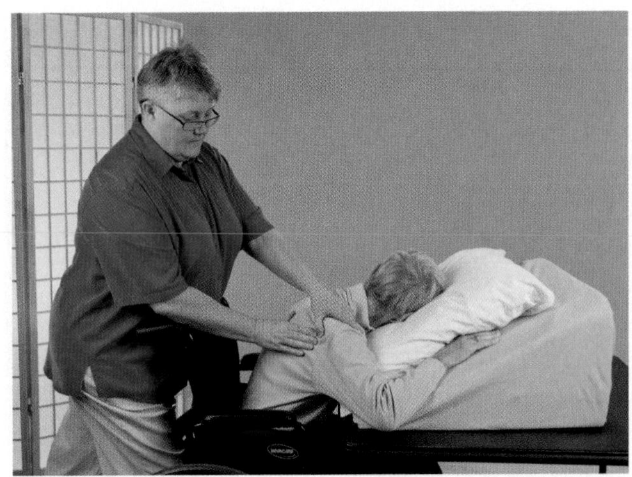

FIGURE 2-3 Propping with a foam rubber bolster.

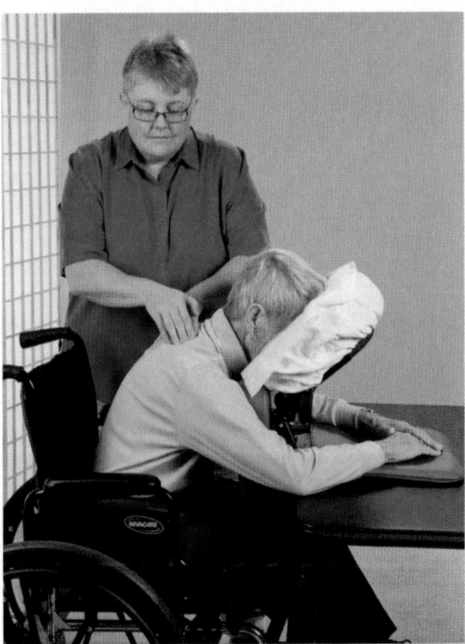

FIGURE 2-4 Client in wheelchair being massaged using a desktop massage support.

The most expensive option is the professionally manufactured massage chair. However, it provides the most comfort for the widest variety of clients, can be transported to many different types of locations, and, if properly maintained, will provide years of service.

CHOOSING A MASSAGE CHAIR

History of the Massage Chair

As discussed in Chapter 1, David Palmer and Serge Bouyssou designed the first massage chair in 1984. In 1986,

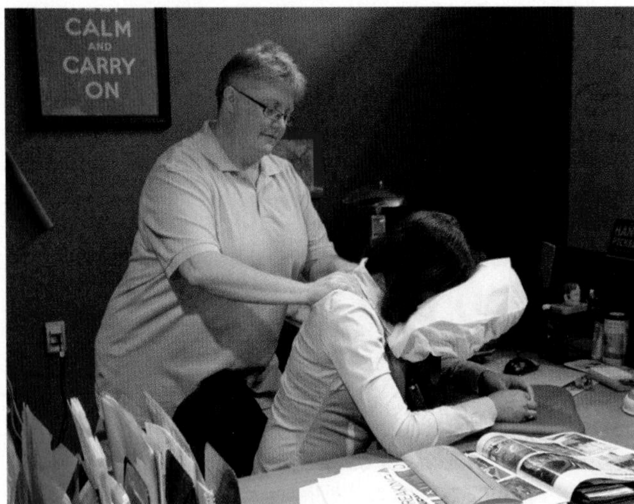

FIGURE 2-5 Client at a desk being massaged using a desktop massage support.

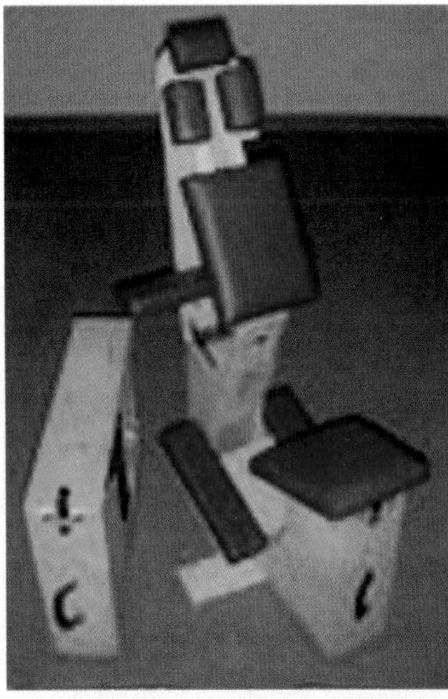

FIGURE 2-6 Wooden Stronglite chair from the early 1980s. (Courtesy Stronglite.)

Living Earth Crafts introduced the first production version of this chair. It was heavy by today's massage chair standards (28 pounds), was made primarily of wood, and resembled a large suitcase when it was folded. Figure 2-6 shows a wooden Stronglite Chair from the early 1980s.

In 1989, the Quicklite Massage Chair was introduced by Golden Ratio Woodworks. It was designed and developed by one of David Palmer's students, Scott Breyer, and by John Fanuzzi. At 14 pounds, it was the first lightweight massage chair, had a metal frame, and operated with quick and easy adjustments (Figure 2-7).

Since 1989, more and more companies have produced massage chairs. Although these chairs differ from each other in certain respects such as their adjustment methods or available options, they all provide the way to position clients properly to receive the most effective massage possible.

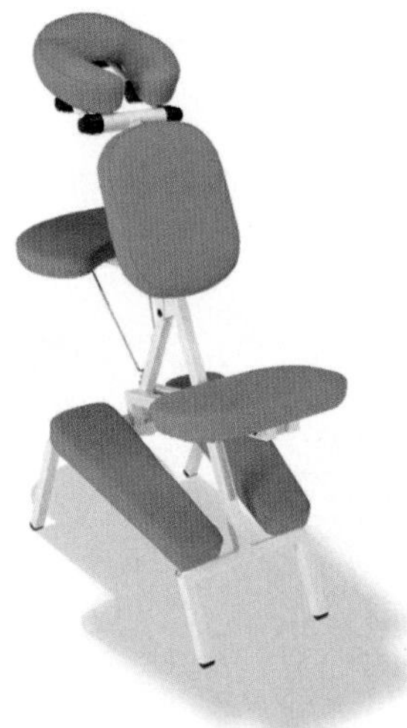

FIGURE 2-7 The Quicklite massage chair, the first metal-framed, lightweight massage chair. (Courtesy John Fanuzzi.)

Finding the Right Chair

Because there are many different massage chairs currently on the market, it is up to individual practitioners to decide which chair will fit their needs as well as their **equipment personality** (i.e., the qualities a person prefers when using equipment). For example, some practitioners like to have a lot of adjustment options on a massage chair, whereas other practitioners may have a no-nonsense approach, preferring not to deal with lots of "bells and whistles" when setting up or taking down a chair.

If the chair will be used primarily for on-location treatments, a lightweight chair with wheels is a good choice. If the chair will be used to complement a massage and bodywork office setting, then a heavier chair with many adjustments may be more appropriate. If the treatments will be done in both types of settings, then the practitioner needs to decide what is most important in terms of mobility and weight of the chair, adjustment options, and so forth.

Features of Massage Chairs

Because massage chairs serve a similar function as massage tables, it is important to consider their individual features as seriously as the features of a massage table when deciding on which chair to purchase. Also, the cost of massage chairs generally ranges from about $200 to $600, which can make some of them equal to the cost of a massage table. When choosing a massage chair, it is important to keep the following overall considerations in mind:

- *How heavy is the chair?* Generally, most massage chairs weigh anywhere from 15 to 22 pounds. When deciding between chairs that weigh almost the same, a few pounds can really make a difference. For example, if two chairs have virtually the same features but one weighs 18 pounds and the other weighs 20 pounds, the odds are those extra 2 pounds can be felt after a long day of lifting the chair in and out of a vehicle, carrying the chair around, and performing many massages.

- *How durable is the chair? Is it well made?* For example, are there any exposed adjustment mechanisms? These are potentially unsafe for both clients and practitioners—fingers and hair can get caught in exposed gear teeth, adjustment levers that do not lock can be accidentally knocked out of place, resulting in slipping face cradles or armrests, and so forth. Well-made chairs may cost more, but they may be safer and, in the long run, more cost-effective as they are less likely to need repair and tend to last longer.
- *How stable is the chair?* It needs to be stable enough to accommodate different body sizes and shapes and to ensure the safety of clients.
- *How easy is it to set up?* Some chairs are relatively simple to set up, whereas others may require more steps. Individual practitioners need to decide for themselves how much time and effort they want to spend setting up the chair.
- *What adjustment options are included? How easy is it to make adjustments?* For the practitioner to access the client's tissues effectively while maintaining proper body mechanics, the chair needs to be adjustable to fit different client body sizes and shapes, as well as the practitioner's body size and shape. Adjustment options on chairs can range from just a few to quite an array. No matter which chair is chosen, practitioners need to be able to make the adjustments quickly and easily and should choose a chair that allows them to do so.
- *What special options does the chair have? Does it come with any accessories?* These can include the following:
  - Wheels on the chairs (for easier transport)
  - Adjustable face cradles and armrests
  - Sternum pads
  - Removable knee pads (necessary for clients whose knees are sensitive and so cannot press against the pads; once the pads are removed, the client places his feet flat on the floor)
  - Pouches to hold client glasses and jewelry
  - A place for drops of aromatherapy oils
  - Instructional DVDs that demonstrate how to set up, adjust, and take down the chair
  - Carrying case (If a carrying case is not included with the chair, it would be worthwhile to purchase one. A case not only protects the chair from damage, it adds to the practitioner's professional look when entering the setting where the massage sessions will take place. Some carrying cases have wheels on them, which makes a wheel-less chair easier to transport. If neither the chair nor the carrying case has wheels, the practitioner may consider buying a separate wheeled cart to ensure ease of movement.)
- *Does the chair come with a warranty?* Warranties can range anywhere from one year to lifetime, with some lifetime warranties being limited. They vary from manufacturer to manufacturer.
- *What choices in vinyl and color are available?* Some manufacturers offer only a few choices in vinyl types and color, and some have quite a variety from which consumers can choose.

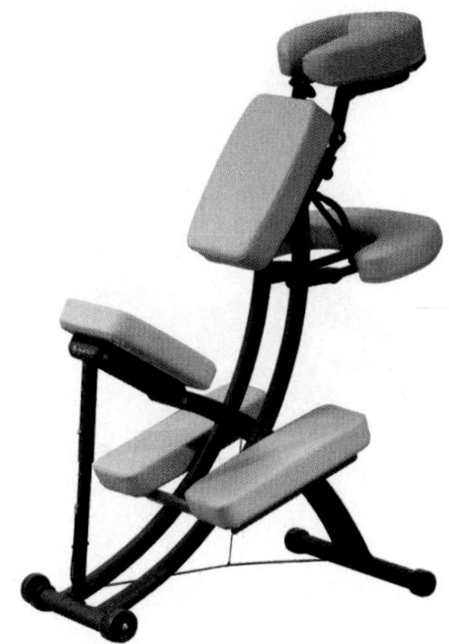

FIGURE 2-8 The Oakworks Portal Pro. (Courtesy Oakworks.)

Massage Chair Manufacturers and Distributors

There are quite a few manufacturers and distributors of massage chairs and desktop massage supports. They are located in the United States, Canada, China, and other countries. However, a few companies dominate the market and are, therefore, the best known. Some of them have been in the business of making and distributing massage and bodywork equipment for some time and so have proven records of quality workmanship and consumer satisfaction. Practitioners may want to consider exploring these companies first before buying from lesser-known businesses.

Oakworks. Figure 2-8 shows the Oakworks Portal Pro. Oakworks has been in business since 1977 and is located in New Freedom, Pennsylvania. In addition to massage tables, chairs, and accessories, the company manufactures medical tables, electric lift spa tables, physical therapy tables, and athletic training tables. Its equipment is sold throughout the United States and in 35 countries worldwide (www.oakworks.com).

Living Earth Crafts. Figure 2-9 shows the Living Earth Crafts Avilla II. Living Earth Crafts has been a provider of equipment and supplies in the massage and spa industry since 1973. It sells throughout the world and is located in Vista, California (www.livingearthcrafts.com).

Stronglite, Inc. Figure 2-10 shows the Stronglite Ergo-Pro massage chair. Stronglite is located in Salt Lake City, Utah. It focuses exclusively on the manufacture of massage therapy equipment and accessories and has been doing so

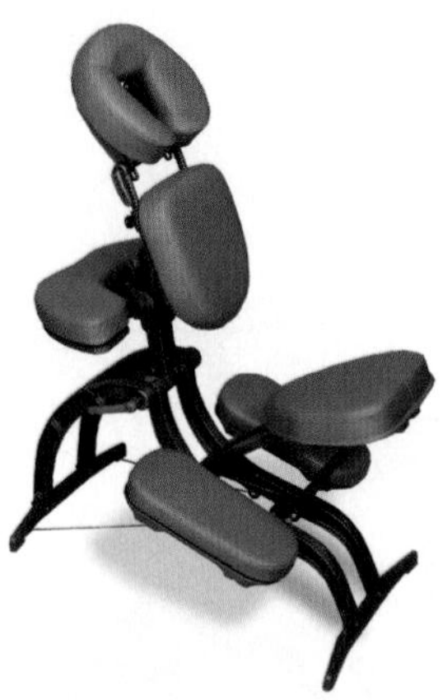

FIGURE 2-9 The Living Earth Crafts Avilla II. (Courtesy Living Earth Crafts.)

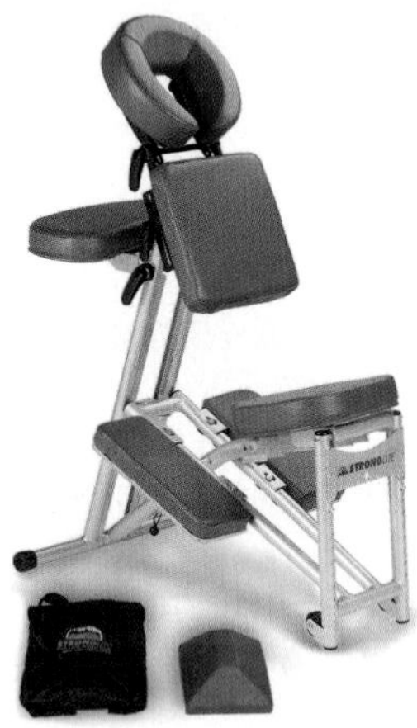

FIGURE 2-10 The Stronglite Ergo-Pro massage chair. (Courtesy Stronglite.)

since 1986. Distributors are located throughout the United States and Canada (www.stronglite.com).

Earthlite. Earthlite, founded in 1987 by a massage therapist, is also located in Vista, California. In addition to massage tables, chairs, and accessories, it also manufactures spa and salon tables. Earthlite sells the Avilla II, the same chair sold by Living Earth Crafts (www.earthlite.com).

Pisces Production. Figure 2-11 shows the Pisces Dolphin II massage chair. Pisces Production was founded in 1977 by a massage therapist. Located in Sebastopol, California, it manufactures massage tables, chairs, and accessories. The company makes the only massage chair that can position the client from a standard sitting position to completely horizontal (www.piscespro.com).

Touch America. Figure 2-12 shows the Touch America (Golden Ratio) Quicklite Massage Chair. Located in Hillsborough, North Carolina, Touch America has been manufacturing spa and massage therapy equipment and furniture since 1983. In 2007, it became the exclusive manufacturer and marketer of products originally developed by Golden Ratio Woodworks (a company started in 1982), including the Quicklite massage chair (www.touchamerica.com).

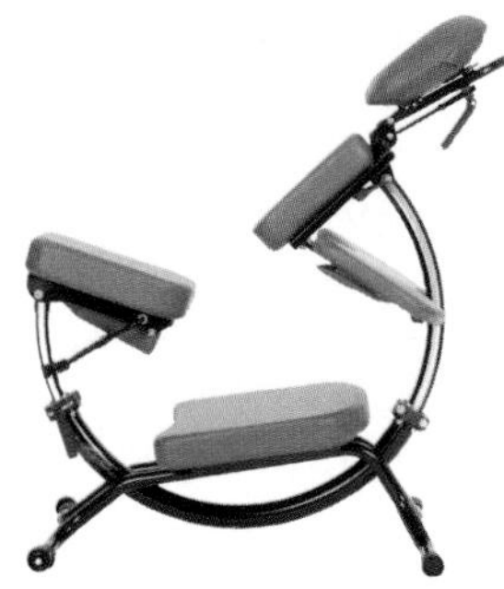

FIGURE 2-11 The Pisces Dolphin II massage chair. (Printed with permission Pisces Productions. *www.piscespro.com.*)

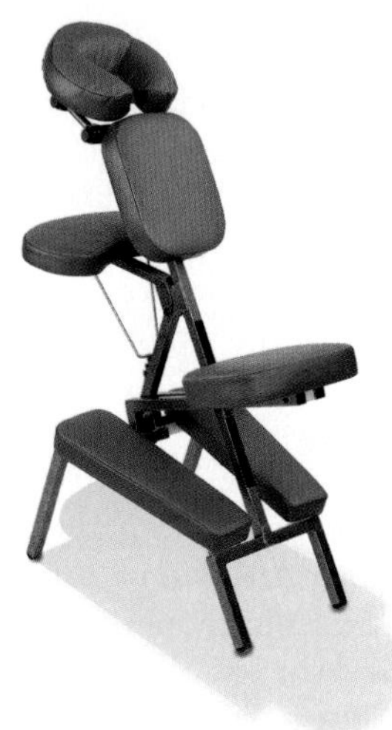

FIGURE 2-12 The Touch America Quicklite™ massage chair. (Courtesy Touch America.)

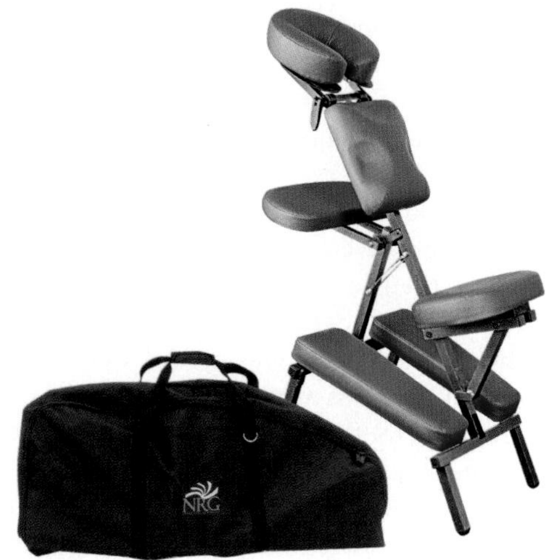

FIGURE 2-13 The NRG Grasshopper portable massage chair. (Courtesy Massage Warehouse.)

NRG Energy Massage Tables. Figure 2-13 shows the NRG Grasshopper portable massage chair. The NRG Grasshopper is the massage chair manufactured by NRG Energy Massage Tables. Although there is not a website to contact NRG directly, the Grasshopper can be purchased through distributors of other massage therapy equipment. Suggested websites to search include, but are not limited to, the following:

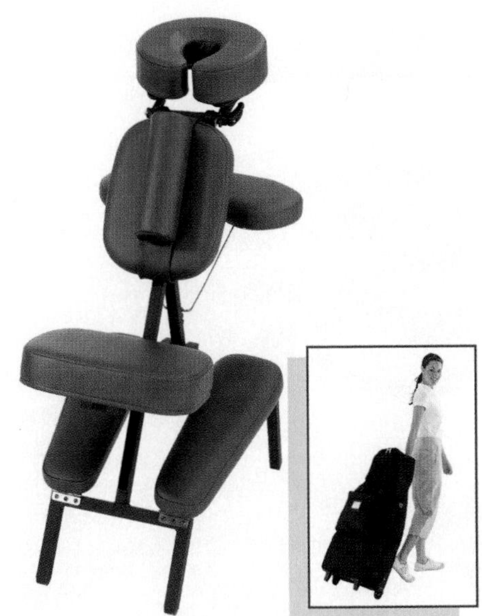

FIGURE 2-14 Costco's portable professional massage chair. (Courtesy Master Massage Equipment.)

www.massageking.com
www.massagewarehouse.com
www.midasmassage.com

Membership Warehouse Clubs. Figure 2-14 shows Costco's Portable Professional massage chair. Membership warehouse clubs carry a wide variety of products–everything from food to office supplies to electronics. Two of these clubs that carry massage tables and chairs are Costco (www.costco.com) and Sam's Club (www.samsclub.com).

Another option for practitioners to buy lower-cost massage chairs is to buy them used from other practitioners or through the Internet on such sites as craigslist (www.craigslist.com) and eBay (www.ebay.com). However, it may be somewhat risky to do this unless the chair can be personally inspected to ensure that it is in good working order.

HANDLING THE MASSAGE CHAIR

Body Mechanics

One of the most common reasons massage therapists and bodyworkers leave the profession is because of work-related injuries. These can usually be traced directly to improper body mechanics and posture. Because handling a massage chair to perform techniques onsite not only involves setting it up and taking it down but also lifting, carrying, and setting it down, it is important that practitioners use good **body mechanics** while performing these actions. Good body mechanics are, of course, also essential during the performance of techniques on clients who are receiving seated massage, and these body mechanics are discussed in detail in Chapter 3.

According to Sandy Fritz on page 213 of Mosby's *Fundamentals of Therapeutic Massage*, 4th edition, published by Mosby Elsevier, 2009, "Body mechanics allow the massage practitioner's body to be used in a careful, efficient and deliberate way. They involve good posture, balance, leverage and use of the strongest and largest muscles to perform the work." This is especially important for practitioners of chair massage who are not only performing techniques on their clients, they are physically transporting their equipment as well.

There are three main elements to body mechanics that practitioners should keep in mind when handling their massage chairs:

- Keep the back straight.
- Use larger muscles to do the work.
- Remember to breathe.

Keeping a straight back provides stability from the core of the body, and it keeps the torso open so that efficient breaths can be taken. If the back is not kept straight, unnecessary strain will be placed on the small muscles of the back, such as the paraspinals, leading to back pain and possible injury. Also, the strength for lifting and carrying the massage chair will then come from the shoulder and arm muscles, causing fatigue and possibly muscle strain and injury to these muscles as well, and the size of the thoracic cavity decreases, which prevents the lungs from expanding to their best capacity.

As most massage therapists and bodyworkers know, the larger the muscle, the stronger the muscle, and therefore the less chance of injury compared to a smaller muscle doing the same work. Therefore, when lifting, carrying, and setting down a massage chair, practitioners should use their larger muscles–their leg and hip muscles. Lifting from the legs cannot be emphasized enough. Figures 2-15 and 2-16 show improper and proper ways to lift and carry a chair. The carrying strap should cross over the practitioner's body so that the weight is distributed more evenly on the practitioner's body, and the shorter strap should be used as a handle. If the strap is placed on one shoulder, all the weight of the chair will be on that shoulder, increasing the chance of injury. As was discussed under the "Features of Massage Chairs" section, having a chair with wheels, a carrying case with wheels, or a wheeled cart to transport the chair will mean considerably less strain on the practitioner's body (Figure 2-17).

Moving a massage chair often involves turning movements of practitioners' bodies, such as placing the chair into and taking it out of the trunk of a car. When placing the chair into and taking it out of the trunk of a car, practitioners should make sure the carrying strap crosses over the practitioner's body. Keeping the back straight and lifting with the legs, the practitioner should use the shorter strap as a handle to maneuver the chair. Figure 2-18 shows the improper and proper ways to grip the case and lift it in and out of a car.

Most low back injuries involve twisting movements of the spine, so practitioners should take particular care when turning while handling their chairs. They should lift and then turn, pivoting on the feet, not twisting with the back.

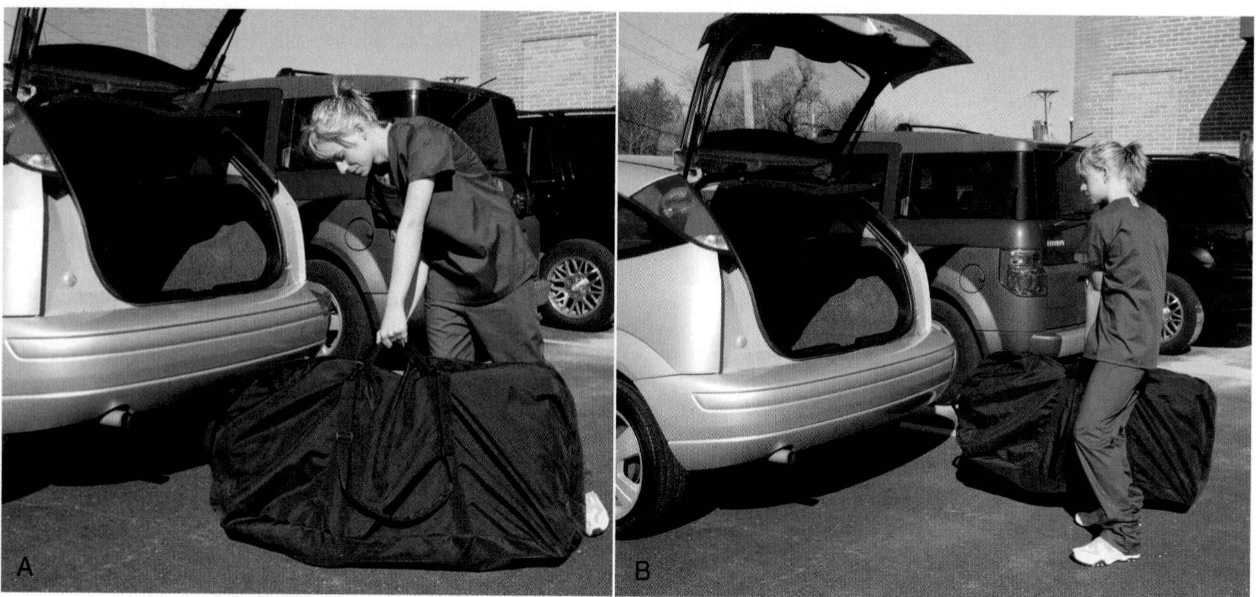

FIGURE 2-15 **A,** Improper way to lift a massage chair. **B,** Proper way to lift a massage chair.

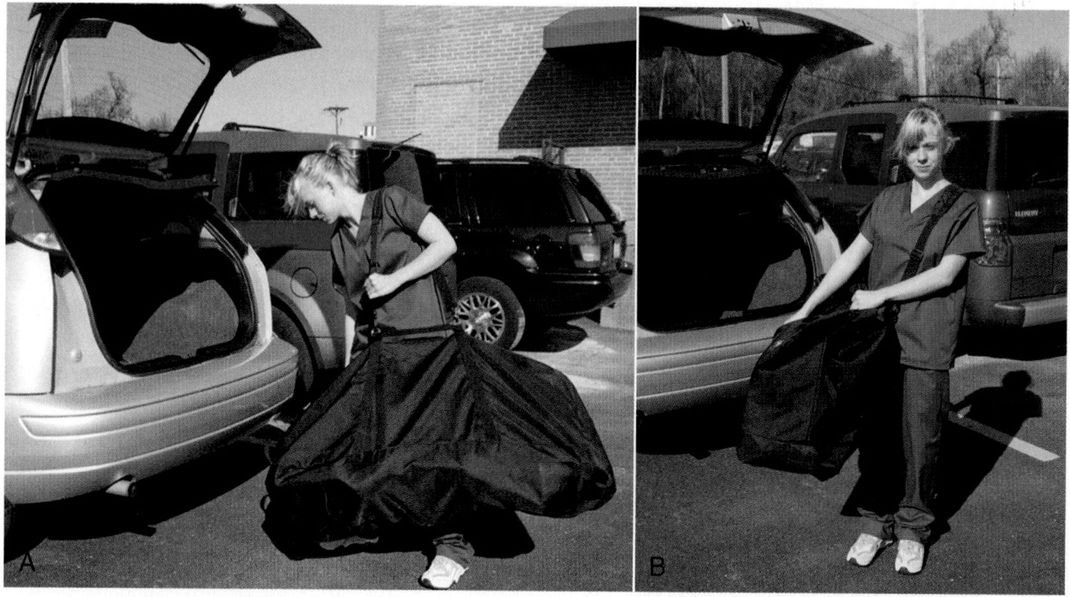

FIGURE 2-16 **A,** Improper way to carry a massage chair. **B,** Proper way to carry a massage chair.

Figure 2-19 shows improper and proper ways to turn while handling a massage chair.

Setting down a massage chair basically involves controlled drop movements, but the chair itself should never be dropped as this can damage it.

While the chair is set smoothly on the ground, certain muscles are shortening to create the downward movement, and their antagonistic muscles are elongating to counteract the rate of downward movement so that a smooth, controlled action is performed. As muscles elongate, the tension within them increases. Again, larger muscles that have more strength, such as the hip and leg muscles, can tolerate this increase in muscle tension better than smaller muscles, such as the shoulder, arm, and low back muscles. Figure 2-20 shows improper and proper ways to set down a massage chair.

Remembering to Breathe

Handling a massage chair is a physical activity. It is important to remember to take efficient breaths while moving the chair (as well as during the performance of techniques on seated clients) to ensure that a continual supply of oxygen is being sent to the cells of the body. Controlled, even breaths help prevent fatigue, maintain focus, and decrease unnecessary tension in the body. As with weight-bearing exercises (e.g., lifting weights), practitioners should exhale on exertion (as they lift the chair) and inhale when their muscles relax.

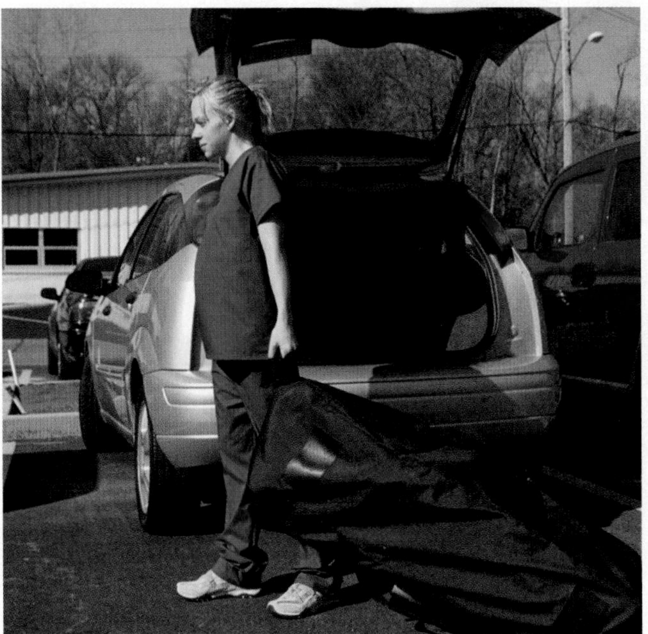

FIGURE 2-17 Moving a chair with wheels.

Setting Up the Massage Chair

When one purchases a chair, it will likely come with a manual that will describe how to set it up, make adjustments for client comfort, and take it down. Some companies also include an instructional DVD. However, all massage chairs have similar structures and set up in a similar fashion.

The first step is to remove the chair from the carrying case properly. It may seem easiest to lay the case on the floor, bend over and unzip it, then pick the chair up out of the case. As Figure 2-21 A shows, this method puts unnecessary strain on the practitioner's low back as she is mainly using her paraspinals and erector spinae muscles, not her stronger hip and leg muscles, to **dead lift** the chair up from the floor. (Dead lift is a weight-lifting term meaning to lift weight from the floor to hip level.)

The method that uses the most efficient body mechanics involves placing the chair upright, unzipping the case, then lifting the chair just enough to remove it from the bag. The practitioner is better able to keep a straight back and use mostly hip and leg strength for lifting. This method is shown in Figure 2-21 B.

The basic structures include a seat, face cradle, sternum pad, and armrest. There are mechanisms that can be loosened in order to reposition the different components, then tightened to ensure they stay in place (Figure 2-22). Once the chair is set up, the practitioner should sit in it to make sure it is stable and that all the necessary cam locks and

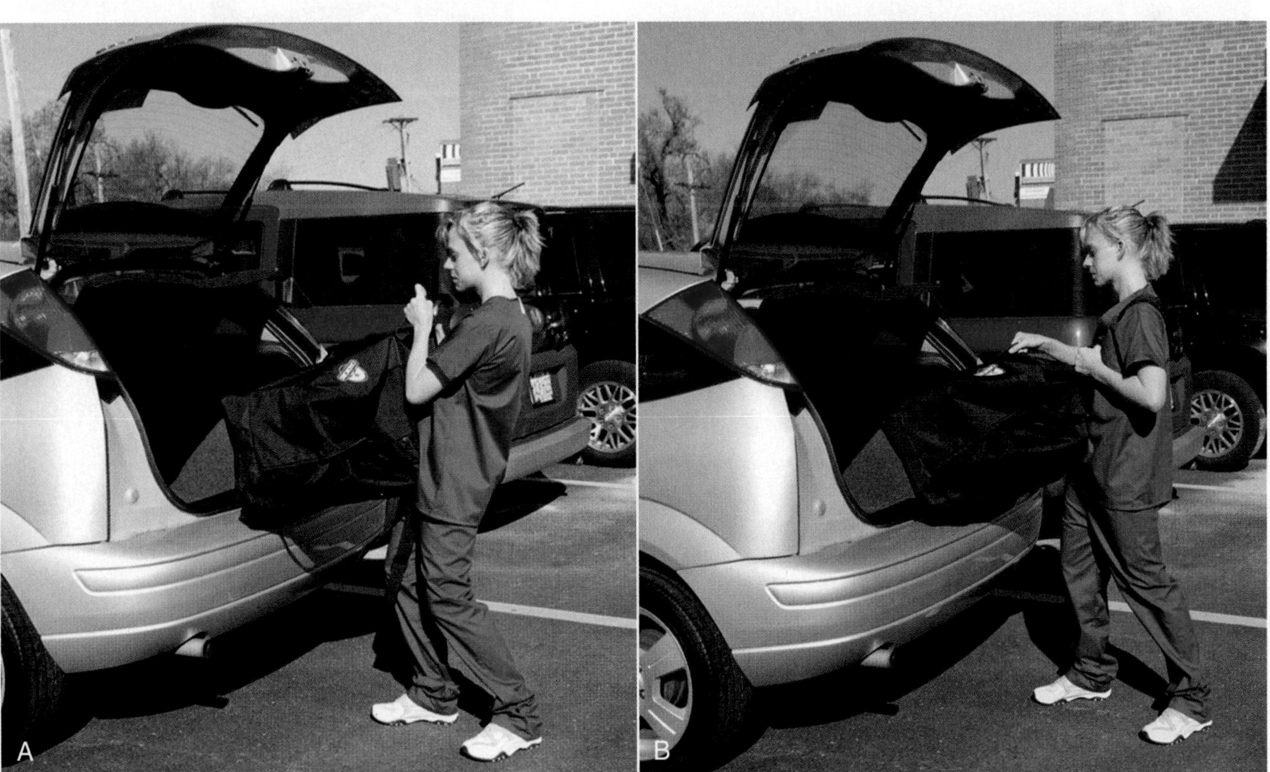

FIGURE 2-18 **A,** Improper way to grip the case and lift it in and out of car. **B,** Proper way to grip the case and lift it in and out of car.

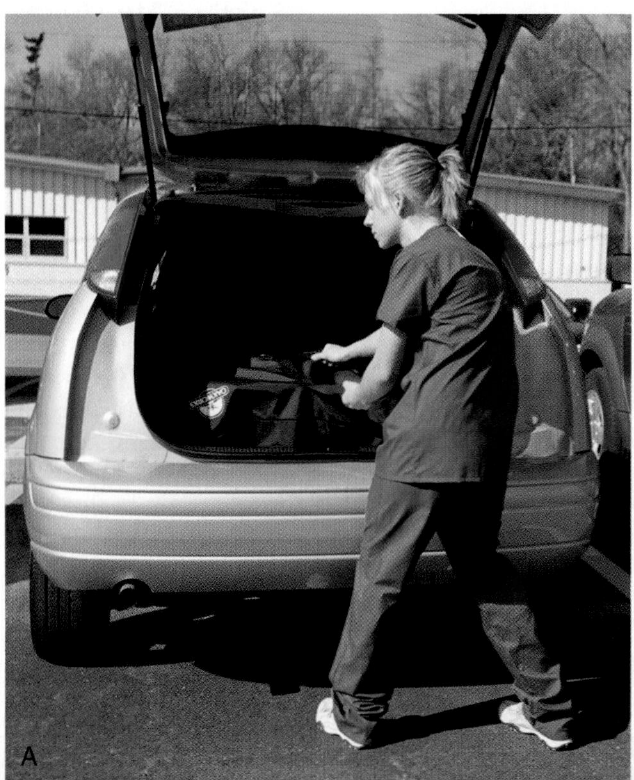

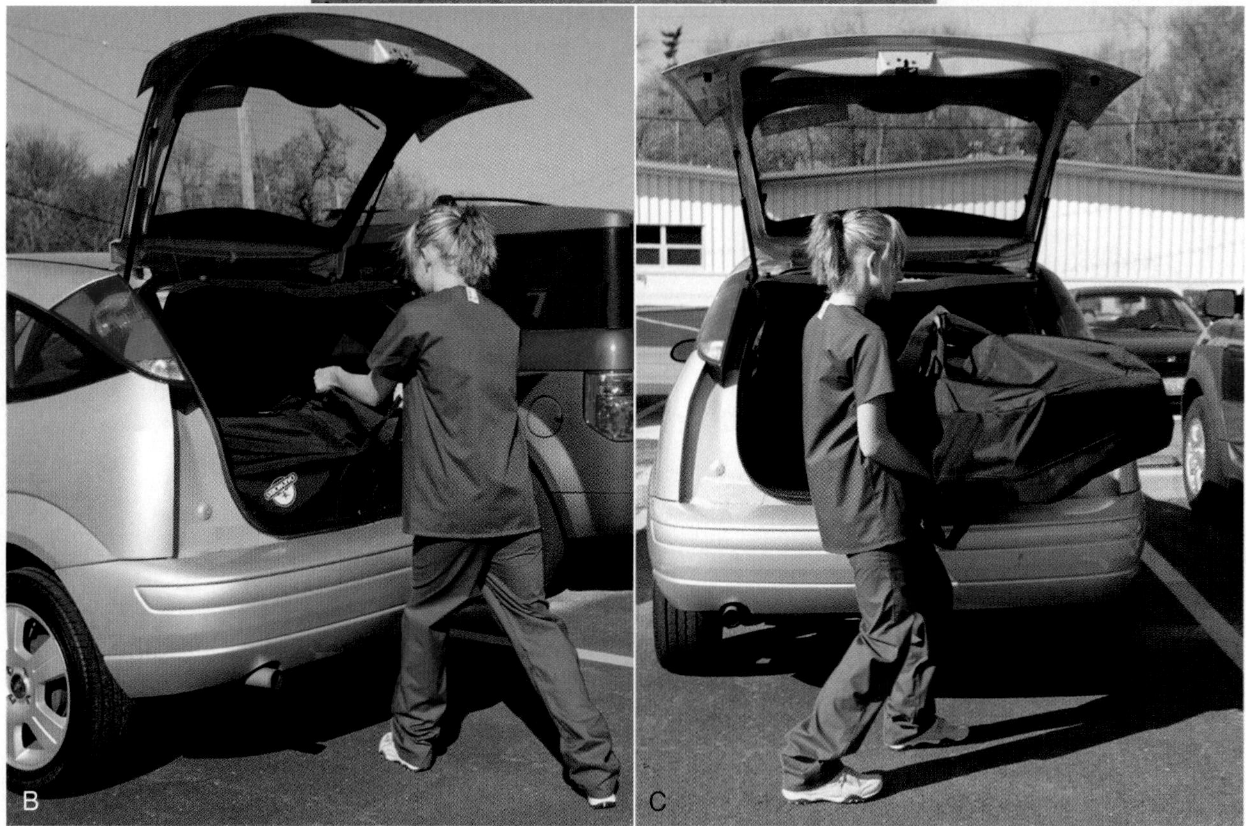

FIGURE 2-19 **A,** Improper way to turn while handling a massage chair. **B** and **C,** Proper way to turn while handling a massage chair.

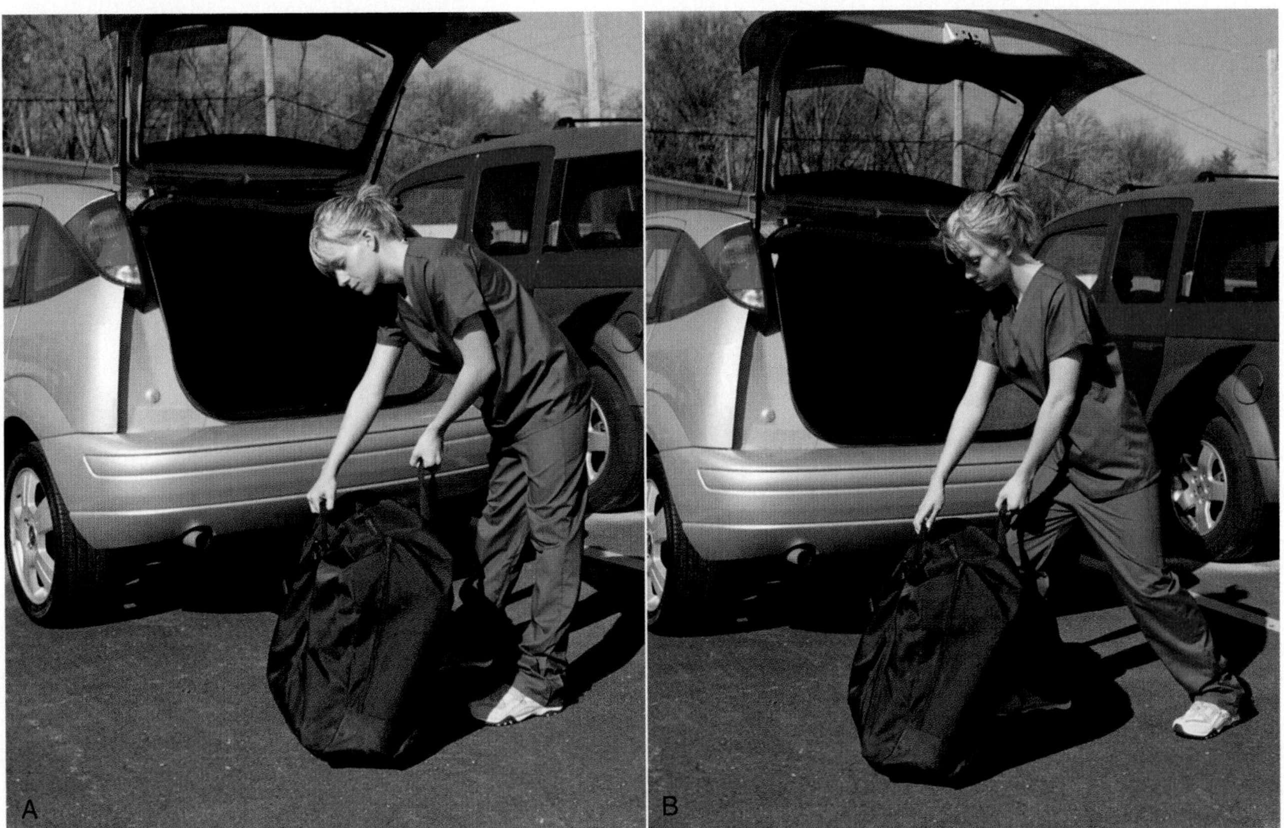

FIGURE 2-20 **A,** Improper way to set down a massage chair. **B,** Proper way to set down a massage chair.

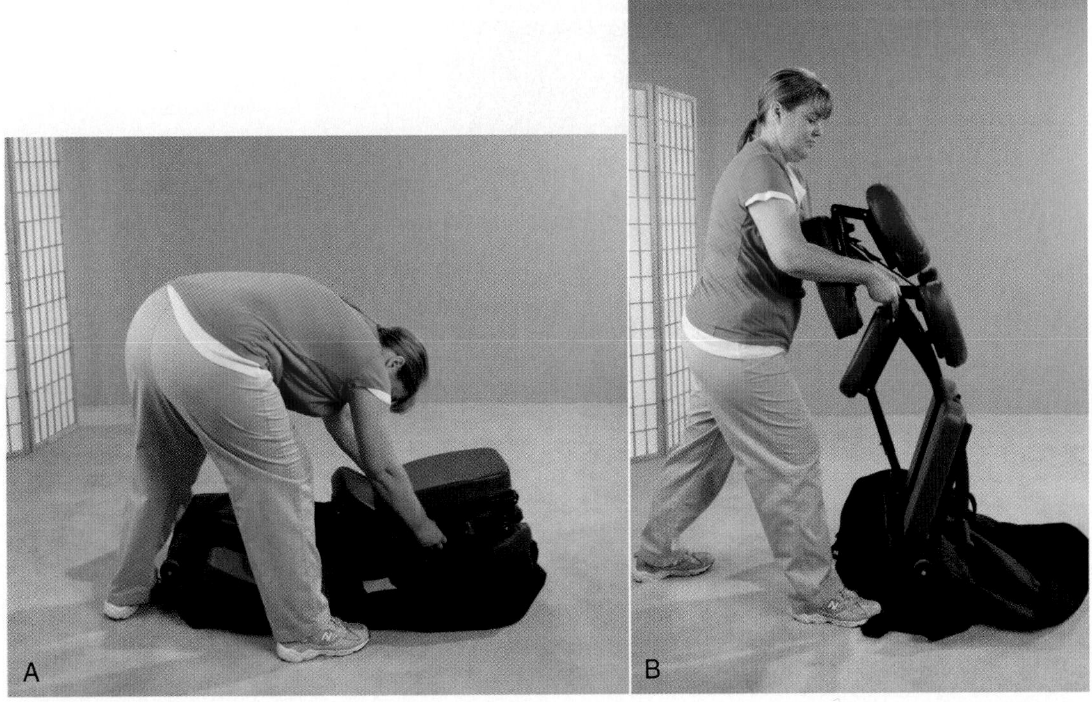

FIGURE 2-21 **A,** Improper way to take the chair out of the case. **B,** Proper way to take the chair out of the case.

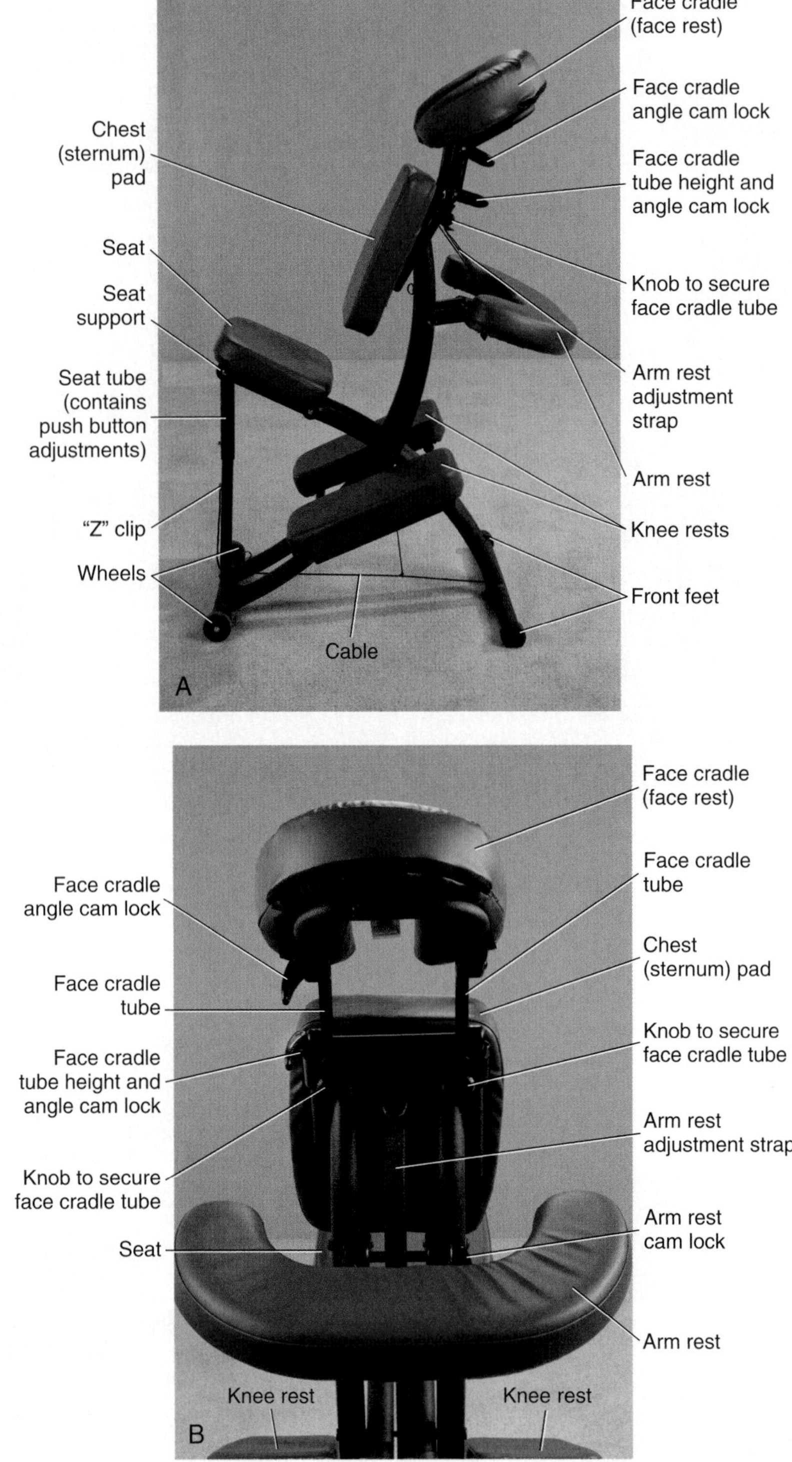

FIGURE 2-22 **A,** Side view of massage chair with labeled parts. **B,** Front of massage chair with labeled parts.

knobs are tightened so that the chair does not collapse and the seat, face cradle, sternum pad, and arm do not slip out of place, possibly injuring the client.

Start setting up the chair by creating a firm foundation at the base of the chair. Most chairs have a folding mechanism that creates an A-frame when unfolded. Move the seat of the chair outward to create the solid base of the structure (Figures 2-23 A, B, and C). Elevate the face cradle into position, then lock it in place using the face cradle angle cam lock (Figures 2-23 D and E). Elevate the armrest into position (Figure 2-23 F). The armrest can be adjusted by pulling on the armrest adjustment strap (Figure 2-23 G), then locked into place using the armrest cam lock (Figure 2-23 H).

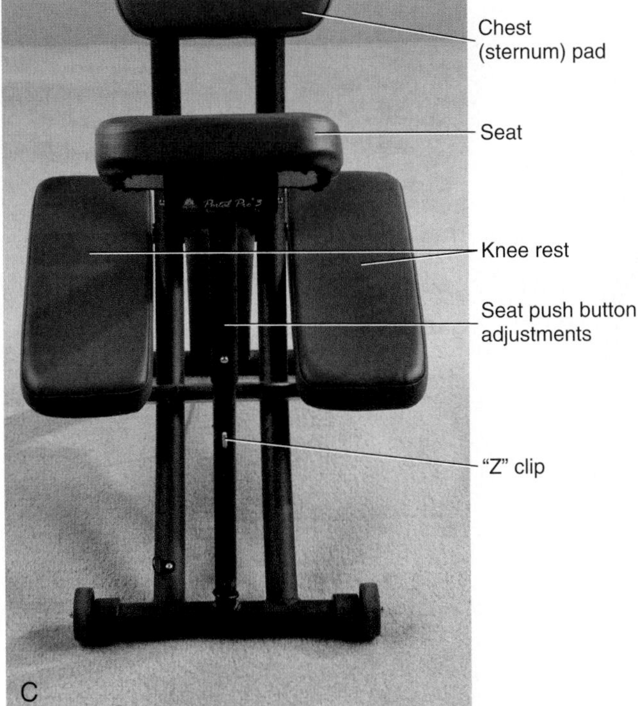

FIGURE 2-22, cont'd **C,** Back of massage chair with labeled parts.

The width of the base chair can be adjusted by removing the Z clip (Figure 2-23 I), changing the width of the base, then replacing the Z clip in the proper hole (Figure 2-23 J). The height of the seat can be changed by using the push button adjustments on the seat tube (Figure 2-23 K). Press the button in and raise or lower the seat tube as needed; the button will automatically pop into the appropriate hole.

To change the angle of the face cradle, release the face cradle angle cam lock, adjust the angle, then secure the face cradle by tightening the angle cam lock (Figure 2-23 L). The height of the face cradle can be changed by releasing the face cradle tube height and angle cam lock, adjusting the height of the face cradle tubes (Figure 2-23 M), then securing the face cradle tubes in place by tightening the cam lock and tightening the knob to secure the face cradle tube (Figure 2-23 N).

Adjusting the Massage Chair

Once the base of the chair is set and the seat is in place, the sternum pad, face cradle, and armrest need to be adjusted so that the client can sit comfortably and the practitioner can use proper body mechanics while working.

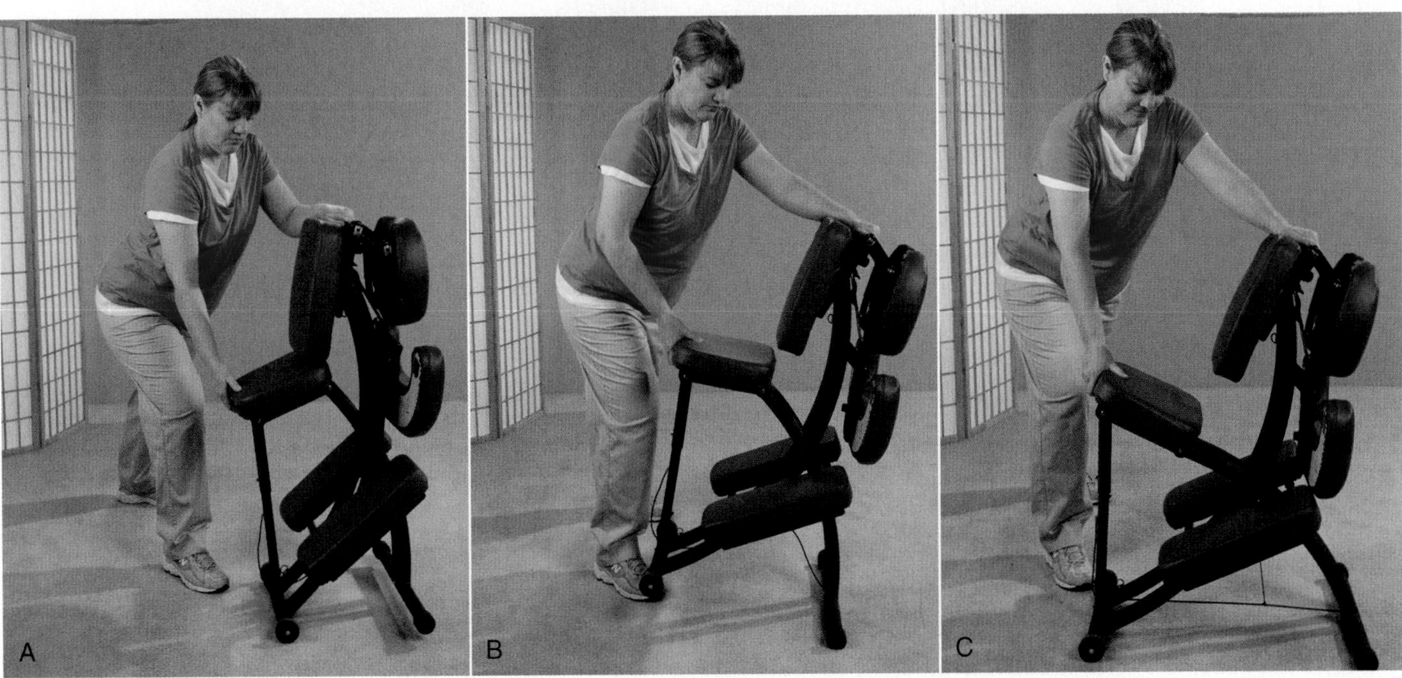

FIGURE 2-23 **A, B,** and **C,** Move the seat of the chair outward to create the solid base of the structure.

Continued

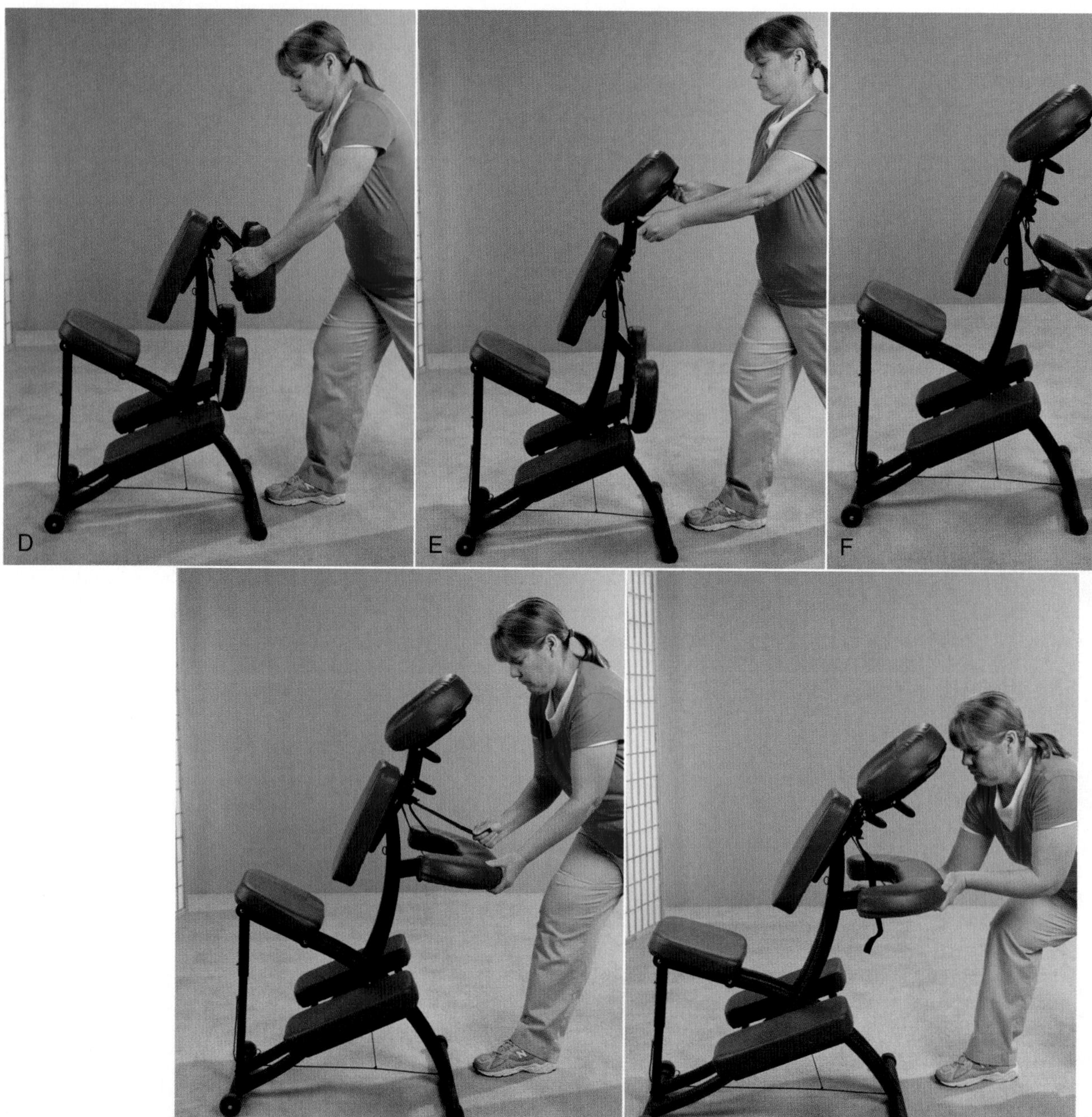

FIGURE 2-23, cont'd **D,** Elevate the face cradle into position. **E,** Lock the face cradle in place using the face cradle angle cam lock. **F,** Elevate the armrest into position. **G,** Adjust the armrest by pulling on the armrest adjustment strap. **H,** Lock the armrest in place using the armrest cam lock.

One of the most common mistakes practitioners make is to have clients positioned in the chair at an incorrect height or angle, thus impairing their ability to use proper body mechanics when working.

Massage chairs have a variety of settings to accommodate many body types. It is best to take a few extra moments to ensure the client's comfort at the onset of the treatment, rather than start the session and then notice the client is not at an optimal position for an effective treatment. Here are some general guidelines to use when adjusting the chair for individual client comfort:

- Visually assess the client's height and raise or lower the seat to a level that accommodates the length of the client's torso as well as allow for the legs to be comfortable in the kneeling position. The seat is generally positioned to allow the client ample room for the knees when in a kneeling position, and there should be enough space between the seat and the face cradle for comfortable

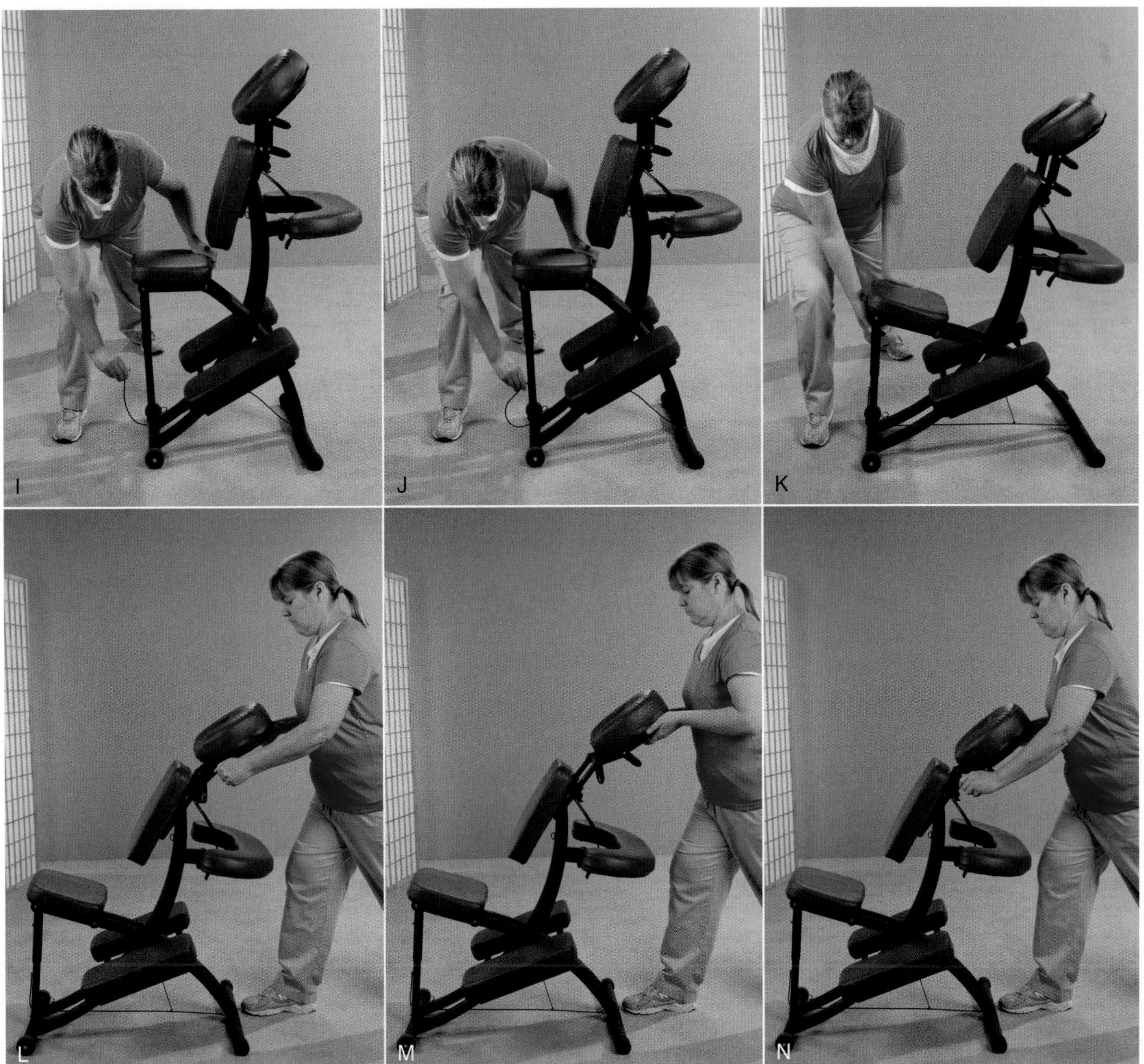

FIGURE 2-23, cont'd **I,** Prepare to adjust the base of the chair to the proper width by removing the Z clip. **J,** Place the Z clip in the proper hole. **K,** Adjust the height of the seat using the push button adjustments on the seat tube. **L,** Release the face cradle angle cam lock, adjust the angle of the face cradle, then secure the face cradle by tightening the angle cam lock. **M,** Release the face cradle tube height and angle cam lock, and adjust the height of the face cradle. **N,** Secure the face cradle tubes in place by tightening the cam lock and tightening the knob to secure the face cradle tube.

extension of the client's back. Taller clients should not have cramped knees (Figure 2-24 A), and shorter clients should not have their legs overly extended so their knees are pressing directly into the knee pads and their feet are on the floor (Figure 2-24 B). The taller the client, the lower the seat; the shorter the client, the higher the seat. Figure 2-24 C shows the seat placed at a comfortable height for the client.

Sometimes clients think that that they should be on the chair with all their weight in the kneeling position and sitting on just the front edge of the seat. Practitioners should encourage these clients to sit all the way back on the seat and just rest their lower legs on the kneeling pads.

- The sternum pad allows the client to lean forward comfortably in the chair with full support of the chest. Adjust the sternum pad so that it rests comfortably below the

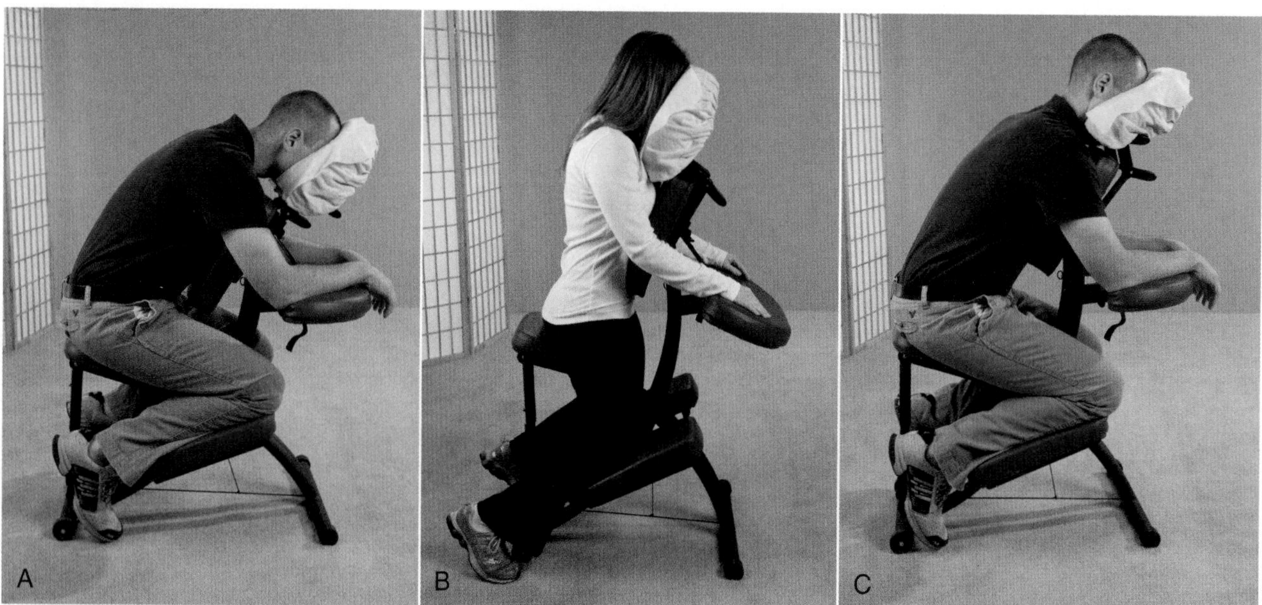

FIGURE 2-24 **A,** Seat placed too high for a taller client. **B,** Seat placed too low for a shorter client. **C,** Seat placed at a level that is comfortable for the client.

clavicles. As the client leans forward, the sternum pad should not press into the client's trachea, breast tissue, or abdominal region (Figure 2-25). Some chairs are designed to be moved from a vertical position to a horizontal position to accommodate the client's comfort. Triangle-shaped sternum pads that provide more comfort are also available for purchase. These pads can be changed from vertical (Figure 2-26 A) to horizontal (Figure 2-26 B). This is a helpful feature as it allows for more options when working with clients who have a larger body size or for pregnant women (Figure 2-26 C).

- The face cradle should be adjusted so that there is a comfortable, slight extension of the client's neck. If the face cradle is too high, the client's neck will be hyperextended; if it is too low, the neck will be uncomfortably "scrunched" down into the shoulders.

There are two methods that can be used to determine if the face cradle is in the proper placement. One is a visual assessment. The client's neck should not have any wrinkles or folds of the posterior tissue. Figure 2-27 A shows proper placement of the face cradle; Figure 2-27 B shows improper placement of the face cradle. If these appear, the face cradle is too low and needs to be raised. If the client is left in this position for the duration of the treatment, it could cause a headache because of a lack of proper blood flow to the brain, or muscle spasms because of improper alignment of the neck muscles.

Another quick assessment tool involves palpation. If the practitioner can grasp and get good lift of the muscle tissue of the posterior neck while kneading it, the client's neck is not hyperextended and the face cradle is in the proper position (Figure 2-28).

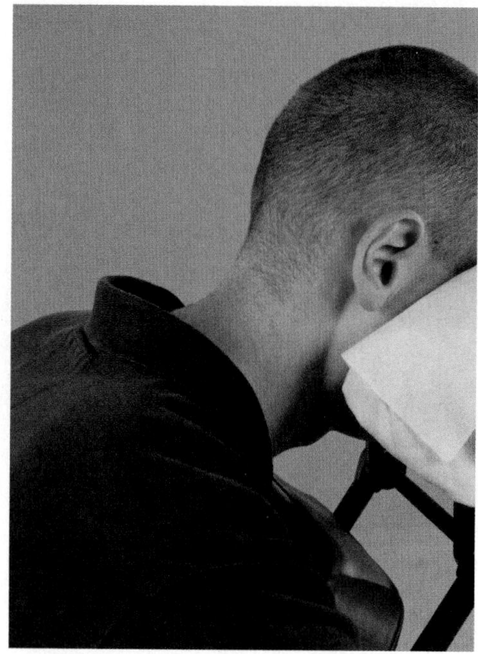

FIGURE 2-25 Proper placement of the sternum pad.

The cushion of the face cradle should not be in a position to interfere with the client's ability to breathe. The client's chin should not rest on any part of the cradle, such as the support bar, that would cause discomfort while

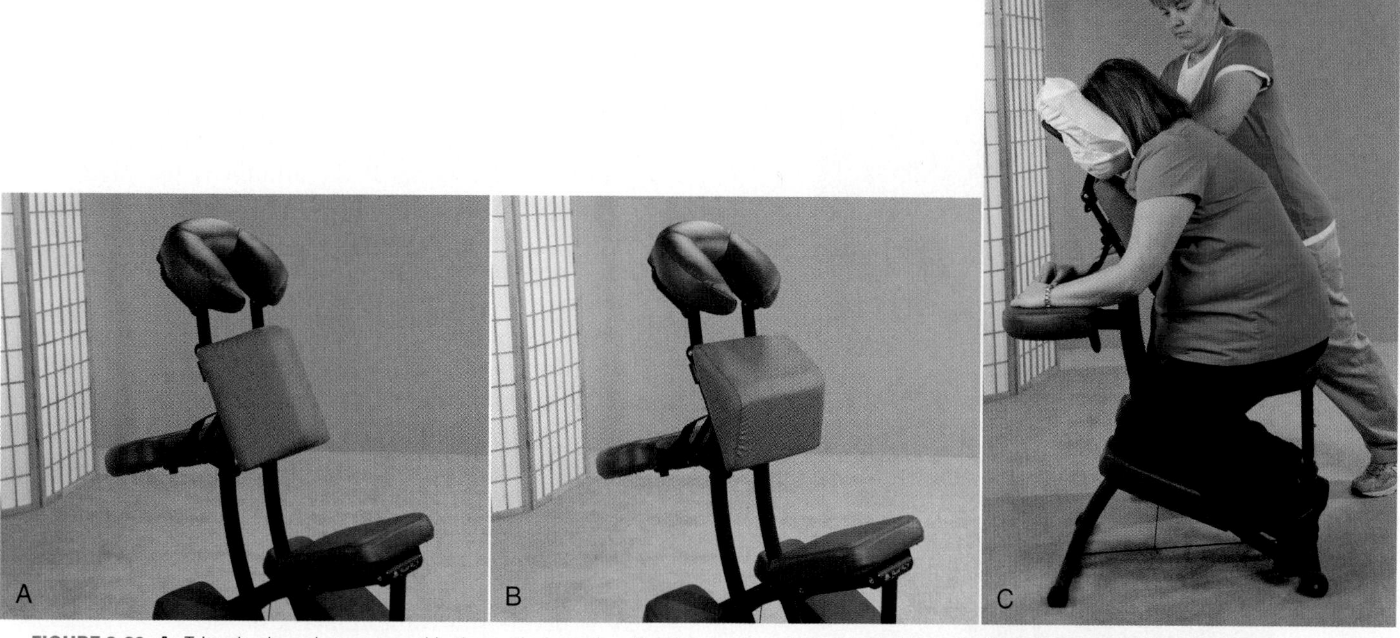

FIGURE 2-26 **A,** Triangle-shaped sternum pad in the vertical position. **B,** Triangle-shaped sternum pad in the horizontal position. **C,** Triangle-shaped sternum pad in the horizontal position with a pregnant client.

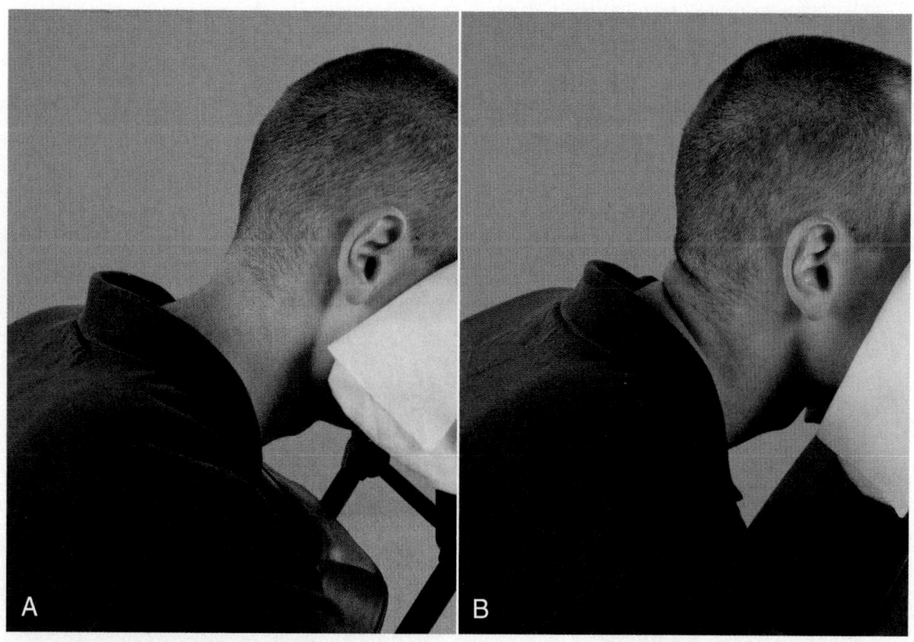

FIGURE 2-27 **A,** Proper placement of the face cradle. **B,** Wrinkles or folds in the client's posterior neck indicating improper placement of the face cradle.

receiving the treatment, nor should the cheeks rest on any part of the metal structure of the face cradle frame. Also, the face cradle cushion should not be low enough to touch the client's upper trapezius muscles; this interferes with the practitioner's ability to use the forearm on this area of the client's body. Face cushions are kept in place with Velcro, which makes it is easy to adjustment them.

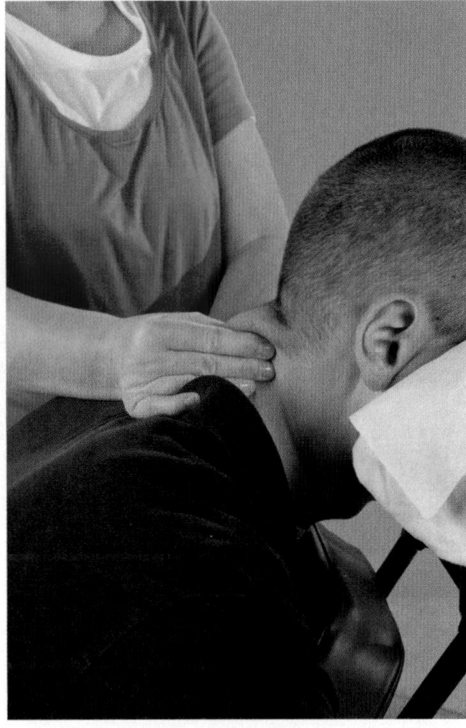

FIGURE 2-28 Grasping a portion of posterior neck tissue to check if the client is in proper alignment.

- The armrest allows the client to rest the arms comfortably when receiving the treatment. The armrest should be placed in a position that allows for slack in the upper trapezius muscles (Figure 2-29 A). If the armrest is placed too low, shoulder and arm muscles will be elongated, making it difficult to grasp the muscle tissue while performing kneading. If the armrest is too high, the shoulders will be elevated, possibly leading to nerve compression, which can manifest as numbness and tingling down the client's arms, and it will be difficult to knead the tissue as well.

To check for proper position of the armrest, grasp the upper trapezius bilaterally. If there is good lift of the tissue, then the armrest is in an appropriate position (Figure 2-29 B).

It should be noted that these are universal suggestions for proper set up and adjustment of a massage chair. It is important to ask, each time a client sits in the chair, "Are you comfortable?" No matter how much the practitioner knows about adjusting the chair, it is ultimately up to the client to decide how comfortable he or she is.

Part of professionalism is being able to set up, adjust, and take down the massage chair efficiently. Because chair massage appointments are usually kept on a tight schedule, it is better not to waste valuable treatment time handling the chair. This can be noticeable to clients, and they may get frustrated with any delays, thus starting the treatment off poorly.

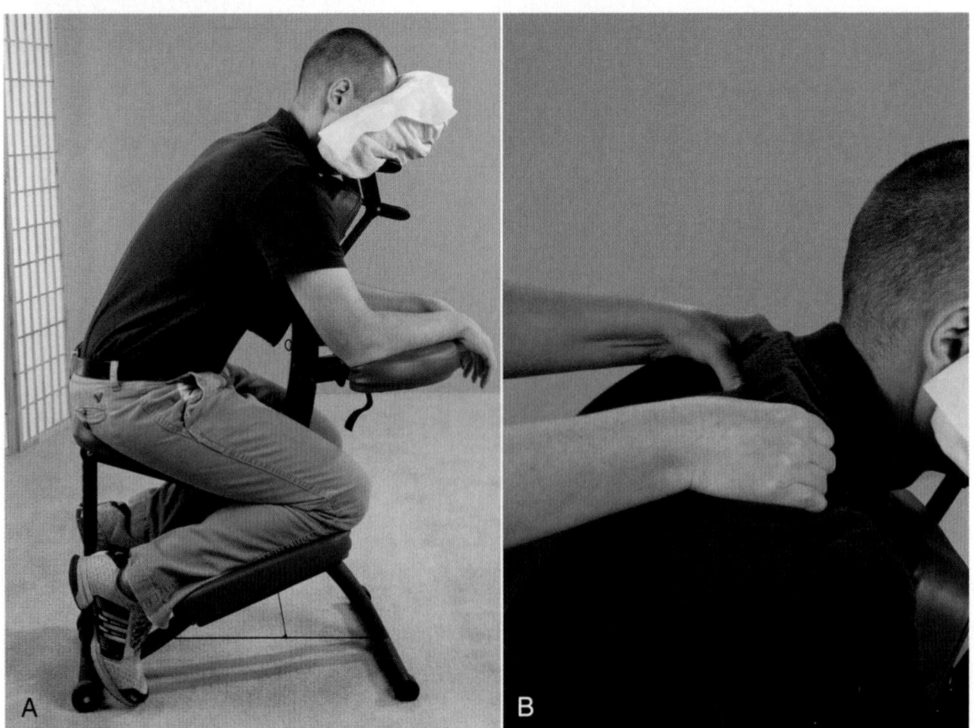

FIGURE 2-29 **A,** Armrest placed in proper position for client. **B,** Good lift of the upper trapezius muscle.

With practice, all of the adjustments will take just a few seconds. One way to become proficient is to practice setting up the chair and making client adjustments many times before performing the first treatment. Enlisting family and friends of all body sizes and shapes can be good practice. Over time, the practitioners will be able to assess a client's height as they are greeting the client and immediately know the basic adjustments to make.

Taking Down the Massage Chair

Taking down the chair involves reversing the steps involved in setting it up. Close the base of the chair first by bringing the seat down and closing together the two parts of the chair that create the foundation. The face cradle and sternum pad should then be put in their lowest setting and secured by tightening the cam locks. The armrest pad is placed downward (flat against the chair), and then the chair can be placed in its carrying bag.

SANITATION AND HYGIENE

The success of a bodywork practice depends on, to a large extent, the equipment and supplies that the practitioner uses. Once a massage chair has been chosen and purchased, it is essential that the chair be kept in excellent working condition, that all supplies be clean and well kept, and that appropriate sanitation measures are taken. In addition to equipment and supplies that are clean and fully functional, practitioners need to pay attention to personal hygiene. All of these details not only ensure the health and safety of clients, they demonstrate professionalism and inspire confidence, in both clients and the practitioner.

As with all services that involve human-to-human contact, practitioners need to be aware of the dangers of pathogen transmission. **Pathogens** are disease-causing organisms such as fungi, yeast, molds, viruses, and bacteria. Sometimes the term **microorganism** is used instead of pathogen. Microorganisms are any life forms that are microscopic.

Even though practitioners are working with clients who are clothed while receiving chair massage, there is still risk of passing pathogens from practitioners to clients and from clients to practitioners. There is also a risk of practitioners transferring pathogens from one client to another. This is because microorganisms can be transferred from client clothing and skin (such as bare arms and legs, if the client is wearing a short-sleeved top and shorts) to the vinyl of the chair. If the chair is not sanitized between clients, then the microorganisms can be passed to another person. If practitioners do not clean their hands and arms, they can also pass the microorganisms onto another person. Aside from the human factor, pathogens can also be found on supplies and equipment.

Hygiene and **sanitation** involve methods that ensure good health and cleanliness and are a necessary part of bodywork practice routines. Personal hygiene is an essential component of professionalism. It plays a role in maintaining both practitioner and client health. Although it is unlikely that practitioners of chair massage would come into contact with client body fluids regularly, there is always the possibility that blood, mucus, saliva, vomit, urine, and even semen from clients can contaminate equipment and can come in contact with practitioners' skin and clothing. For example, the client's skin, nasal excretions, and saliva may contact the face cradle. Accidents happen. Blood from wounds or menstruation, urine, or fecal material from clothes or hands may contact parts of the chair. Although it may be uncomfortable to think about, or perhaps some practitioners think it will never happen to them, all of these body fluids have been known to contaminate bodywork equipment, including massage chairs. It is better to plan for the unexpected than to be confronted with a situation for which the practitioner is completely unprepared.

Hygiene Guidelines

The following sanitation and hygiene guidelines are useful for all bodywork practitioners:

1. Take care of personal hygiene by bathing daily.
2. Keep fingernails short and clean, and do not wear nail polish. Long nails and cracked nail polish provide places for pathogens to grow. Long nails can also injure the client.
3. Do not wear rings, bracelets, or wristwatches during treatments. These have a lot of small crevices that provide places for pathogens to grow. They might also injure the client or be distracting if the bracelets make noise as they move.
4. Wear a clean uniform or clean clothing each day. If the uniform or clothing comes in contact with body fluids, it needs to be changed immediately.
5. Thoroughly wash hands, forearms, and elbows before and after each treatment, using soap, hot water, and paper towels. Liquid soap in a pump dispenser is best, as bar soap can become contaminated by direct contact. Massage soapy hands (making sure to include the areas between the fingers), forearms, and elbows for 30 seconds, then rinse them until all lather is gone. Wipe dry with paper towels, and use the paper towels to turn off the taps to prevent re-contamination. Paper towels are more sanitary because they are disposed of after one use. Cloth towels that are used over and over provide a place for pathogens to grow.

When performing chair massage onsite, it may not be practical to wash the hands before and after each treatment. For example, if many treatments are being given and there are only a few minutes in between each treatment, there may not be enough time to visit a washroom. Or if the treatments are being given in an outdoor setting, such as in a park or parking lot, washing facilities may not be available. In situations like these, the practitioner will need to bring hand sanitizer. One option is rubbing alcohol, which can be wiped over the skin and other surfaces (and so can also be used to sanitize equipment). It evaporates quickly and destroys a wide variety of pathogens. Rubbing alcohol is most useful when combined with water; 70% isopropyl alcohol is, in fact, more effective than 95% alcohol. Seventy percent isopropyl alcohol is inexpensive and easy to obtain. It can be diluted to a solution that is half 70% isopropyl alcohol and half water and transported to the treatment site in a spray or squirt bottle. However, alcohol can be very drying to the skin, especially if it is used repetitively. Also, the scent of alcohol can be objectionable, although alcohol scented with wintergreen, cherry, or citrus is available.

Another option is witch hazel. It is also useful for cleaning the hands and equipment, can be diluted 50/50 with water, and can be transported in a spray or squirt bottle. Some people, though, dislike or are allergic to the scent of witch hazel.

A third option is commercial hand sanitizers; there are many currently on the market. Many have alcohol in them, which is why they evaporate quickly, and so they may be drying to the skin if used quite often. Some hand sanitizers have aloe or other skin moisturizers in them to combat the dehydration.

6. Disposable gloves should be worn any time the practitioner has a cut or broken skin on the hands, needs to handle contaminated supplies, or is cleaning any equipment that has come in contact with body fluids. If the wound or cut is on a finger, a finger cot may be used instead.
7. Do not perform treatments if ill because of the danger of passing on pathogens to clients and coworkers.
8. Do not perform treatments under the influence of alcohol or recreational drugs. These impair judgment and increase the chance of making poor decisions about infection control, as well as other poor decisions. It is also extremely unprofessional.

In some areas of the country, state laws or employers may require or highly recommend that practitioners be vaccinated against certain diseases such as rubella, tuberculosis, poliomyelitis, and hepatitis. Practitioners should do research to determine what the immunizations are required for their particular municipalities.

Sanitation

Just as important as personal hygiene is proper sanitation for equipment and supplies. Proper sanitation involves the use of **disinfectants** and **antiseptics**. Disinfectants are used on nonliving objects to destroy microorganisms; antiseptics kill microorganisms on living tissue. It is important that equipment and supplies that came in contact with the client's skin are cleaned between clients. Many good antibacterial sprays and disinfectants are on the market; practitioners should research them to find the ones that work the best for them.

As discussed under "Hygiene Guidelines," rubbing alcohol (70% isopropyl alcohol) is a good, all-purpose disinfectant because it can be wiped over surfaces, evaporates quickly, destroys a wide variety of pathogens, is inexpensive, and is easy to obtain. Of course, many other sanitizers and disinfectants are available as well.

Because of chemical sensitivities some clients may have, using "green" or environmentally safe products is also highly recommended. Citrus products made from citrus essential oils such as orange, lemon, or grapefruit can be purchased. These disinfectants are safe, nontoxic, and environmentally friendly. Other natural products and commercial cleaning agents are also available. Manufacturer's instructions on all products should be followed to ensure they disinfect properly.

Household bleach is the one of most effective disinfectants available. It is mandated by the Centers for Disease Control and Prevention (CDC) for cleaning up blood and

First-Aid Kits

Many locations in which seated massage is performed may have first-aid kits available for minor emergencies. If, however, practitioners feel more comfortable having their own kit readily available in case either they or clients receive an injury, an option would be to purchase a commercial first-aid kit. Another option is to make one. A simple kit could include just adhesive bandages and an antiseptic solution such as hydrogen peroxide. More complex kits could include some or all of the following:

- A first-aid manual
- Sterile gauze
- Adhesive tape
- Adhesive bandages in several sizes
- Elastic bandage
- Antiseptic wipes
- Soap
- Antibiotic cream (triple-antibiotic ointment)
- Antiseptic solution (like hydrogen peroxide)
- Hydrocortisone cream (1%)
- Acetaminophen and ibuprofen
- Tweezers
- Sharp scissors
- Safety pins
- Disposable instant cold packs
- Calamine lotion
- Alcohol wipes or ethyl alcohol
- Plastic gloves (at least two pairs)
- A mouthpiece for administering cardiopulmonary resuscitation (CPR) (can be obtained from the local Red Cross)

Additionally, it is highly recommended that massage and bodywork practitioners become certified in first aid and CPR, and maintain that certification. In some municipalities, this may be a requirement for massage and bodywork licensure.

other body fluid spills in healthcare settings, and because it is inexpensive and easy to obtain, it should be used for body fluid decontamination in the bodywork setting. A 10% solution (1 part bleach to 9 parts water) is recommended.

Universal (Standard) Precautions

Universal (standard) precautions are protocols established by the Centers for Disease Control and Prevention (CDC) to reduce the chance of spreading contagious diseases within healthcare settings. These protocols are designed to protect both the patient and healthcare provider. They are required to be followed when healthcare providers are performing medical procedures that involve puncturing or penetrating the body or when dealing with body fluids. The reason these are called universal precautions is that they are applied universally to all patients, not just to certain ones. Because *universal* is sometimes misunderstood to mean that these precautions protect patients and healthcare providers from all pathogens universally and perfectly, which they do not, the term *standard precautions* is sometimes used instead.

For healthcare providers these precautions include, but are not limited to, the following:

- Wearing protective equipment such as masks, gowns, gloves, goggles, and face shields
- Specific methods of disposal for needles and other sharps and for linens
- Specific decontamination techniques for instruments and supplies as well as for blood spills
- Frequent and thorough hand washing

Not all universal precautions that apply to the healthcare profession apply to the bodywork profession. There are several, though, that are particularly relevant. Although practitioners may not come into contact with body fluids regularly, there is always the possibility that blood, mucus, saliva, urine, and semen from clients can contaminate linens and equipment and can come in contact with practitioners' skin and clothing. The hygiene and sanitation methods outlined in this chapter are based on the CDC's universal precautions.

The CDC issued universal precautions in 1987, and they are updated as necessary. It is recommended that practitioners update their information on sanitary procedures every six months. The website address is www.cdc.gov.

Although bleach can be stored and used in bodywork offices, it is not practical to carry it onsite. However, commercial, professional-grade germicidal wipes to sanitize equipment are available to purchase. These are not the general-purpose, household-grade cleaning wipes found in grocery and department stores. Instead they are found in medical supply stores and online. There are several different brands and types from which to choose. The best choice would be one that kills a wide spectrum of pathogens including some of the most common and potentially deadly:

- The tuberculosis (TB) bacterium
- Hepatitis viruses
- *E. coli* bacteria
- MRSA (methicillin-resistant staphylococcus aureus bacterium)

At approximately $10 plus shipping for a container of 160 wipes, they are affordable. As with alcohol, these wipes can be dehydrating to the skin, so practitioners may want to consider wearing latex gloves when cleaning surfaces with the wipes. If there is an allergy to latex, gloves made of nonlatex materials such as vinyl or nitrile rubber are also available. Here are some websites to research for germicidal wipes:

http://medrepexpress.com/store/supplies/antibacterial.htm
www.keysan.com/ksu1729a.htm
www.nextag.com/SANI-CLOTH-PLUS-GERMICIDAL

Equipment Maintenance and Sanitation Guidelines

As discussed previously, it is essential to maintain equipment and follow sanitation procedures to ensure the health and safety of clients. There are sanitation guidelines to follow during treatment sessions as well as general equipment maintenance and sanitation guidelines.

The following are sanitation guidelines to follow during treatment sessions:

1. Massage chairs and desktop systems need to be cleaned and disinfected before the first client, in between each client, and after the last client. This includes the face cradle, sternum pad, armrest and leg rests, and any other part of the chair the client may have breathed on or touched. Use rubbing alcohol, witch hazel, or the professional-grade germicidal wipes. As discussed previously, rubbing alcohol and professional-grade germicidal wipes are drying to the skin, so practitioners may want to consider wearing latex, vinyl, or nitrile rubber gloves when sanitizing equipment.
2. Any thumb-saving tools used should also be sanitized before the first client, in between each client, and after the last client.
3. After sanitizing the face cradle, place a clean cover on it for each client. There are several options for covering face cradles:
   - *Paper towels.* This is the most inexpensive option. The paper towels should be flat and not textured; if they are textured, the design will be pressed into the client's face during the course of the treatment. Paper towels can be used in one of two ways. If the individual sheet is large enough to cover the face cradle, measure out one sheet and tear it halfway up the middle, then place on the face cradle (Figure 2-30 A). The tearing allows room for the client's nose and mouth so he or she can breathe comfortably. Another option is to measure out two sheets (do not separate

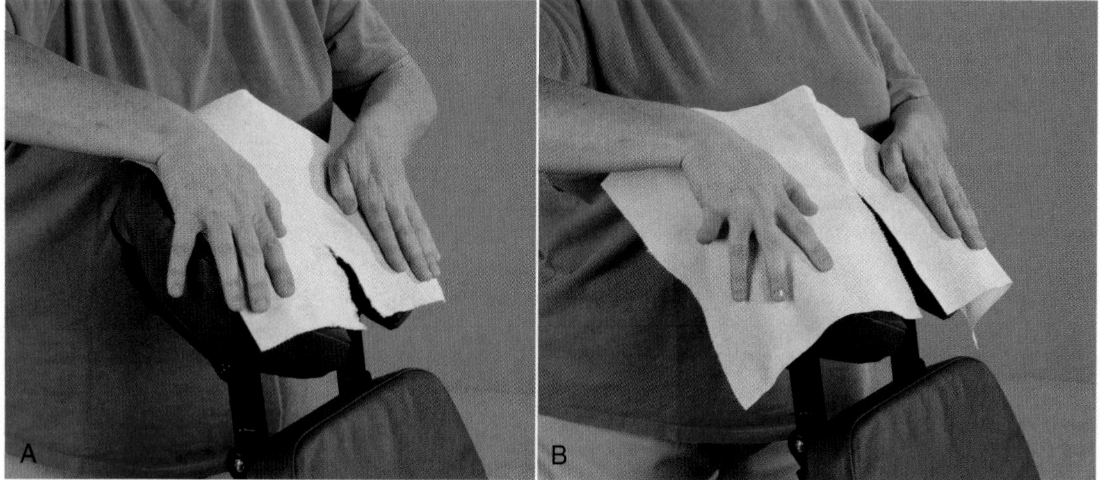

FIGURE 2-30 **A,** Single sheet of paper towel used as a face cradle cover. **B,** Double sheets of paper towel used as a face cradle cover.

them) and tear them off the roll. Then separate the two sheets halfway up the perforated seam. Place the sheets over the face cradle, with the seam running vertically, and the separation on the bottom (Figure 2-30 B).

- *Commercial disposable face cradle covers.* These are designed for single-client use and are made of soft, thick paper or soft, fabric fibers. They come in two main styles: those that are flat pieces (Figure 2-31 A) and those that resemble the shape of the face cradle and may have elastic around the perimeter to secure it to the cradle (Figure 2-31 B). They are available from several companies, such as some of those that sell massage chairs, and from massage supply companies.
- *A washable cloth face cradle cover that stays on throughout the treatment session.* The most comfortable and long-lasting ones are made of 100% cotton and have an elastic band around the perimeter to secure it to the cradle (Figure 2-31 C). New paper towels or disposable face cradle covers are placed over it for each client (Figure 2-31 D), unless the cloth cover becomes contaminated, in which case it would need to be removed and replaced with a clean cover.

  Here is a list of some websites for practitioners to explore for disposable and washable cloth face cradle covers:
  Massage Warehouse, www.massagewarehouse.com
  Massage King, www.massageking.com
  Massage Depot, www.massagedepot.com
  Massage-Tools, www.massage-tools.com
- *Washable cloth face cradle covers that are replaced for each client.* Practitioners should keep in mind that this not only means cost for a stock of the cloth face cradle covers, it means increased laundry as well.

4. Place a clean cover on bolsters and pillow covers used for each client.

The following are general equipment maintenance and sanitation guidelines for bodywork practitioners:

1. Follow all manufacturer's instructions to clean and maintain equipment properly. Improperly maintained equipment can endanger client and practitioner safety, as well as be potential havens for pathogens. Inspect the massage chair or desktop system regularly for cracks or damage; travel is hard on equipment. Also keep the carrying bag in good working order, such as by fixing broken zippers or tears in the fabric and cleaning it regularly. A clean, intact bag not only protects the equipment, it is a sign of professionalism.
2. Use only clean face cradle covers, bolster, and pillow covers. All cloth covers that come in contact with the client's skin should be used on only that client and laundered between uses. Wash them in hot water with detergent, and then dry them in a dryer with hot air. An option is to use disposable face cradle covers, such as paper towels or commercial covers. These are discussed in more detail in "Other Necessary Equipment and Supplies."
3. Uniforms or other clothing used while performing treatments should be laundered separately from cloth equipment covers. They should be washed in hot water with detergent and hot-air dried between wearing.
4. Replace any thumb-saving tools used as soon as they show signs of wear. Cracks and crevices in the surfaces of these items are ideal for pathogen growth.

Decontamination Protocol

If any of the coverings such as face cradle covers and covers for bolsters and pillows should become contaminated with body fluids, practitioners should wear disposable gloves to remove them from the treatment area and place them in a secure container separate from containers that hold other used coverings or linens. When working onsite, gallon

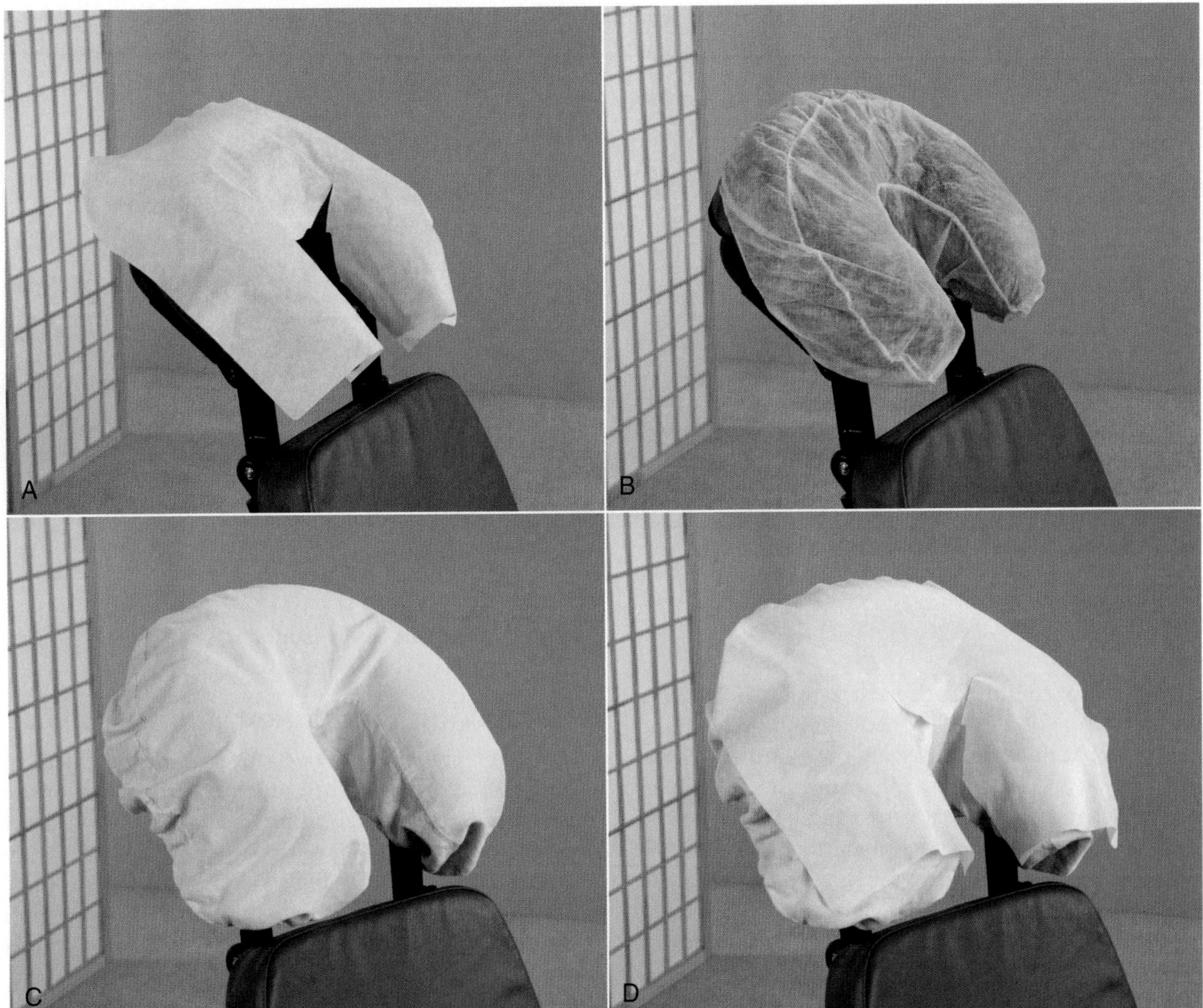

FIGURE 2-31 A, Flat, paper disposable face cradle cover. **B,** Fiber disposable face cradle cover that resembles the shape of the face cradle. **C,** Washable cloth face cradle cover. **D,** Washable cloth face cradle cover with a disposable face cradle cover placed over it.

plastic bags that can be sealed or a garbage bag that can be tied securely can be used as secure containers.

The contaminated items should be laundered separately from any other items. Hot water, detergent, and one fourth of a cup of chlorine bleach should be used, and then the coverings should be hot-air dried. This procedure should also be used for contaminated uniforms or other clothing worn to perform treatments.

Disposable gloves should be worn while using paper towels to wipe up any body fluids that have come in contact with equipment, the floor, or other surfaces. The paper towels should then be discarded in a secure container separate from other waste. Using fresh paper towels, the area should then be cleaned with soap and water, and these paper towels should also be discarded in the separate, secure container. The area should next be disinfected with a 10% bleach solution. After thoroughly cleaning and disinfecting the area, the disposable gloves should be removed and discarded in the separate, secure container, and the hands should be washed using soap and water.

As discussed previously, it is not practical to carry bleach to locations in which chair massage is performed. Should contamination from body fluids occur while performing treatments, some practitioners may instead feel more comfortable having an emergency spill kit with them. It can include the following (Figure 2-32):

- Professional, commercial-grade germicidal wipes
- Paper towels
- At least two sets of latex, vinyl, or nitrile rubber gloves
- Gallon plastic bags that can be sealed or garbage bags that can be tied securely

OTHER EQUIPMENT AND SUPPLIES

When providing massage treatments, there are additional supplies that practitioners may want to consider. Some of

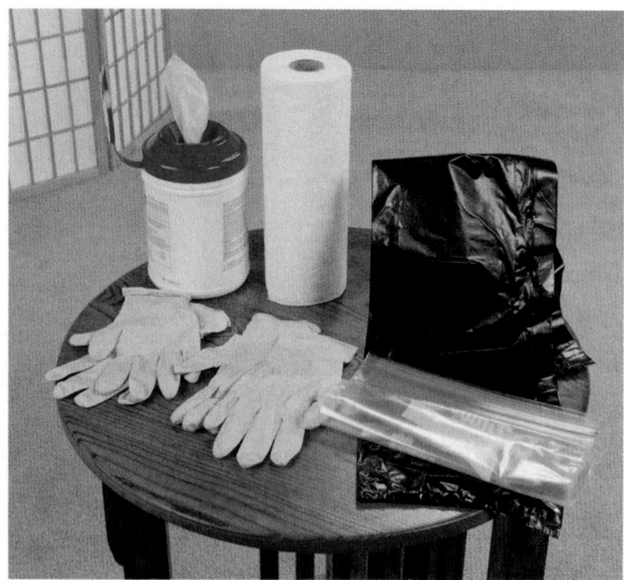

FIGURE 2-32 Emergency spill kit.

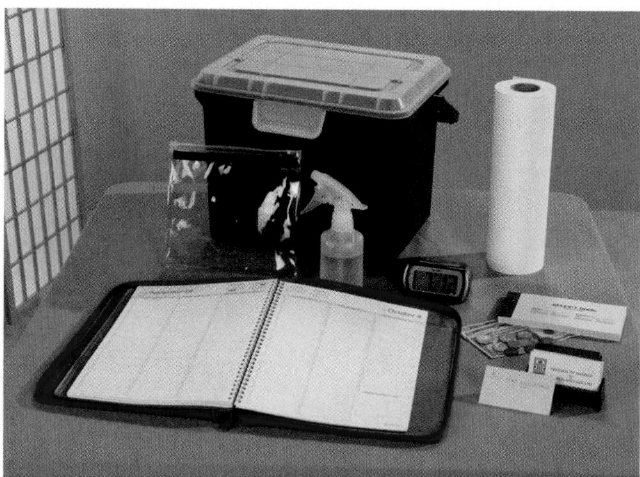

FIGURE 2-33 Minimum kit of supplies practitioners need to take.

these are for client comfort, such as extra props and bolsters or a small mirror for clients to check their face, hair, and makeup (if applicable) after receiving the treatment. Some of these are business items for the practitioner such as a clock to keep track of treatment lengths, receipts and change for clients who pay the practitioner directly, an appointment book, and business cards. Yet other items can be for advertising that chair massage treatments are available or the practitioner's business. These can be items such as banners, DVDs, PowerPoint displays, and price lists.

When deciding what supplies are needed, practitioners need to again consider their "equipment personalities." Some people like to have many different items with them because it makes them feel more prepared for any contingency. Others may be more minimalist and prefer to travel as lightly as possible. Other factors that the practitioner should take into account when deciding what to travel with include the following:

- *Size of the transport vehicle.* Obviously, the more room in the vehicle, the more equipment and supplies can be transported.
- *Location of the treatment session.* If many items are brought, is there enough space to store or display them? Where does the practitioner need to park? If it is a far distance from the treatment location, the practitioner may want to carry everything to the treatment location in one trip, necessitating fewer items.
- *Setup time and takedown time.* If there will be plenty of time to set up and take down the treatment space, more items can be brought in and set up, then taken down and carried away after the treatment session. If setup and takedown time is limited, fewer items should be brought.
- *Financial investment.* Practitioners with limited funds may be able to only invest in a few, but necessary, items at first, then add more supplies later on when realizing profits from their businesses.

Organizing Equipment and Supplies

A little planning and organization of equipment and supplies goes a long way when providing treatments onsite. By being organized, practitioners use their time and energy more efficiently, and it can cut down on the stress of traveling to locations. Practitioners should first decide what is absolutely essential to bring for treatments, then they should decide what additional items they would like to bring if logistics allow. They should then assemble the items in one place so that everything is ready when the practitioner needs to travel to provide treatments.

What follows are some suggestions for ways to assemble equipment and supplies. These are designed as kits practitioners can take along with their massage chair or desktop support.

Minimum Kit (Figure 2-33)

These are the basic, essential items a practitioner needs for onsite treatment sessions:

- Hand and equipment sanitizer: rubbing alcohol or witch hazel (diluted 50/50 with water) in a spray or squirt bottle
- Nontextured paper towels
- Clock
- Receipts for clients who pay the practitioner directly (as opposed to situations where the practitioner is paid by a company to perform treatments)
- Change for clients who pay in cash
- Appointment book, pen, and appointment cards to book clients either for more chair massage treatments or for table massage if the practitioner performs that as well
- Carrying case for all the supplies

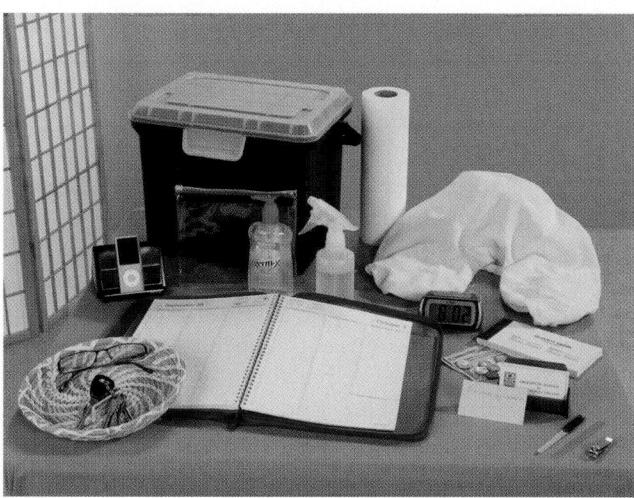

FIGURE 2-34 Medium kit of supplies practitioners may want to take.

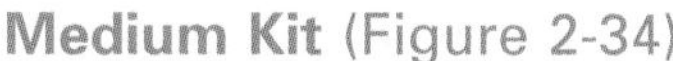

Medium Kit (Figure 2-34)

In addition to the items in the minimum kit, these additional items will enhance the onsite treatment session experience:

- A washable cloth face cradle cover—the practitioner can then just replace paper towel face cradle covers in between each client and does not have to sanitize the face cradle each time
- Commercial hand sanitizer
- Nail clippers and nail file to groom the practitioner's nails if needed
- A small basket in which clients can place their glasses and items from their pockets such as keys, coins, wallet, pens, and cell phone
- Music, either on a portable CD player or a portable digital audio player such as an iPod or MP3 player with speakers; the digital audio player has the advantage of being much smaller than a CD player and can be programmed to play hundreds of songs as opposed to the one to five CDs the average portable CD player can play

Deluxe Kit (Figure 2-35)

The deluxe kit is so named because this includes supplies that may be considered luxury items to take on location. However, they can greatly enhance the chair massage session treatment and setting. These supplies are in addition to all the items in the minimum and medium kits:

- Folding chair or stool if the practitioner prefers to sit while working on client arms and hands; sitting while working on client arms and hands is covered in more detail in Chapter 3, "Basic Sequence"
- Disposable face cradle covers or washable face cradle covers
- Blanket or beach towel to wrap around clients who become chilled while receiving the treatment or to lay across the lap of clients who wear short skirts to the treatment

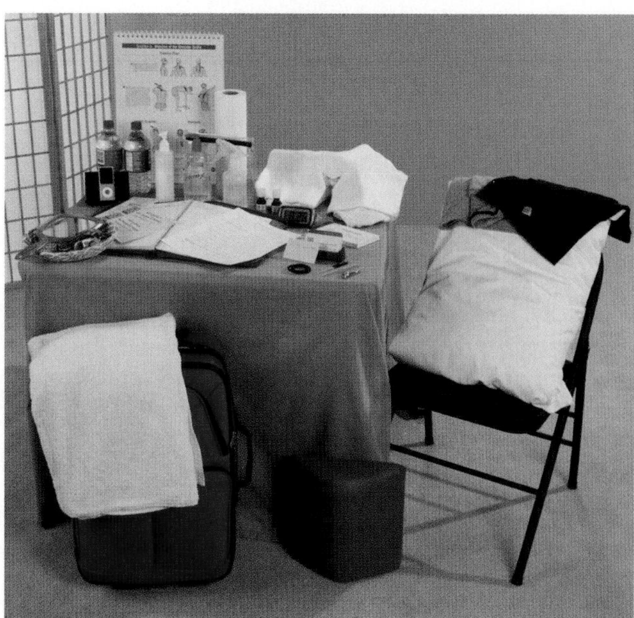

FIGURE 2-35 Deluxe kit of supplies practitioners may want to take.

- T-shirts in various sizes; clients who are concerned about their shirts or blouses can wear these during the treatment instead
- Washable/disposable hair ties for clients with long hair that may interfere with the treatment
- Small mirror for clients to check themselves after receiving the treatment
- Client intake forms; these are discussed in more detail in Chapter 6, "Essentials of Business"
- Props:
  - Additional triangle-shaped sternum pad for pregnant clients, large-breasted women, larger body sizes
  - Pillow for clients to rest on if they do not want to put their faces in cradle
- Aromatherapy; practitioners should be aware that clients may be allergic or have sensitivity to certain scents, so they should always check in with clients about any possible allergies or sensitivities before using any aromatherapy
- Lotion or oil to massage areas of the client not covered by clothing, such as arms and hands, if desired by the client
- Promotional items:
  - Business cards
  - Brochures
  - Gift certificates
  - Client gifts, such as water bottles or magnets with the practitioner's business name and business phone number on them
- Tools for client education:
  - Small, portable flip charts showing, for example, the bones and muscles of the body, or trigger points
  - Handouts of stretches/exercises clients can do for themselves to continue the benefits of the chair

massage; practitioners should have their business name and business phone number on any and all handouts as reminders to clients
- Price list

Kit for Exhibitions, Tradeshows, and Fairs

When working at exhibitions, tradeshows, and fairs such as health fairs, practitioners may have the opportunity to provide chair massage in a designated treatment area or booth that lends itself to more sophisticated marketing and promotion for the practitioner. In addition to the items in the minimum, medium, and deluxe kits, practitioners might also consider bringing the following:

- Signs or banners promoting the business
- Large posters or display boards listing the benefits of chair massage and showing pictures of people receiving chair massage
- DVD or PowerPoint display showing pictures of people receiving chair massage and discussing the benefits of chair massage
- Bottled water and refreshments such as candy, fruit, or cookies
- Waste basket

LOGISTICS OF TRAVELING TO LOCATIONS

There are several logistical factors practitioners should keep in mind when traveling to locations to perform chair massage. The most important one is to be flexible. For example, practitioners may be given unclear or incorrect directions to the location. Perhaps practitioners have been told that there will be plenty of parking at the location but find that the only spots available are a great distance away. The treatment space may turn out to be tiny and hot, or maybe the contact person at a business forgot to tell workers about the treatment session and practitioners arrive to find they have no clients. Being able to remain calm, professional, and think on their feet will help practitioners sort out just about any unfavorable situation they find themselves in.

Before Traveling to the Location

As stated previously, a little planning and organization goes a long way. To prevent as many mishaps and misunderstandings as possible, there are some things the practitioner can do before traveling to the location. One of the most important is for the practitioner to communicate with the people at the location, such as a company or event representative. By determining what to expect ahead of time, practitioners will know what equipment and supplies to take, what the treatment space will be (although this could end up being radically different from what the practitioner envisions), how the payment will be handled, how many clients they will have, and how much time out of the day they need to plan for.

When communicating with the company or event representative, practitioners should be sure to discuss the following:

- How many treatment sessions of what length will be given? Treatments can be 10, 15, 20, or 30 minutes long. Practitioners need to determine for themselves how many treatments of what length they are able and willing to do. For example, if 30 employees each receive a 15-minute treatment, that is 7½ hours of massage with no breaks. On the other hand, 5 employees receiving 10-minute treatments is 50 minutes of massage, which some practitioners may decide is not worth their time and effort.
  - Practitioners should keep in mind what they need to do in between each treatment. For example, 15-minute treatment blocks may include the pretreatment interview, assisting the client out of the chair at the end of the treatment, sanitizing the chair and preparing for the next client, and practitioners getting a drink of water for themselves. The actual treatment time may, out of necessity, be 12 minutes. Otherwise, clients may start backing up, which can be frustrating for both practitioners and clients.
- Who creates the signup sheet, the practitioner or the representative? It can be as simple as a piece of paper on which people write their names or a typed schedule denoting client names and treatment times. A signup sheet is useful for several reasons. It creates an order in which clients will be seen, it lets practitioners know how many clients they will be working on and what order they will be seeing them, and it is a reference tool for payment.
  - If possible, the signup sheet should also include client contact phone numbers (for no-shows), how long each session lasts, and the cost of the treatment (if applicable).
  - The practitioner and representative should also clarify how the clients will be signed up. Will the signup sheet be circulated to the employees before the treatment session? If so, who will circulate it, how will it be circulated (email, paper copy sent around, etc.), and how far in advance will it be circulated? Will it be sent to the practitioner ahead of time? If so, how? By fax, email, or regular mail? Or will the signup sheet be posted outside the treatment area just before the treatment session begins, giving clients the opportunity to sign up then?
- How is the practitioner being paid? Is it hourly or per treatment? This can determine treatment length and fee structure. For example, if the practitioner is hired to perform 15-minute treatments for two hours and works on only 5 people, she will be waiting around a lot. The practitioner could then decide to charge for only the 5 treatments but needs to keep in mind that she had allotted two hours of her time, not including travel time, to perform the treatments.

- What will the treatment space be like? Will it be, for example, at a company in its conference room, small office, or the lobby? Or will it be performed on employees as they sit at their desks? Will it be at a bridal shower in the spare bedroom of someone's home? Will it be in a designated booth at a craft fair in the park?
- How much setup and takedown time is available? Some companies want as little disruption to their business as possible, and so the practitioner is given little time to set up and take down equipment. On the other hand, a health fair, for example, may give exhibitors and practitioners quite of bit of time.
- Where is the available parking and how far is it from the treatment location? Are there any special considerations for parking? These can include, for example, needing a code to get into a parking structure or only being able to park in special sections of a parking lot or street.

There are also some other things practitioners can do before traveling to the location to help ensure as smooth an experience as possible. These include the following:

- Map out the route to the treatment location ahead of time, using a paper map or online mapping site. If the area is unfamiliar and it is practical, practitioners may consider driving the route a day or two before the event.
- Allow plenty of time to arrive at the location. Ideally, practitioners should allow 20 to 30 minutes for setup time after arriving, then add the amount of time it will take to drive to the location. Practitioners should also factor in delays in travel, such as traffic accidents.

If the practitioner has the signup sheet ahead of time and there are contact phone numbers for the clients, she can give the clients reminder calls about the upcoming treatment session to help avoid late and no-show clients. She could also give clients tips on what to wear for the treatment. For example, short skirts can make it difficult for clients to get onto the massage chair, so longer skirts or pants are recommended. Clients could choose to wear shirts and blouses that they do not mind being wrinkled during the course of the treatment. Sometimes clients plan ahead and bring a camisole shirt or tank top to change into, or wear one underneath their work shirts, so can they can get specific work in the neck, back, shoulder, and scapular areas.

Arriving at the Location

Once arriving at the location, practitioners have several logistical considerations to address:

- Allowing time to do the following:
    - Park and find the building or space in which the event is being held
    - Find the treatment space within the location
    - Meet the representative and get the signup sheet, if it was not given to the practitioner ahead of time
    - Set up
- Being able to work within the allotted treatment space. Treatment spaces can run wide a wide gamut, including these:

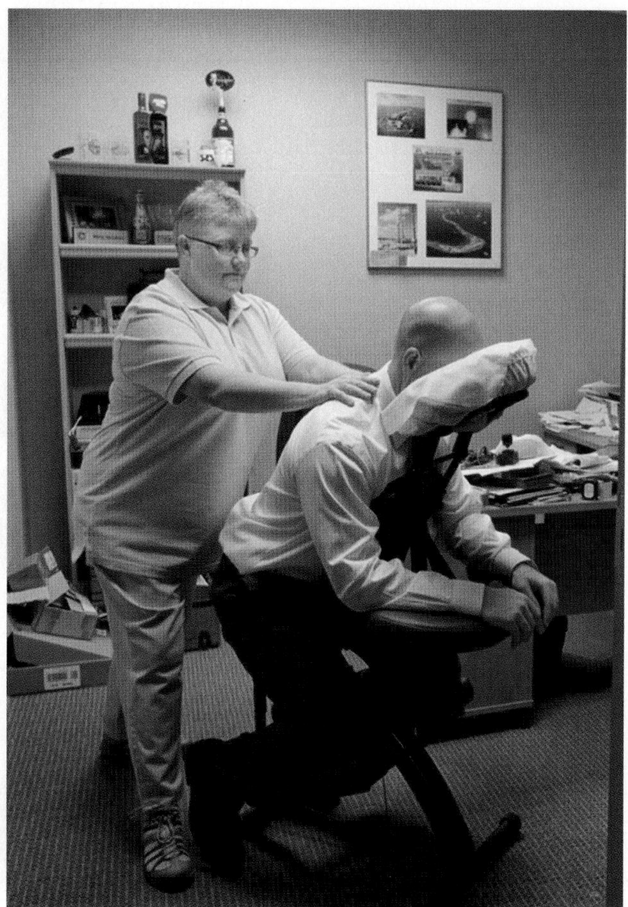

FIGURE 2-36 Performing massage in a cluttered office.

- Closets
- Boardrooms
- Cluttered offices (Figure 2-36)
- In a cubicle, using a massage chair or desktop system; practitioners may even be required to work on clients in their chairs as the clients talk on the phone
- In a spacious office (Figure 2-37)
- In a lobby; people may be walking by staring at the practitioner and client while the treatment is being performed, so if practitioners are not comfortable with this, they may want to reconsider offering onsite massage treatments
- In industrial settings (Figure 2-38)

The practitioner should set up the chair in a clean, safe area. All supplies should be arranged neatly, and the carrying case should be folded neatly and placed out of the way. The area around the chair should be clear so that proper body mechanics can be used while working and so that there are no obstacles that can cause accidents or injuries. If there are unavoidable risks, such as extension cords or sharp cabinet corners, let clients know about them as they are entering the space. If at all possible, avoid setting up in direct sunlight or under a heating or cooling vent. Sometimes this is not possible, so practitioners should be aware

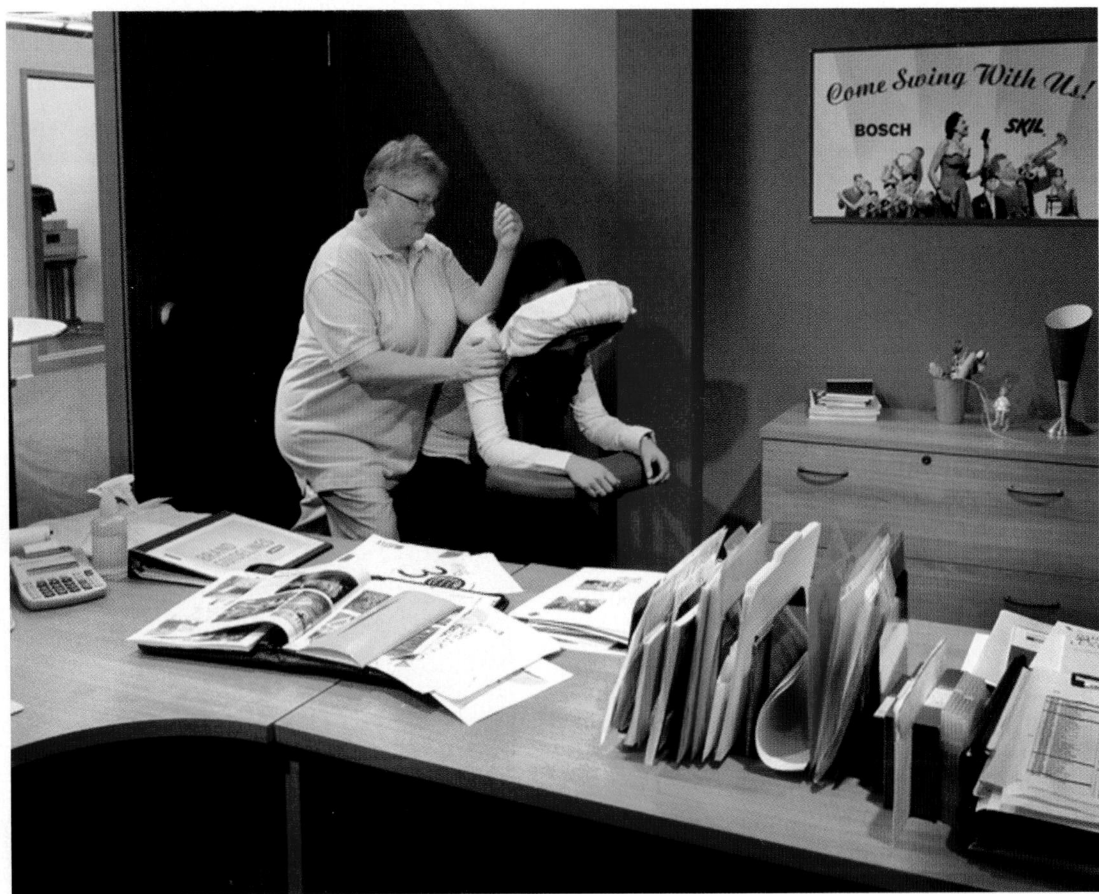

FIGURE 2-37 Performing massage in a spacious office.

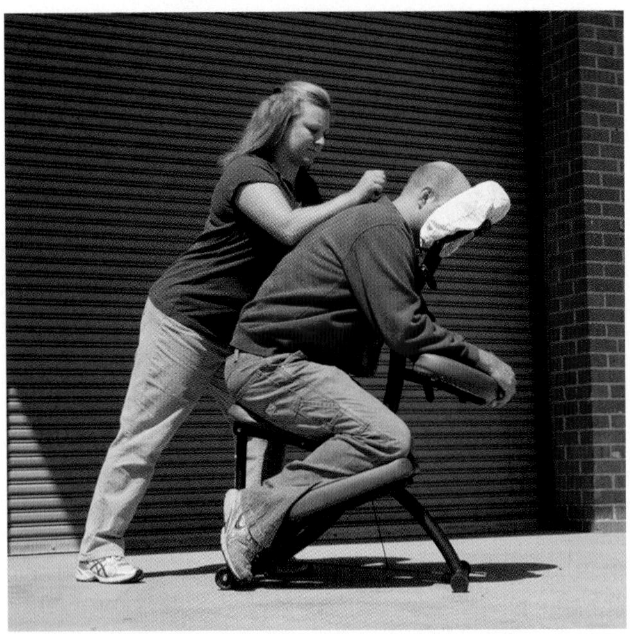

FIGURE 2-38 Chair massage outside a warehouse.

that they may be performing treatments in overly hot or cold conditions.

Client Considerations

Clients, of course, come in all shapes and sizes. Additionally, there are other aspects that practitioners need to keep in mind when working with the public performing chair massage. Practitioners need to be accommodating and professional, adapting to client needs while giving them the best treatment possible.

Certain clients may be claustrophobic and therefore uncomfortable placing their face in the face cradle. An adaptation could be to use pillows or bolsters to help support the client in an upright position in the chair. The same is true for clients who are wearing makeup they do not want to be smudged, or clients who do not want the creases on their face that can result from placing their faces in the face cradle.

A typical chair massage treatment will include scalp massage. However, practitioners should not assume that all clients will want this, especially as it can mess up the client's hair. Practitioners should check in with each client about scalp massage and not perform it if clients do not want it. If clients are concerned about the effect placing their face in the face cradle will have on their hair, they can be supported in an upright position with bolsters or pillows in the chair.

Clients will show up for chair massage treatments in every type of clothing imaginable, even if given tips beforehand on what to wear. If the client has on, for example, an expensive silk blouse, the practitioner will need to let the client know that performing the treatment will wrinkle it and ask the client if that is acceptable. If not, it would be handy for the practitioner to have a T-shirt to offer the client (and have them change in private), or perhaps the treatment will need to be rescheduled.

On the other hand, the client may wear a thick sweater, making specific work difficult or impossible. The practitioner needs to give the client this information and offer the client a T-shirt, if the practitioner has one, to change into. Otherwise, a treatment with nonspecific work can be performed, or perhaps the treatment will need to be rescheduled.

Sometimes male clients will want to take their shirts off and receive the treatment that way. This should never be done because, in addition to it being unsanitary, the client's skin can stick to the vinyl of the chair and be extremely uncomfortable.

SUMMARY

The initial investment in onsite massage equipment can be relatively low. The most inexpensive method of providing seated massage is by using a straight-backed chair with pillows or other bolsters for support. The next step up in onsite massage equipment is a desktop massage support. The most expensive, and the most versatile, option is the professionally manufactured massage chair. When choosing a massage chair, practitioners need to consider features such as the chair's weight, durability, stability, ease of set up, adjustment options, special options and accessories, warranty, and vinyl and color options. There are many manufacturers and distributors of massage chairs; practitioners should research each company carefully before deciding on which chair to purchase.

Practitioners use good body mechanics while setting up, taking down, lifting, carrying, and setting the chair down. These include keeping the back straight, using larger muscles to do the work, and remembering to breathe. The steps involved in setting up the massage chair are removing the chair from the case, moving the seat of the chair outward to create the solid base of the structure, elevating the face cradle into position then locking it in place, and elevating the armrest into position then locking into place. To adjust the chair for individual client comfort, changes can be made to the width of the base of the chair, seat height, height and angle of the face cradle, and the placement of the sternum pad. An optional triangle-shaped pad can be purchased for additional client comfort.

Hygiene and sanitation methods are essential to the practice of bodywork. This includes personal hygiene as well as proper sanitation for equipment and supplies. In addition to maintaining equipment and supplies in good working order, practitioners should use appropriate sanitation methods between each client and follow the decontamination protocol should contamination by body fluids occur.

Other supplies that practitioners may want to consider taking to onsite treatments are divided into the categories of minimum kits, which include the basic essentials needed to perform treatments onsite, medium kits with additional items to enhance the onsite treatment session experience, and deluxe kits with supplies that can greatly enhance the chair massage session treatment and location.

When traveling to locations to perform treatments, the most important factor is for practitioners to be flexible. To prevent as many mishaps and misunderstandings as possible, the practitioner should communicate with the company or event representative about the treatment sessions, signup sheet, payment, treatment space, setup and takedown time, and parking. Practitioners should allow time to park and find the treatment space within the location, get the signup sheet, and set up. Also important is that practitioners be aware that treatment spaces can vary in size, location, amount of clutter, temperature, and so forth. Clients come in a variety of sizes and shapes, and some will be wearing clothing that may be inappropriate for receiving a chair massage treatment. Practitioners need to be able to adapt to varying client needs.

STUDY QUESTIONS

Answers to Study Questions are on page 227.

Multiple Choice

1. Which of the following is a consideration when deciding which massage chair to purchase?
   a. Weight
   b. Durability
   c. Stability
   d. All of the above

2. What is the first step in setting up the massage chair?
   a. Adjusting the face cradle
   b. Moving the outward to create a solid base
   c. Sliding the sternum pad into place
   d. Raising the armrest

3. Which of the following is a useful hygiene guideline for bodywork practitioners?
   a. Having neatly polished nails
   b. Washing the hands in soapy water for 10 seconds
   c. Bathing daily
   d. Wearing quiet bracelets

4. Which of the following should be used to disinfect blood and other body fluid spills in healthcare settings?
   a. Household bleach
   b. Soap and water
   c. Witch hazel
   d. Rubbing alcohol

5. Which of the following is essential for the chair massage practitioner to have when performing treatments?
   a. Music
   b. Hand and equipment sanitizer
   c. Small basket for client items
   d. Appointment book

Fill in the Blank

1. Calculating how many treatments need to be performed to make the cost of equipment and supplies worthwhile is known as ______________________________ ______________________________ ______________________________.

2. Most massage chairs weigh anywhere from ______________ to ______________ pounds.

3. ______________ ______________ allow the massage practitioner's body to be used in a careful, efficient, and deliberate way.

4. Methods that ensure good health and cleanliness and are a necessary part of bodywork practice routines involve ______________ and ______________.

5. By remaining ______________, professional, and thinking on their feet, practitioners can sort out just about any unfavorable situation they find themselves in.

Short Answer

1. Describe how seated massage can be performed using equipment and props other than a massage chair.

____

____

____

____

____

STUDY QUESTIONS

2. Describe in detail each of the three main elements to body mechanics practitioners should keep in mind when handling their massage chairs.

3. Explain the factors involved in adjusting the massage chair for clients.

4. Explain the sanitation guidelines to follow during treatment sessions.

5. Discuss the logistical considerations to address once arriving at a location to do chair massage.

ACTIVITIES

1. Choose a massage chair company, and look through its website. Look at the chairs the company offers. Which ones do you find appealing? Why are they appealing? What features do the chairs have? Which chairs do you find unappealing? Why are they unappealing?

2. Practice setting up the massage chair, adjusting it for various body sizes, and taking it down, until you can do it efficiently. Enlist family and friends of all body sizes and shapes to sit in the chair until you are able to make adjustments quickly and easily.

3. Create a chair massage signup sheet. Include treatment lengths, time between treatments, spaces for client names and contact phone numbers. Include anything else you think is necessary.

4. Using the concept of minimal, medium, and deluxe kits, determine what supplies you think are necessary to performing chair massage, and make a list of them. Divide the list into supplies that only need to be purchased once (such as a small basket for clients to place items in while receiving a treatment) and supplies that require ongoing purchase as they are used up (such as hand sanitizer). Price the items in each list, and come up with what your total investment in supplies would be.

Basic Sequence

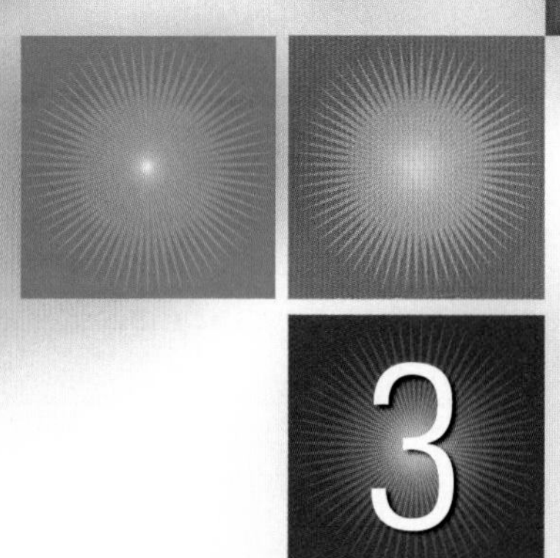

OBJECTIVES

Upon completion of this chapter, the reader will have the information necessary to do the following:

1. Explain the proper body mechanics for performing chair massage.
2. Perform the techniques used in chair massage: compressions, palming, thumb and finger pressure, deep gliding, kneading, friction, forearm work, elbow work, vibration, brush strokes, and percussion.
3. Explain what cautionary sites are and how to apply massage appropriately in these areas.
4. Outline the considerations for working on a clothed client.
5. Perform self-stretching and warm-ups before performing chair massage, and explain the importance of doing so.
6. Discuss the components of a pretreatment interview, and demonstrate how to conduct one.
7. Describe the bony landmarks and muscles of the body covered in the basic sequence.
8. Perform the basic sequence, and demonstrate adjusting pressure appropriately during the treatment.
9. Explain vasovagal syncope, including the definition, causes, symptoms, and appropriate response by the chair massage practitioner.

KEY TERMS

Adhesion
Basic sequence
Brush strokes
Cautionary (endangerment) sites
Contraindication
Compressions
Elbow work
Finger pressure
Forearm work
Friction—circular, deep specific
Indication
Kneeling stance
Lunge stance (archer stance, bow stance)
Palming
Percussion—cupping, hacking, quacking, pummeling, plucking, tapping
Straight stance (horse stance)
Syncope
Thumb pressure
Vasovagal syncope
Vibration

Providing chair massage may be a little daunting at first for practitioners who are not used to the shorter time frame of treatments and for those who are not used to working on fully clothed clients. Being able to help clients with relief from stress and muscle tension, help them increase flexibility and joint range of motion, and give them an overall sense of balance and well-being may seem to be too much to do in a 15- or 20-minute session on a massage chair without the use of lubricants. However, by practicing a set of foundational techniques over and over, practitioners will develop their chair massage skills and become as proficient in using them as they are with table massage techniques.

A basic sequence for incorporating these techniques in a seated chair massage treatment is also presented. The goal of this sequence is to provide a simple yet effective routine that will allow practitioners who are new to this modality to provide an efficient treatment. In addition, this sequence lends itself to creative adaptation by practitioners as they become skilled and comfortable with the various techniques.

The applications of the techniques need to be accompanied by efficient practitioner postures and stances. Learning proper body mechanics reduces the possibility of injury to the practitioner and to the client and increases the effectiveness of the techniques. Therefore, learning the body mechanics pertinent to chair massage is every bit as important as learning the techniques.

The body mechanics for chair massage are, in some ways, different from those for table massage, so they may feel unnatural at first. Just like the proper body mechanics for table massage became natural and even second nature over time, so will those for chair massage.

BODY MECHANICS

Some practitioners may be able to do chair massage for an entire day and not feel tired, whereas others may feel exhausted after just an hour of chair massage, even though they do not get tired after giving a full body table massage. The difference is almost always attributable to body mechanics, which speaks to the considerable value of good body mechanics for practitioners of chair massage.

The same three key elements that are considered when handling massage chairs are to be kept firmly in mind when performing chair massage techniques:

- *Keep the back straight.* Efficient alignment (posture) and use of the body while performing massage will help prevent fatigue, muscle strain, and injury. A properly aligned skeleton will provide the body support necessary for practitioners to do massage techniques without injury to their soft tissues. (Proper posture and alignment keep the abdomen and chest open so the practitioner can take deep, efficient breaths; see "Remember to breathe," which follows.)
- *Use larger muscles to do the work.* Larger muscles are stronger and less prone to injury than smaller muscles. Smaller muscles tend to fatigue more quickly than larger muscles.
- *Remember to breathe.* Deep, relaxed breathing puts the body in parasympathetic mode and helps practitioners have clear, focused thoughts. Overall, breathing should be done slowly and mindfully. It should not be done too fast or too deeply because of the chance of hyperventilating. Practitioners must be able to breathe smoothly and evenly throughout the treatment to ensure enough oxygen to do the work. Running out of breath during the treatment or breathing shallowly can indicate that the practitioner is not focused.

Body mechanics for chair massage are similar to those for table massage in terms of allowing body weight and the force of gravity to apply the pressure rather than using the force of muscular strength to press into the client's tissues. However, there are some modifications in body stances and massage techniques necessary to provide effective pressure into the tissues of a client who is upright and clothed, and because of the seated position, the client is at a different angle than when lying down on a massage table.

Lunge Stance

One of the primary body stances used in chair massage is a **lunge stance**, also known as the **archer stance** or **bow stance**. In this stance, the back is straight, one foot is stepped forward of the other, with toes of both feet parallel, and the hips facing the same direction as the feet. Both feet, as well as the practitioner's entire body, should be in alignment with the area where pressure will be applied.

In this stance, the practitioner's center of gravity drops into the abdomen (where the umbilicus is), thus allowing the practitioner's sense of balance and force of energy to come from the center of the body. This focus allows the practitioner to be stable, and the strength applied is not due to contracted muscles (which can tire quickly) but more from using the force of gravity when leaning forward. This relationship with gravity is important because it allows for the pressure to be applied by simply leaning forward with the practitioner's weight doing the work.

Pressure should be applied in a way that minimizes the compressive force on the shoulder and arm joints (i.e., passing straight through the joint, not at an angle). To accomplish this, the practitioner's arms are at a 90-degree angle from the shoulder, the shoulder is lined up behind the elbow, and the elbow is lined up behind the hand (or, as will be seen later under "Techniques," the fingers or thumbs).

The practitioner has relaxed elbows and neutral wrists, and the hands are placed forward onto the client. Relaxed elbows means that they are not locked in extension. Instead, the joints are in soft or unforced flexion and then in extension when the practitioner applies pressure. Wrists are in a neutral position (not overly hyperextended), but straight forward with a slight extension upon meeting the client's back. Neutral wrists are important because repetitive stress injuries (RSIs) can occur if the wrists are kept in a chronically hyperextended position throughout the treatment. (There will some applications of strokes in which the wrists are not in a 100% neutral position; however, these strokes are applied briefly and without undue pressure.) The practitioner's shoulders should not be lifted upward, but instead be in a relaxed, neutral position.

When using the lunge stance to apply pressure to the client's body, the practitioner starts with most of the body weight on the rear foot. The practitioner's strength comes from the rear leg; when pushing forward off the rear foot, the front knee flexes somewhat but the majority of the weight is transferred through the arms and hands to the client's body (Figure 3-1 A). The more the practitioner flexes the front knee, the more weight is transferred to the client's body (Figure 3-1 B). Thus, the practitioner controls the amount of weight (pressure) placed on the client's body by adjusting the movements of the legs. Taller practitioners will need to lunge more deeply to ensure they have proper body mechanics, whereas shorter practitioners will need to lunge less (Figure 3-2).

The key to this stance is the practitioner becoming adept at easily shifting the weight backward and forward, with pressure being applied on the forward movement and pressure being released on the backward movement. This creates a sense of rhythm in applying pressure as well as allowing for body weight and not arm muscles to provide the pressure. The pressure should be applied and released evenly and steadily. As the practitioner moves forward to apply pressure, he or she should exhale; moving backward to release pressure, he or she should inhale. This ensures that the practitioner is not holding his or her breath while working and also helps establish rhythmic movement.

Playing rhythmic music during the treatment can help the practitioner provide a graceful application of pressure. The beat of the music acts as a cue for when to lean forward and when to lean back. In many respects, bodywork is a beautiful dance around the client's body. Practicing getting in touch with the rhythmic nature of the work as well as gaining comfort with the lunge position will enhance the practitioner's ability to provide a smooth and flowing treatment. More important, it will also ease stress on the practitioner's joints and allow for a tireless session. In addition,

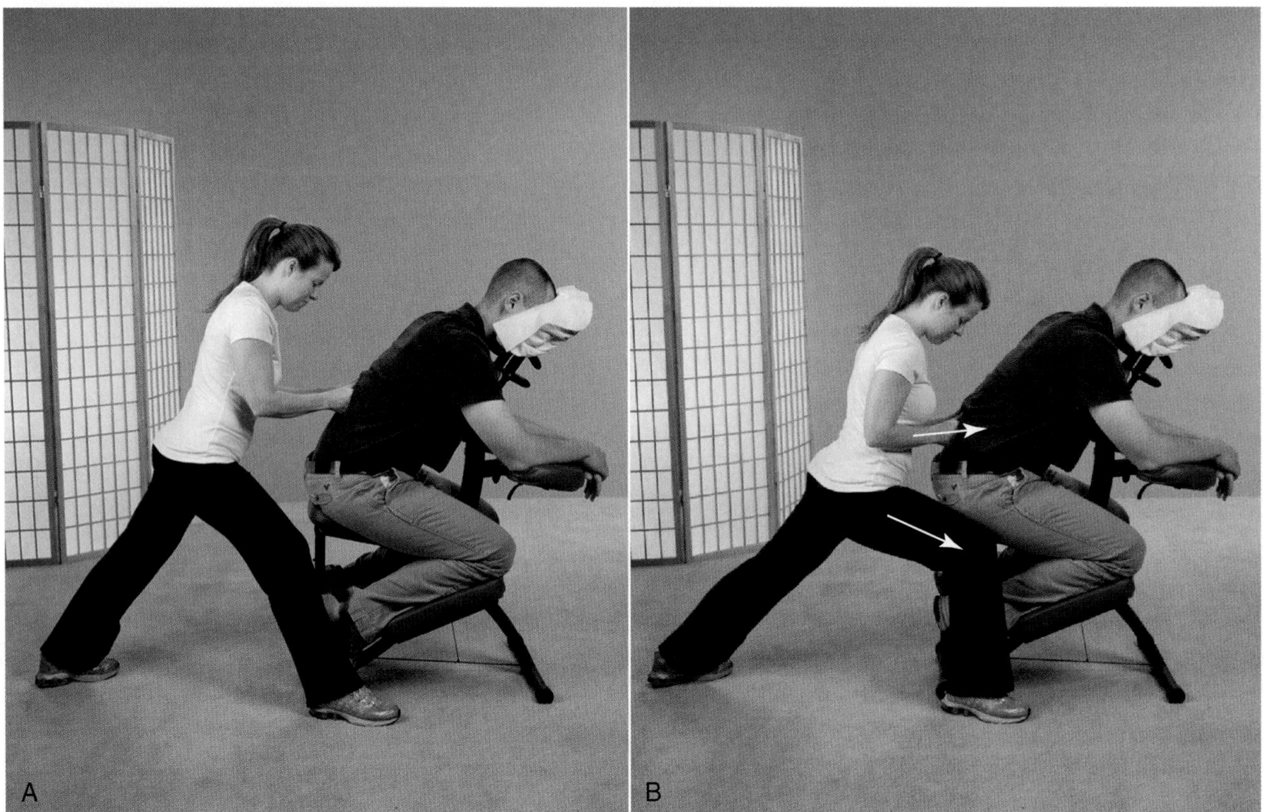

FIGURE 3-1 **A** and **B,** Leaning forward to apply more pressure in the lunge stance.

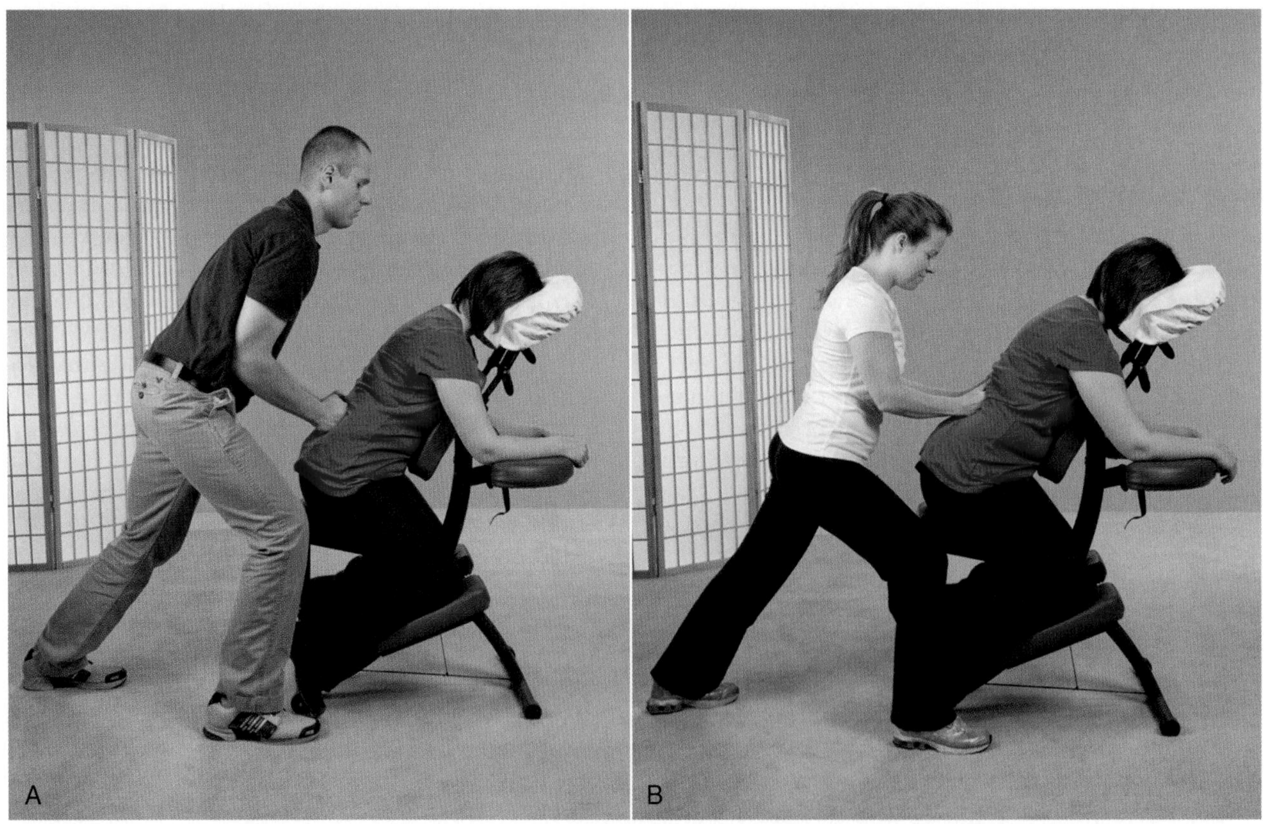

FIGURE 3-2 **A,** Lunging stance of a tall practitioner. **B,** Lunging stance of a short practitioner.

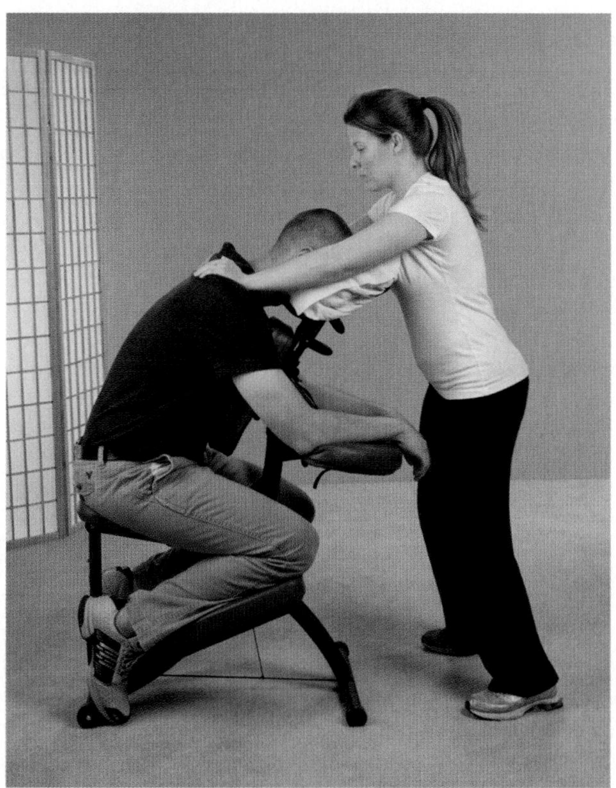

FIGURE 3-3 The straight stance.

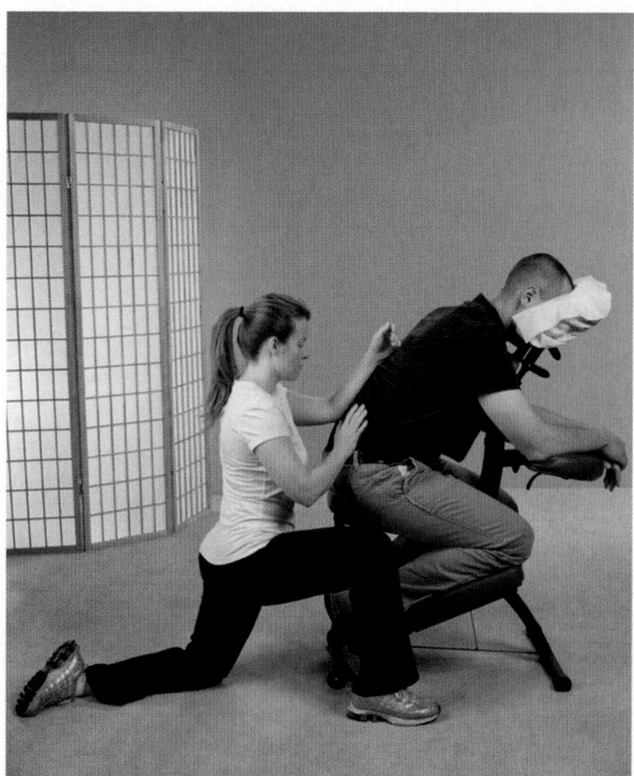

FIGURE 3-4 Kneeling on one knee to apply techniques.

the client will also benefit, and experience a graceful as well as relaxing treatment.

Straight Stance

Some techniques require precision but not necessarily a lot of pressure. In these instances, the practitioner can use the **straight stance** (also called the **horse stance**) (Figure 3-3). With a straight back, the practitioner faces the area being working on. The feet are parallel about shoulder width apart, with the weight evenly distributed. The practitioner's knees are extended but the joints are soft, not locked.

As the practitioner places the hands forward onto the client, the shoulders are relaxed, the elbows are relaxed (soft joints that are not locked into position), and the wrists are neutral. Pressure is applied by rocking forward on both feet. To change direction of movement during the application of techniques, the practitioner should move the pelvis and feet slightly to turn. If a greater change in movement is needed, the practitioner should use the lunge stance to prevent overstressing the paraspinal muscles of the back by twisting. Also, the elbows should not be rotated outward or raised above the practitioner's shoulders, because these positions prevent good leverage and weight transfer from the practitioner to the client.

Kneeling Stance

To address the client's arms and forearms, the practitioner may choose to kneel on one knee, which is a **kneeling stance** (Figure 3-4). In this case, the practitioner's center of gravity is dropped even lower into the abdomen. The back is straight, and the entire body is facing the area of the client's body she is working on. The practitioner should avoid kneeling on both knees to apply techniques. As Figure 3-5 shows, the stance is not as stable as kneeling on one knee, and the practitioner's center of gravity is no longer in the abdomen. There is increased strain on the deep paraspinal and erector spinae muscles as they increase in tension to keep the practitioner upright. Because leg movements cannot be adjusted as pressure is applied, strength comes mostly from the shoulder and arm muscles, increasing the risk of injuring them. The practitioner should also avoid sitting on the floor because reaching may be necessary to apply the techniques, making them less effective and possibly straining the back muscles.

Using a Stool

Some practitioners choose to use a stool or exercise ball when applying certain techniques, such as those for the arms and forearms (Figure 3-6). The stool should be placed close enough to the client so that the practitioner is not reaching to work on the client. If the stool has wheels, the practitioner should make sure it stays firmly in place while the practitioner is working; this will keep the client's arm from being pulled suddenly should the practitioner slide on a moving stool. The practitioner has a straight back while sitting on the stool and is directly facing the area of the client's body being worked on.

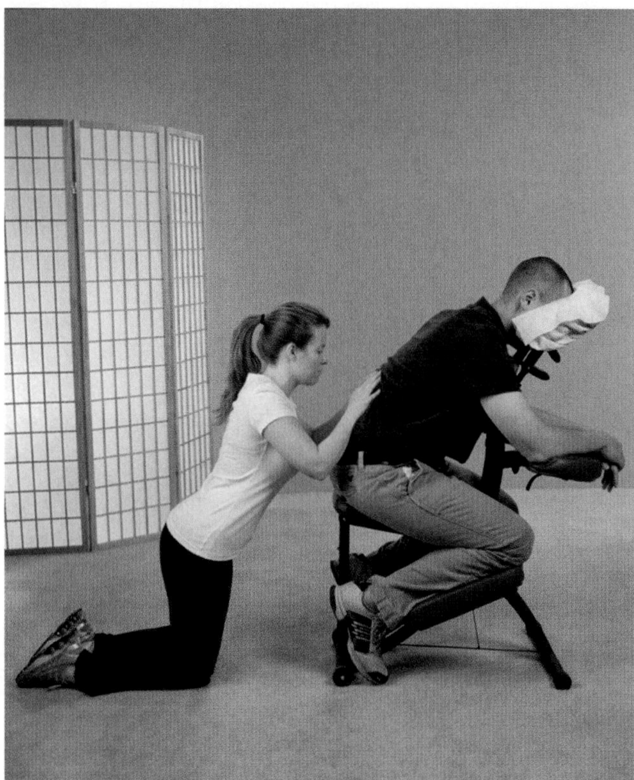

FIGURE 3-5 Kneeling on both knees to apply techniques.

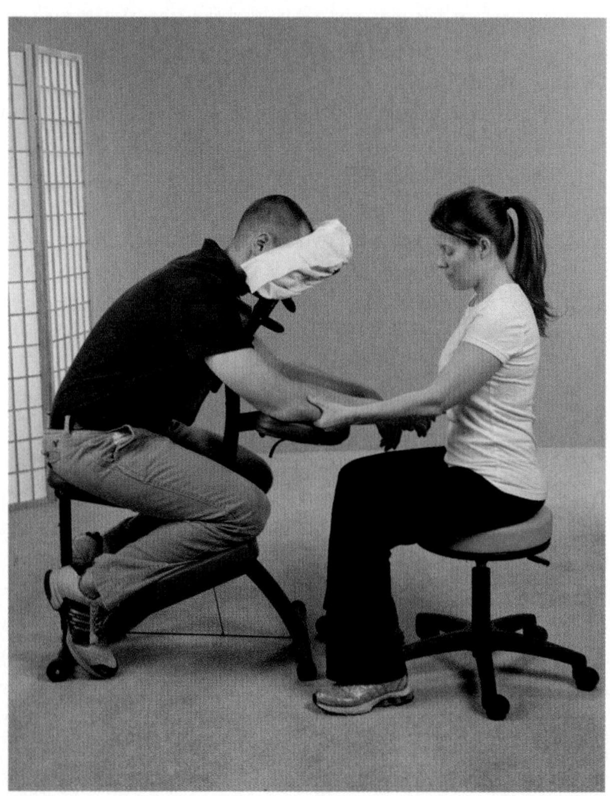

FIGURE 3-6 Sitting on a stool to apply techniques.

TECHNIQUES

There are a variety of techniques used in seated chair massage. The practitioner chooses the type of stroke as well as the use of each stroke specifically to meet the needs of the client. Some of the techniques covered in this section are taken from table massage, and some are from shiatsu. All of them are adjusted for use in chair massage. They include the following:

- Compressions
- Palming
- Thumb and finger pressure
- Deep gliding
- Kneading
- Friction—circular, deep specific
- Forearm
- Elbow
- Vibration
- Brush strokes
- Percussion

Practitioners who are new to bodywork in general, as well as practitioners who are familiar with some or all of these techniques from performing table massage on unclothed clients, need to be aware of considerations for working on clothed clients. The same techniques performed on skin and through clothing can feel vastly different to both the practitioner and the client. Additionally, the clothing itself presents the need for practitioners to adjust their performance methods.

Individual Techniques

The client will best receive massage if the superficial tissues are addressed first. As they soften, the deeper muscles become more receptive to being worked. Skeletal muscle tissue connects to the skeletal framework, of course. There are also associated tissues, such as the dense connective tissue that makes up ligaments (attaching bone to bone), joint capsules, tendons (attaching muscles to bones), aponeuroses (attaching muscles to muscles or muscles to bones), and the myofascia that surrounds and protects each individual muscle. Overlying these tissues are adipose tissue, the subcutaneous layer, then the skin, which is the outermost, or most superficial, layer. By addressing these layers from superficial to deep, optimal effects of the massage treatment can be achieved.

Compressions

Compressions are used to introduce the practitioner's touch to the client, usually on the back. Compressions soften the tissue, bring blood flow to the surface, and prepare the tissue for more sustained pressure and deeper techniques as the treatment proceeds. Compressions can also be performed on the client's shoulders, arms, and thighs.

The compression stroke is performed by placing one or both palms on an area over the soft muscle tissue and

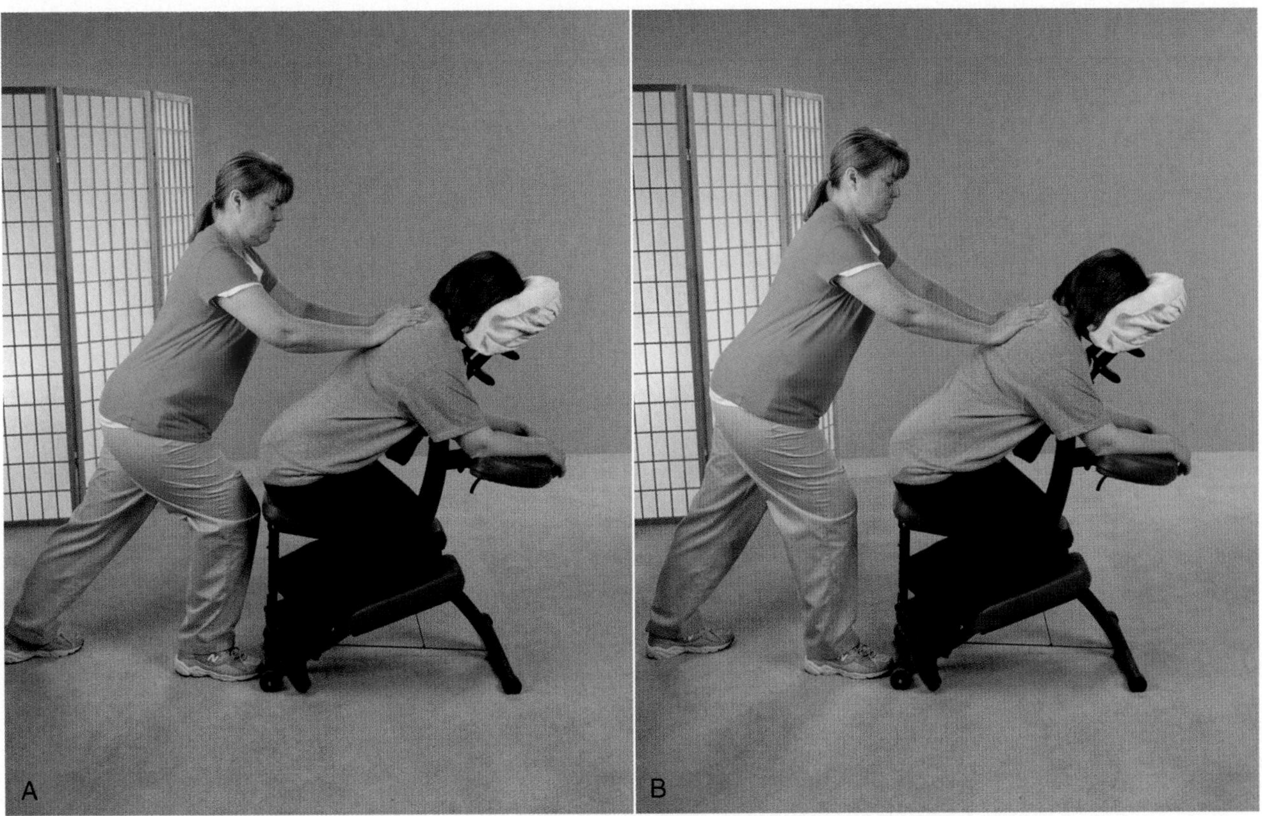

FIGURE 3-7 **A,** Applying pressure during compression. **B,** Releasing pressure during compression.

pumping into the tissue toward the bone, then releasing but not lifting the hand(s) off the body (Figure 3-7). Compressions can be performed bilaterally on the body, with one hand on top of the other and both pressing downward simultaneously (Figure 3-8 A) with the backs of the hands (Figure 3-8 B) and also incorporating a twist downward into the tissue (Figure 3-8 C).

There is a rhythmic nature to the performance of this stroke, which can be enhanced by inhaling while compressing and exhaling while releasing. By combining this focused breathing with the techniques, the practitioner can also center himself or herself as the treatment begins as well as model for the client taking deep breaths to relax into the treatment.

Palming

Palming is a technique in which the practitioner uses the palm of the hand to apply pressure to the client's body, such as the back, shoulders, arms, and thighs. Although it may sound similar to compressions and can also be used as an introduction to the treatment, the pressure applied does not sink in as deeply as with compressions, and there is no rhythmic pumping action. Pressure is applied by pressing with the palm into the client's body then releasing while keeping the hand connected to the client (Figure 3-9).

Palming should be applied smoothly and evenly through the practitioner's palm, and the fingers should be relaxed. The client's tissues are not grasped or pushed sideways. The practitioner should exhale with the client when applying pressure, then release the pressure gradually when the client inhales.

Thumb and Finger Pressure

The thumbs and fingers are used to work more specifically on the client. For **thumb pressure** and **finger pressure**, pressure is applied with the ball of the thumb and the pads of the fingertips. Practitioners should be careful not to jab or poke the client when performing thumbing and finger pressure. Because only the clients know their levels of comfort, it is important that the practitioner check in about depth of thumb and finger pressure and adjust the pressure as necessary.

The practitioner can perform thumbing in several ways to reduce the risk of hyperextending the thumb. One way is called "spider thumbing," so called because the fingers are spread out like a spider's legs to help stabilize the thumb (Figure 3-10 A). The thumb pad is applying the pressure; the fingers are only touching the body lightly. Flexed-finger thumbing involves the fingers being flexed to support the thumb. Again, the pressure is from the thumb pad; the fingers are only touching the body lightly (Figure 3-10 B).

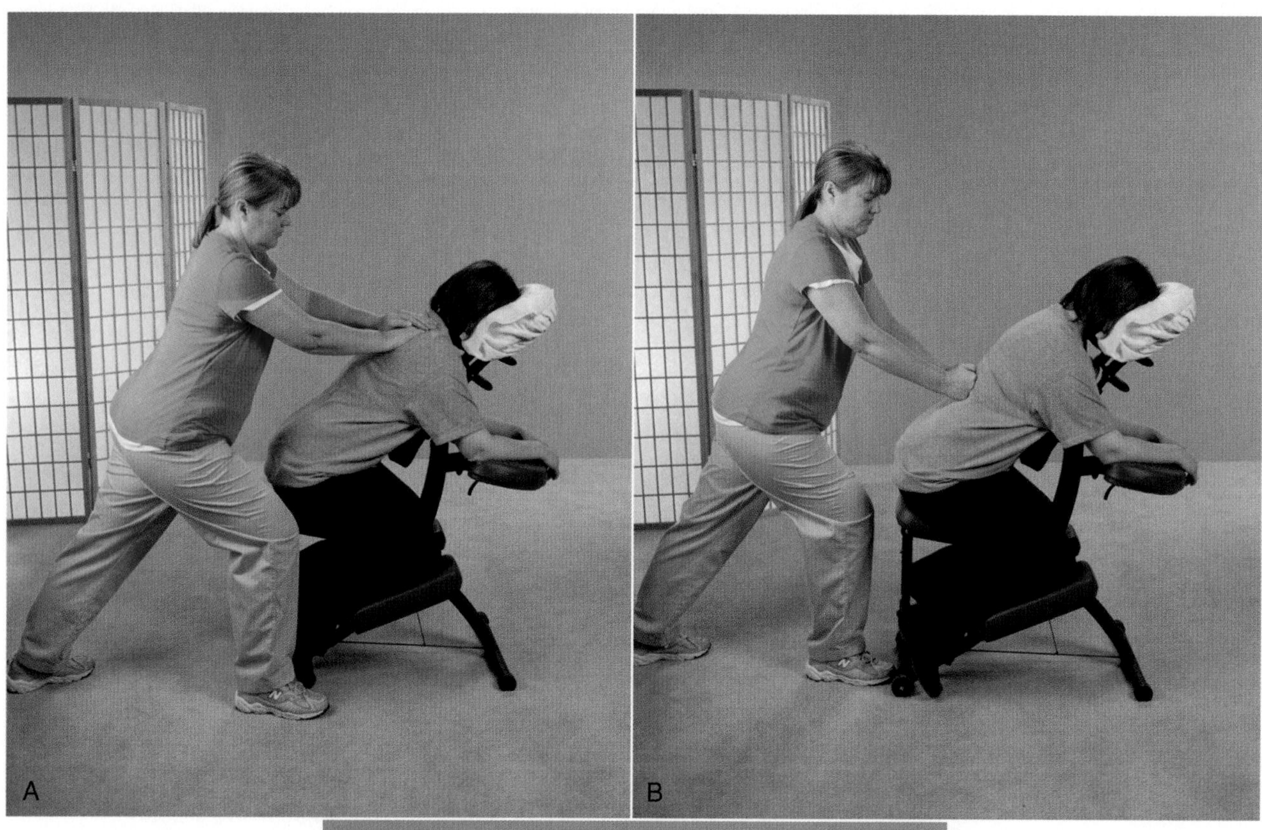

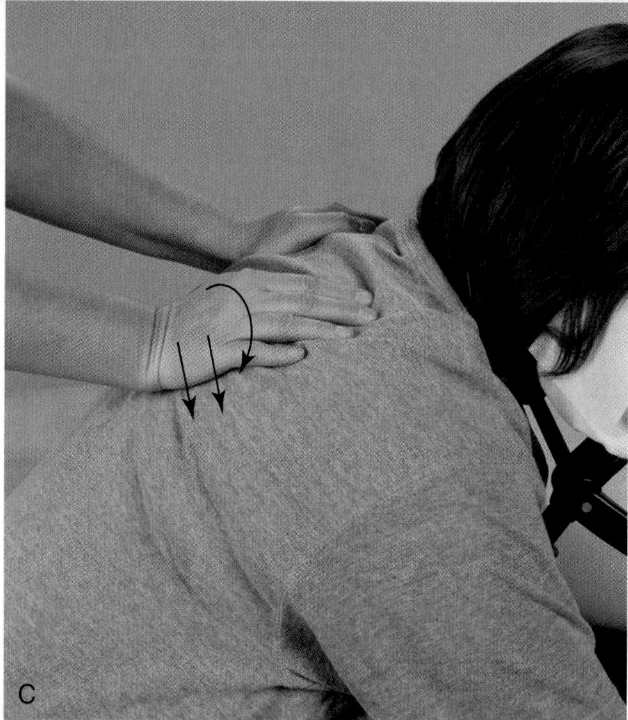

FIGURE 3-8 **A,** Hands stacked on top of each other applying compressions. **B,** Backhand compressions. **C,** Twisting compressions.

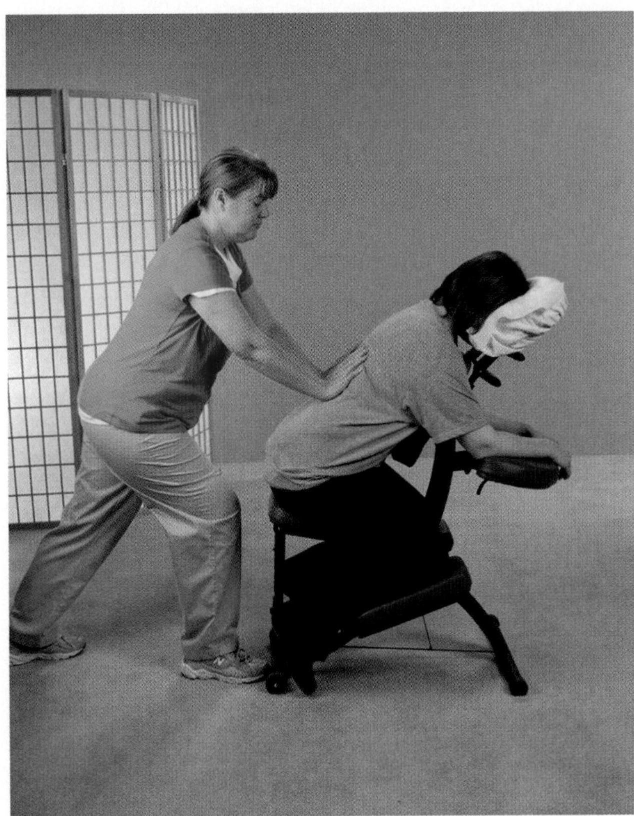

FIGURE 3-9 Palming.

Backhand thumbing means the fingers are flexed at the metacarpophalangeal joint to provide support while the thumb pad applies pressure (Figure 3-10 C).

Thumb pressure can be applied unilaterally, with the practitioner's other hand resting on the client (Figure 3-10 D) or bilaterally as in Figure 3-10 A.

Fingertips can be used to work areas of the body that may be too awkward to reach with the thumbs, such as when working along the medial border of the scapula from certain angles or along the suboccipitals when the practitioner is standing to the front of the client. The practitioner should not strain or hyperextend the fingertips while working (Figure 3-11 A). The fingers can also be placed on top of each other to apply more pressure and to apply deep gliding along muscle fibers (Figure 3-11 B).

Additionally, the thumb pads and fingertips can be used to apply pressure along the channels and points on the channels of qi flow (recall the section "Asian Bodywork" from Chapter 1; more information about the points and channels can be found in Chapter 4 and Appendix A) and to perform deep gliding along muscle fibers.

Deep Gliding

Deep gliding is a stroke that can effectively address the tissue through clothing. The goal is to elongate the tissues along the entire length of the muscle, thus stretching it, relaxing the muscle fibers and increasing blood flow to the area. It is performed with with enough pressure to engage the tissues while slowly moving in the direction of the muscle fibers or across the muscle fibers.

The practitioner stands in a lunge position with soft knees. One of the practitioner's hands can be placed directly on top of the other hand to provide support for the fingers as they deeply glide over the tissue. The finger pads of the bottom hand contact the tissue through the client's clothing to provide the deep gliding movement. During the application of this stroke, the fingers of both hands are slightly curved and relaxed to avoid tension in the finger joints.

One of the areas where this technique is useful is in addressing the rhomboids. Starting at the medial border of the client's left scapula, the practitioner's finger pads apply pressure as the practitioner leans in, and glide deeply from the attachment at the medial border to the attachments at C-7 to T-5. The practitioner may complete two or three passes to effectively treat the area.

Kneading

Kneading is a basic massage stroke that is best described as grasping, lifting, and gently squeezing the soft tissue to promote muscle relaxation and increased flexibility of connective tissue. (The French word for this technique is *pétrissage,* which means "wearing down the stone.") The warmth that results from kneading the tissue is due to increased blood flow into the area. This warmth helps muscles relax and connective tissue to become less rigid. The increased blood flow also assists in ridding the tissue of metabolic waste.

Kneading is performed by grasping the client's tissue using the web of the hand and the digits to scoop the tissue upward (Figure 3-12 A), then releasing but maintaining contact with the client's body (Figure 3-12 B). The client should not feel like he or she is being pinched. Effective kneading feels rhythmic and consistent. Kneading is especially effective on the upper trapezius and can also be used on the deltoid, biceps brachii, and triceps brachii muscles. Pincer-grip kneading is a modification that can be used on the posterior neck (Figure 3-13).

Another modified kneading technique involves the use of soft fists. The fingers are curled but open enough that water or sand could flow through the hands (Figure 3-14 A), not closed tightly (Figure 3-14 B). The two soft fists are used in a simultaneous circular motion (somewhat similar to how a cat kneads). An appropriate use of this stroke would be in the low back along the iliac crest, along the gluteus medius muscles (Figure 3-14 C), and along the iliotibial band on the lateral legs.

The use of kneading should be limited during a chair massage treatment to prevent the practitioner from experiencing repetitive stress injuries. There are other techniques that the practitioner can use to address the deeper muscles, such as with the forearms and elbows (discussed shortly), which can save wear and tear on the practitioner's smaller joints in the wrists, hands, thumbs, and fingers.

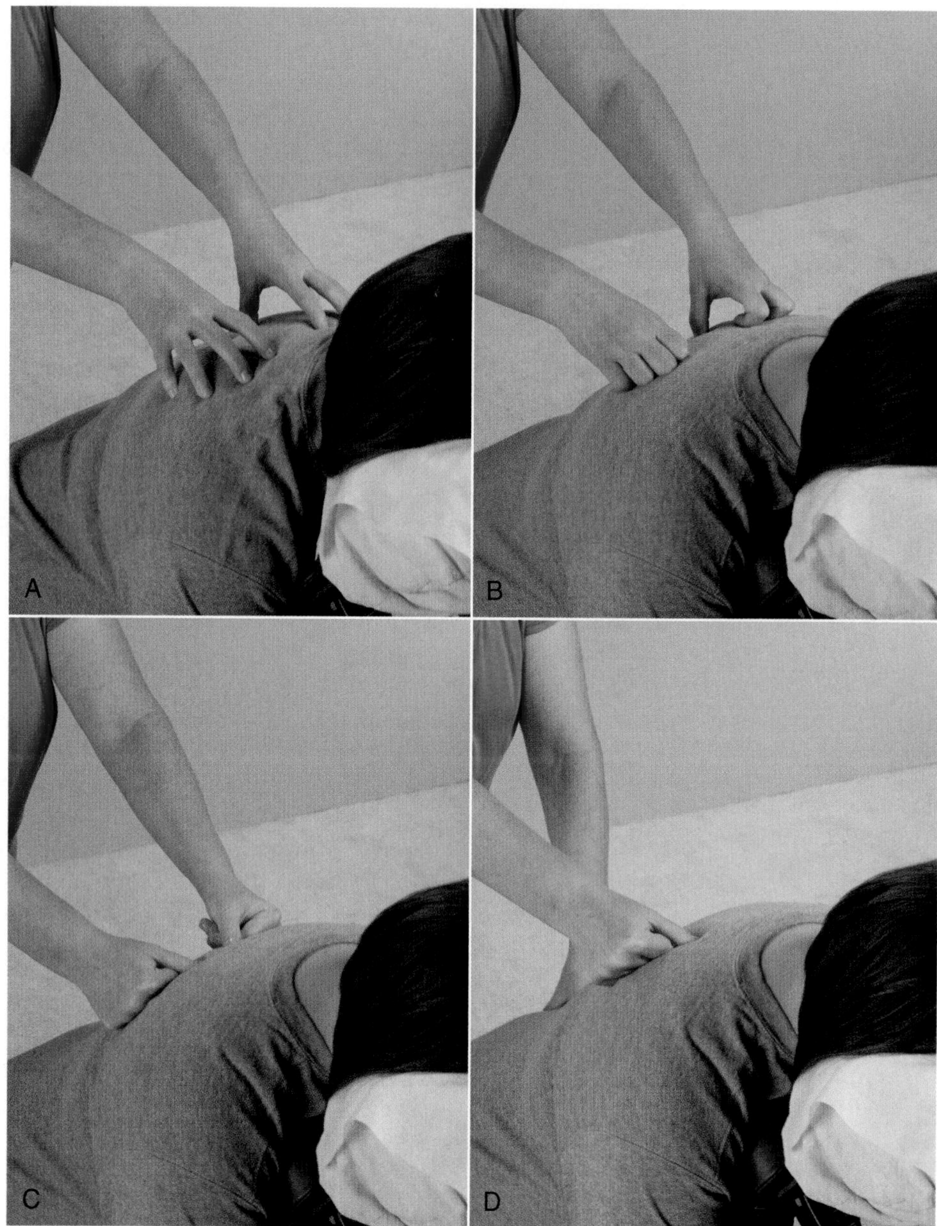

FIGURE 3-10 **A,** Spider thumbing. **B,** Flexed-finger thumbing. **C,** Backhand thumbing. **D,** Unilateral thumbing.

Kneading can also be used quite effectively as a method of transitioning from one section of the client's body to another. For example, if the massage treatment is focusing on the client's upper trapezius, the practitioner may choose to simultaneously knead both the left and right upper trapezius as a way to make the two sides feel connected, as opposed to working each upper trapezius as two separate regions of the body.

Friction

Friction is a massage stroke that incorporates the compression of tissue with movement in different directions, namely, back and forth in a linear fashion, or in a circular direction. The fingers, thumbs, and the ulnar edge of the hand can all be used to apply friction. This technique increases blood circulation, creates warmth in the tissue, and addresses the deeper fascia (myofascia, tendons, and ligaments) by helping the body to realign connective tissue fibers. This increases flexibility in the tissue and can help loosen **adhesions** (abnormal joining of tissues), leading to increased movement of tissues and increased range of motion in joints.

Two types of friction can be used in chair massage: **deep specific friction** and **circular friction**. Deep specific friction is applied by moving in a linear motion back and forth on a specific point in the tissue. The direction of movement

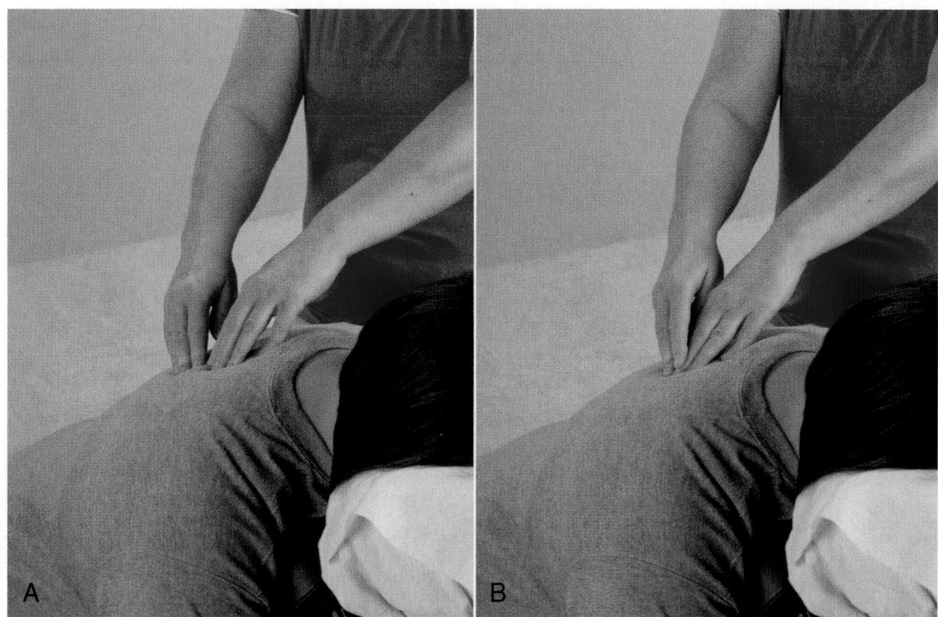

FIGURE 3-11 **A,** Finger pressure. **B,** Fingers placed on top of each other to apply more pressure.

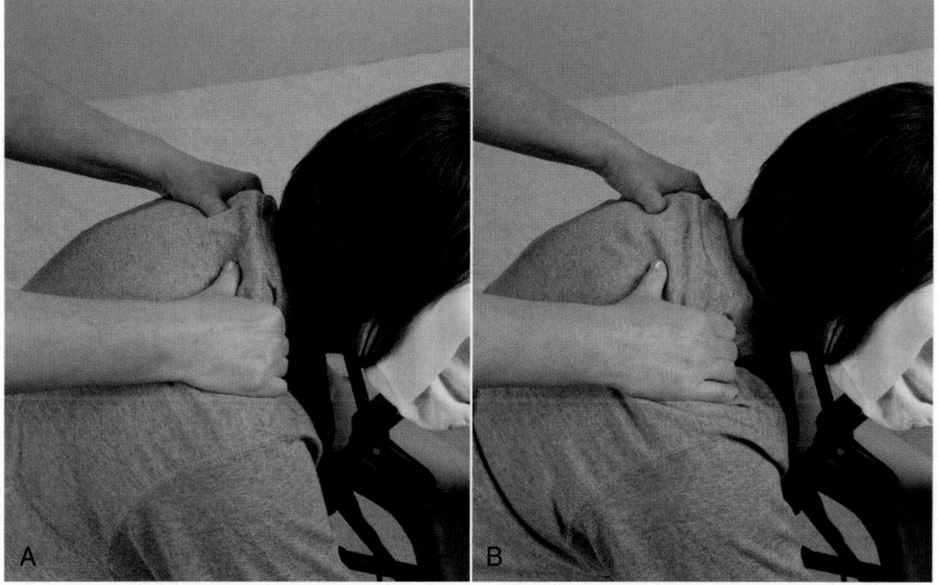

FIGURE 3-12 Kneading by scooping the tissue upward **(A)** then releasing **(B)**.

can be in alignment with the direction of muscle or connective tissue fibers or transversely across the fibers. The technique can be performed with the thumbs or with the fingertips. In Figure 3-15 A, fingertips are placed on top of each other to provide deeper pressure. As its name implies, circular friction is applied by using a circular motion as pressure is applied downward into the tissue (Figure 3-15 B).

This technique is useful in areas that need more specific work to loosen up the muscle at attachment sites such as those of the forearm, the retinacula of the wrists, the rhomboid attachments at the medial borders of the scapula, the posterior neck muscles, and the suboccipitals (Figure 3-15 C). Clients who spend the majority of their workday at a computer can have pain in all of these areas. The tiny minute movements of typing creates tight forearm muscles and wrist pain; long periods of sitting with the arms forward and hands on a keyboard can create tight, overstretched rhomboid muscles. Looking at a computer screen for hours at a time places strain on the posterior neck muscles,

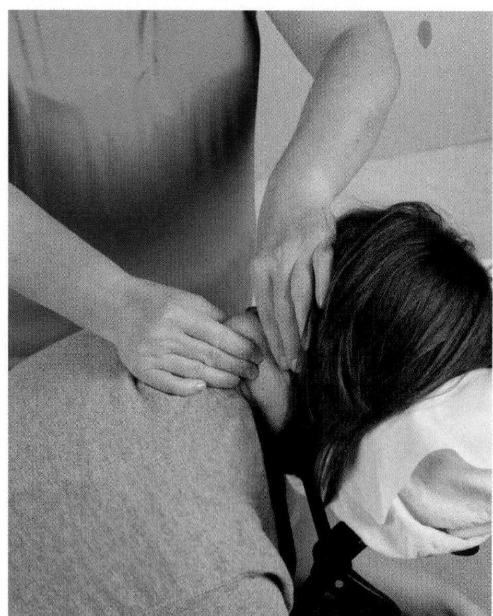

FIGURE 3-13 Pincer-grip kneading on the posterior of the neck.

especially the small, deep ones called suboccipitals near the base of the skull. All of this tightness can eventually interfere with the client's efficiency at work.

Forearm Work

The forearm is an excellent tool for applying deeper pressure during a chair massage treatment. The reason it is so effective is because it has a broad surface that can be applied to dense muscle areas such as the upper trapezius, the shoulder girdle, as well as the low back. The ultimate goal of **forearm work** is to apply broad sweeping strokes to soften the tissue in preparation for receiving deeper work.

When learning to apply forearm work, the practitioner first needs to locate the area of the forearm that is broad enough to be effective and yet does not feel bony. This area is outlined on Figure 3-16. The entire arm, hand, and wrist should all be relaxed. If the forearm muscles are tensed when applying this technique, the pressure may feel uncomfortable to the client, and the practitioner's arm will fatigue easily. Some practitioners may choose to let the wrist and hand hang limply during this technique; others may choose to have the forearm, wrist, and hand stay in alignment (i.e., neutral position) yet be relaxed.

When applying forearm work during a treatment, it is important that the practitioner use appropriate body mechanics that allow for the power of gravity to assist the forearm in its work. For example, when applying the forearm to address the upper trapezius, the practitioner will place the forearm on the muscle, soften the knees, and press downward. The lunge position ensures that the force of the stroke is coming from the weight of the practitioner's body and not from "muscling into" the tissue. The forearm can be applied to many areas of the client's body such as the rhomboids (Figure 3-17 A), the midback, and, as mentioned previously, the upper trapezius, either while standing behind or in front of the client (Figure 3-17 B).

Forearm pressure can also be applied in a gliding motion with pressure directed downward into the tissue. The practitioner's arm and forearm muscles must be fully relaxed so as to not create tension that travels up through the shoulder joint as the technique is applied. Once practitioners become comfortable with using their forearms, they can explore other ways to creatively apply the stroke.

Elbow Work

The use of the elbow, or **elbow work**, allows the practitioner to address the deepest layers of the muscle tissues. The point of the elbow can be used to work specifically, and its effectiveness is dependent on the combination of direct sustained pressure coupled with the force of the pressure coming from the lunge position. Because only clients know their levels of comfort, it is important that the practitioner check in about depth of elbow pressure and adjust it as necessary, being careful at all times not to jab or poke the client with the point of the elbow.

The elbow can be applied at several places along the upper trapezius and upper, middle, and low back (Figure 3-18). (Elbows should not be applied on the low back directly over the kidneys, though, since there is not enough tissue there to protect them from the deep specific work.) It is important that the practitioner palpate the area to be worked before using the elbow so that it is placed on soft tissue and not on bony landmarks such as the medial border of the scapula or the iliac crest. The practitioner should be feeling for the belly of the muscle as well as the attachment sites. Once these are found, the practitioner can then determine the best method to use for the elbow. When applying the elbow during a treatment, the practitioner should use the lunge stance so that the power of gravity assists the elbow in its work. As pressure is applied, the practitioner shifts weight to the front leg, and the back heel should rise off the floor.

The practitioner has two choices as to how to apply the elbow. One method is to start with the forearm extended at the area of application (Figure 3-19 A) and then slowly flex the elbow into full flexion (Figure 3-19 B). Once the elbow is fully flexed, the practitioner leans into the client's body to apply sustained pressure. What the client should feel is a gradual broadening of the tissue as the forearm "scoops" upward with increasing pressure as the elbow comes into full flexion.

When the elbow is in full flexion, a specific area of the tissue is being worked. When the practitioner feels the tissue soften, the practitioner releases the pressure, moves slightly upward, and begins the sequence again. This sequence of movement is repeated throughout the length of the muscle being addressed. This has been compared to "stitching," as in, for example, the practitioner moving in small stitches up the client's rhomboid to provide relief from muscle tension.

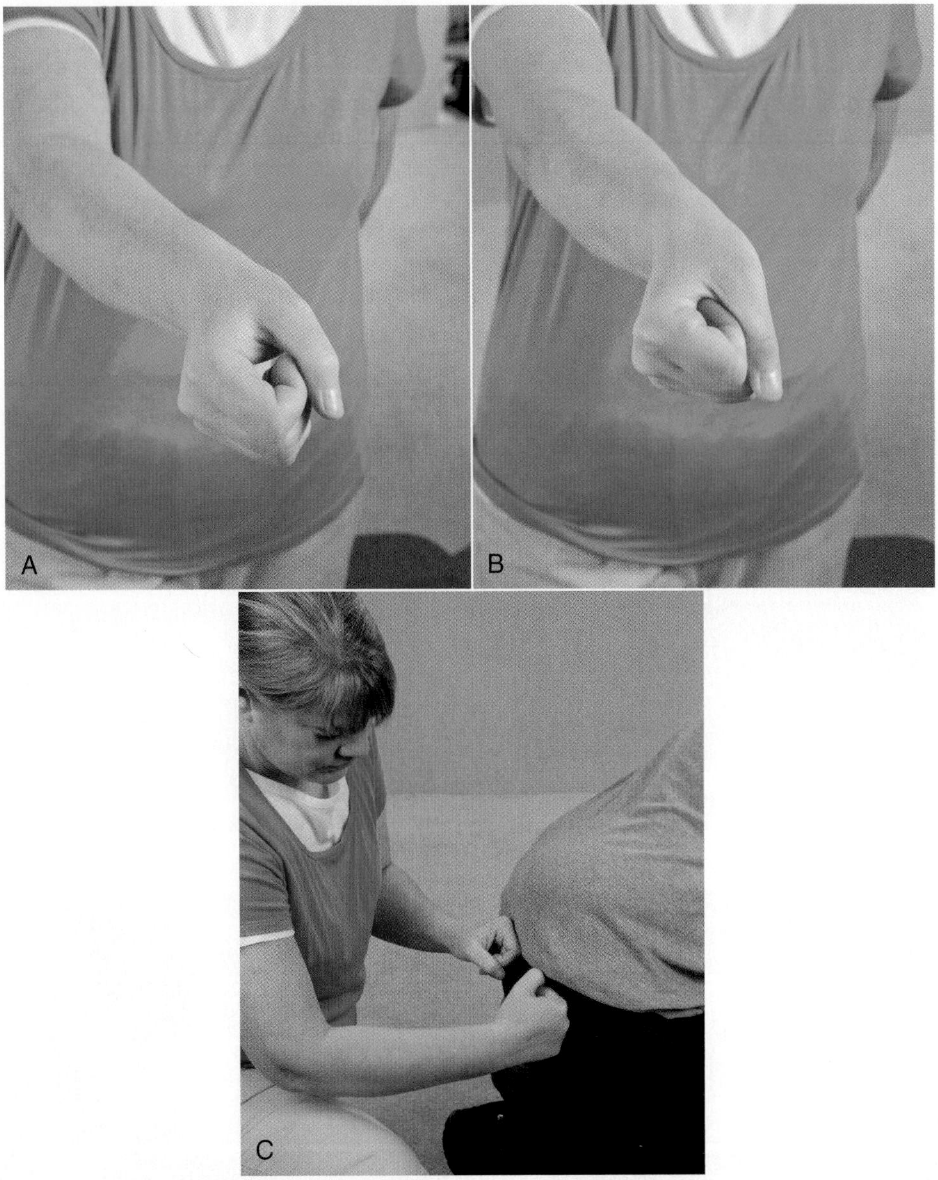

FIGURE 3-14 **A,** Soft fist. **B,** Hard fist. **C,** Fist kneading on the gluteals.

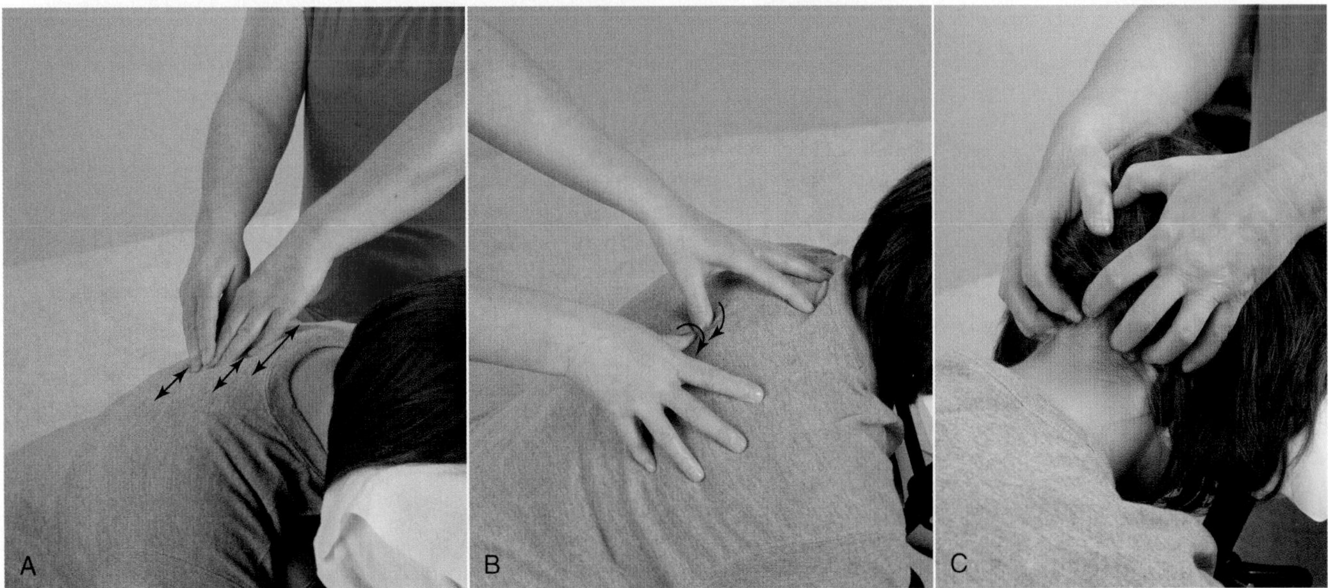

FIGURE 3-15 **A,** Application of deep friction on the rhomboids with the thumbs. **B,** Application of circular friction on the rhomboids. **C,** Application of circular friction with the fingertips on the suboccipitals.

Another method of applying elbow work is to begin the technique with the elbow already fully flexed (Figure 3-20 A). The point of the elbow is then placed on the area of the muscle that needs work, and sustained pressure is applied as the practitioner leans forward into the muscle, then extends the elbow slightly to increase the pressure (Figure 3-20 B).

Practitioners can use one or both of these two methods of applying the elbow as they choose or develop their own methods as they gain expertise. Practitioners should keep in mind, however, the client's comfort level with receiving deep sustained pressure. For clients who are a bit hesitant, the first method discussed may be more fitting as the pressure starts broadly and then gradually gets specific. This

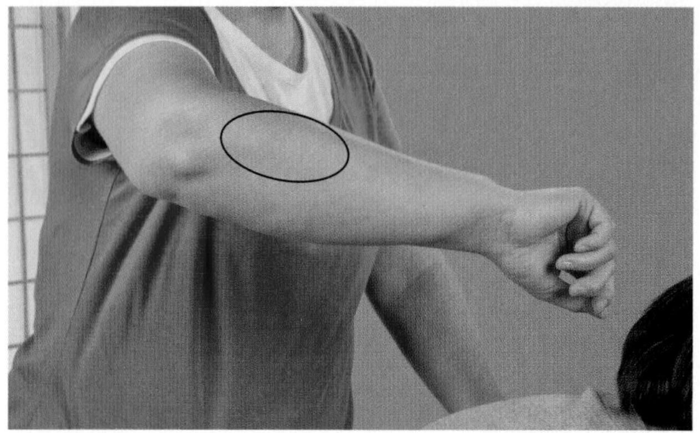

FIGURE 3-16 Area of the forearm that provides the most comfortable and efficient pressure.

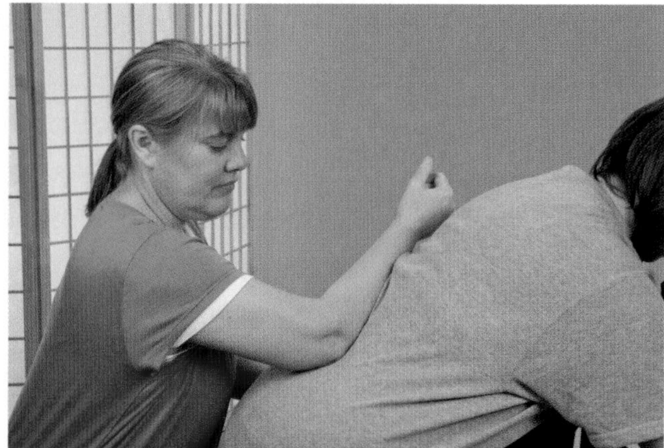

FIGURE 3-18 Elbow being applied in the low back.

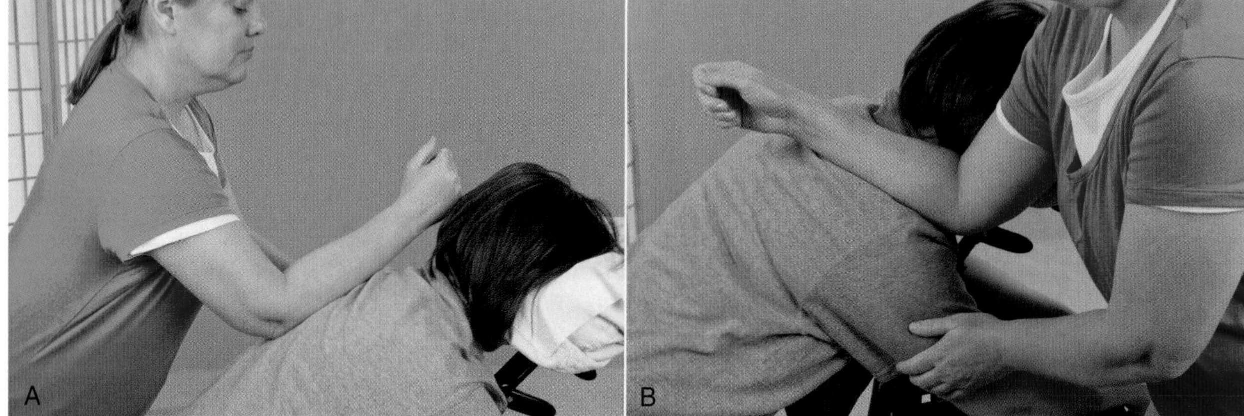

FIGURE 3-17 **A,** Applying the forearm to the rhomboids. **B,** Applying forearm to the upper trapezius while standing in front of the client.

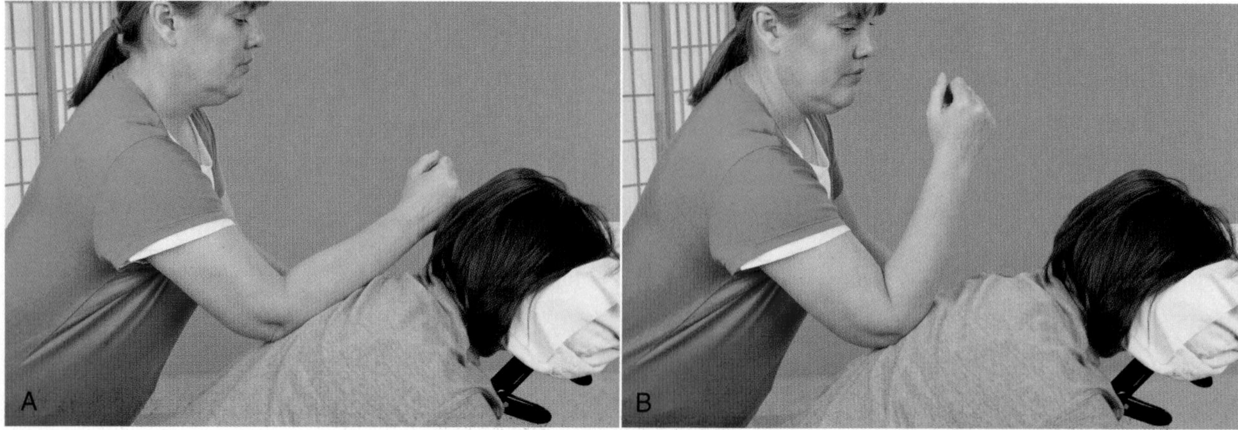

FIGURE 3-19 **A,** Application of the elbow with it initially extended. **B,** Increased flexion of the elbow.

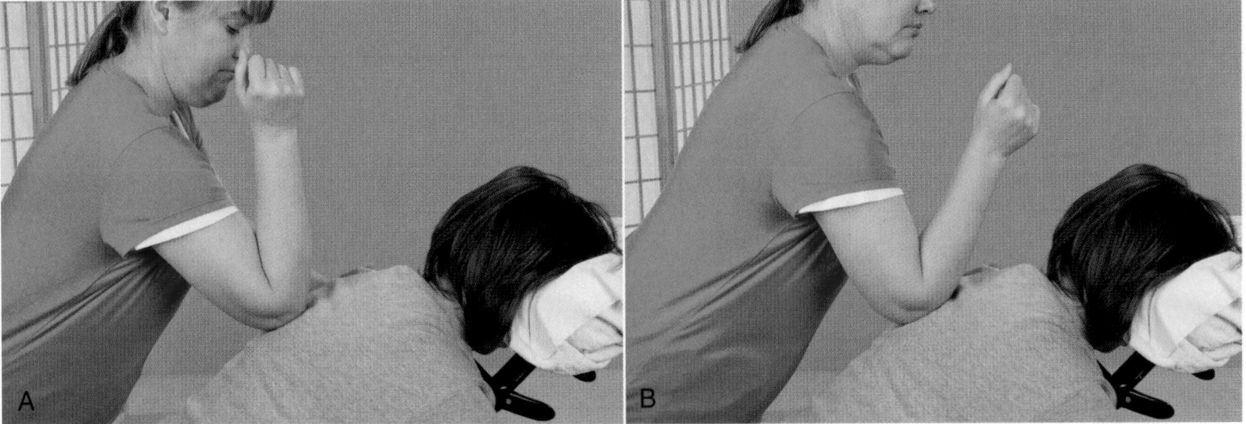

FIGURE 3-20 **A,** Application of the elbow with it initially fully flexed. **B,** Increased extension of the elbow.

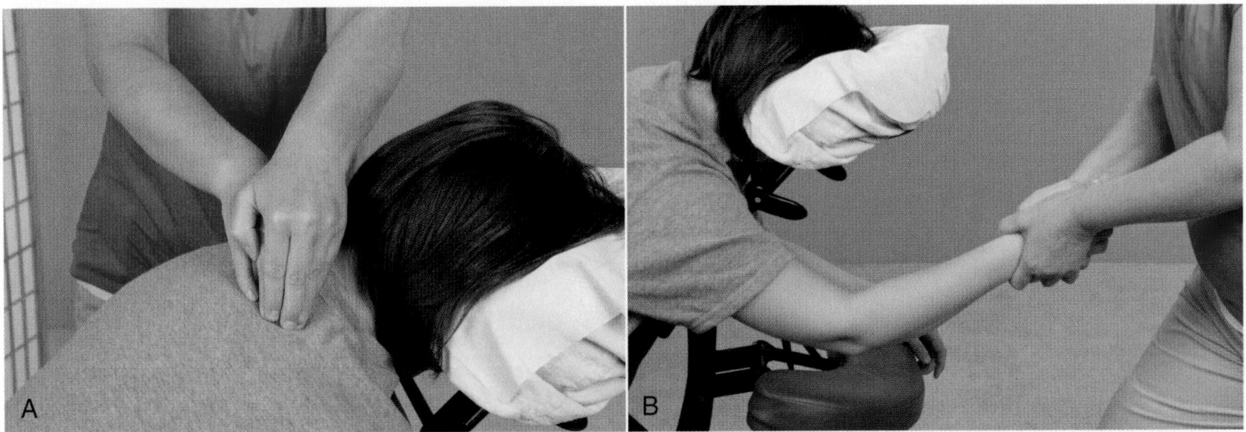

FIGURE 3-21 **A,** Fine vibration performed with the fingertips on the levator scapula. **B,** Vigorous vibration shown as arm jostling.

allows the client to ease into receiving the optimal depth of pressure and for receiving more specific work with the point of the elbow.

Whichever method of applying the elbow is used, it is essential that practitioners become skilled with using their elbow as it gives the smaller joints of their bodies a rest. In addition, client retention increases when the practitioner can provide varying depths of pressure from light to deep.

Vibration

Vibration is a technique that involves rocking, shaking, or jostling the tissue. It can be initially stimulating, and if done for longer periods (more than 15 seconds), it can be sedating, releasing tension and increasing blood flow into the area. It can be used specifically on a muscle or muscle attachments or used generally on a region such as the arm. The rate of vibration can range from fine to vigorous depending on where the technique is being applied. The use of vibration adds a nice variety to the pace and the rhythm of the techniques used in a chair massage treatment.

Fine vibration is applied by placing the fingertips or the palm of the hand on a muscle or joint and shaking it just enough to create a subtle yet definite movement into the tissue. Fine vibration may be used on the attachments of such muscles as the rhomboids or the levator scapula (Figure 3-21 A). When vibration is applied vigorously, the practitioner uses one or both hands to grasp the muscle or body region and shakes or jostles the area for approximately 15 to 60 seconds or longer. Figure 3-21 B shows vigorous vibration being performed on the arm.

Fine vibration can also be incorporated into elbow work by briskly supinating and pronating the hand when the elbow is fully flexed (Figures 3-22 A and B). This form of vibration has sometimes been called "the Queen's wave," as it resembles the type of wave Queen Elizabeth II of the United Kingdom typically performs when greeting her subjects.

Brush Strokes

Brush strokes can be used to connect the different parts of the client's body as each region is addressed individually. They can also be used to give a sense of completion and wholeness as the treatment comes to a close.

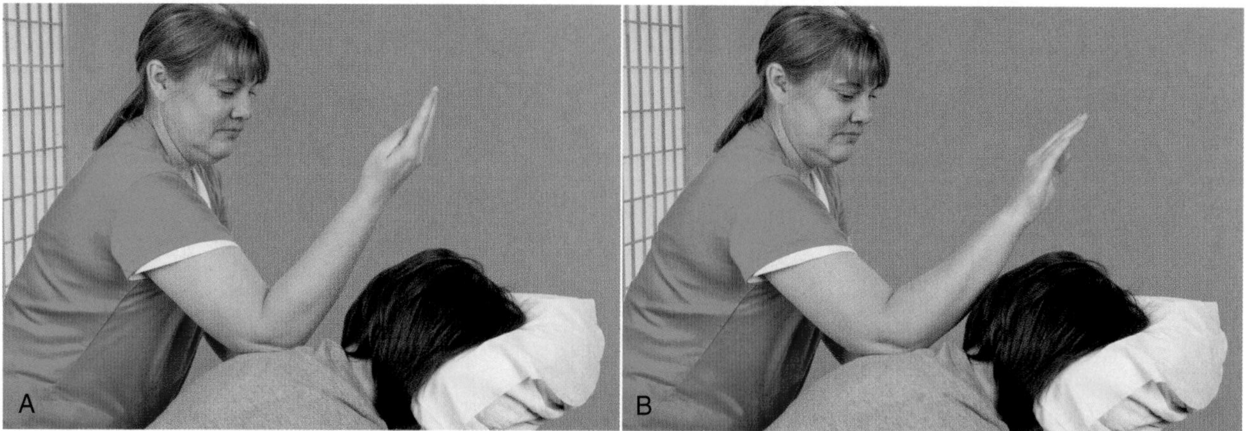

FIGURE 3-22 **A,** Fine vibration incorporated into elbow work, supinated position. **B,** Pronated position.

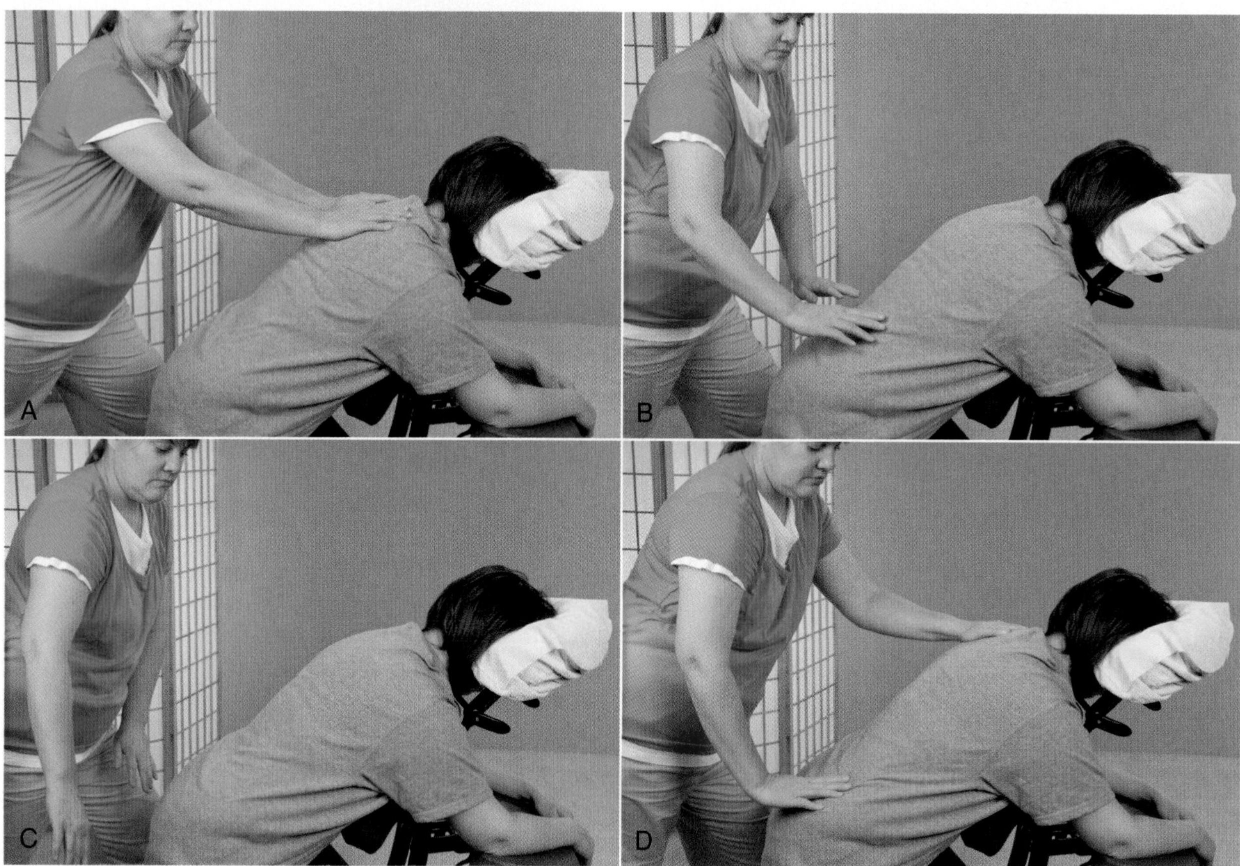

FIGURE 3-23 **A, B,** and **C,** Brush strokes being performed simultaneously in the same direction. **D,** Brush strokes being performed alternately.

Brush strokes are soft, gliding strokes with the fingertips along the entire length of a limb or a region of the body. These strokes have also been called "feather strokes" in reference to the lightness of the touch. The strokes can be done with both hands simultaneously, in the same direction (Figures 3-23 A, B, and C) or in an alternating fashion (Figure 3-23 D). Some practitioners who practice certain types of energy work use this technique as a means to disperse the energy that has been moved out of the body and direct it into the ground to be recharged.

Percussion

In percussion, the practitioner uses various hand positions in repetitive, rhythmic movements that bounce upward off the client's soft tissues. The stroke is performed with relaxed wrists and is short, quick, and springy (as if the tissues were

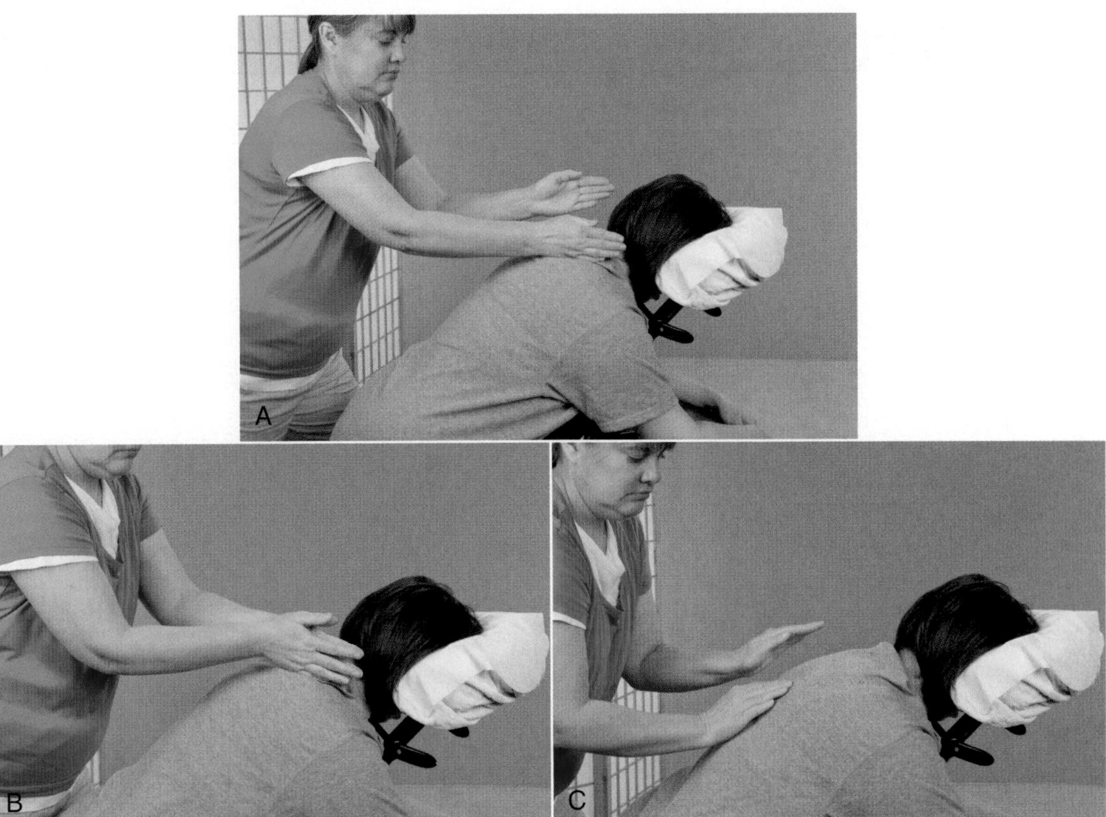

FIGURE 3-24 **A,** Hacking percussion. **B,** Quacking percussion. **C,** Cupping percussion.

a trampoline). The emphasis is on the upstroke. Practitioners should be mindful not to apply percussion over any bony prominences. Percussion increases the contractile power of muscle tissue, increases blood flow in the area, and stimulates the nervous system. It is an excellent technique to use at the end of a treatment to help energize a client who may have become sedated.

There are several types of percussion. **Hacking** is performed with the ulnar sides of both hands striking alternately up and down (Figure 3-24 A). A variation of this stroke can be applied by placing the palms of the hands together in a prayer position with the fingers slightly spread out (Figure 3-24 B). This style is called **quacking** because of the sound it makes as the practitioner's hands strike the client's body.

A third style of percussion that is often used in chair massage is **cupping**. The practitioner creates a slight curve in the palms of the hand as if holding something. The stroke is then applied by using the ulnar edges of the cupped hands, creating a pronounced hollow sound (Figure 3-24 C).

Other styles of percussion include lightly **pummeling** with a loose fist (as though an egg is being held in the hand), **plucking** (as though plucking lint from the client's clothing), and **tapping** lightly with the fingertips (as though playing the piano).

Although a variety of these types of percussion can be used on each client, it is best to keep percussion to a minimum. A small dose of this stroke goes a long way and should not be overdone, especially because some clients do not like the technique. The sound may be too loud and disconcerting, thus taking away from the relaxing effect of the treatment. Other clients may object to the suddenness of the hands striking the body. Practitioners should ask during the pretreatment interview if the client is open to receiving percussion. Even if the client says yes, it is important that the practitioner be aware of any nonverbal cues that the client may project, such as stiffening up, to indicate a dislike of this technique.

CAUTIONARY SITES

Cautionary sites, sometimes called **endangerment sites**, are areas of the body in which there is little tissue protection of nerves, blood vessels, and bony projections, thus significantly increasing the potential for damage and pain from massage techniques. Because of limited tissue protection, techniques performed in these areas warrant caution or are, in some cases, simply contraindicated. A **contraindication** is a factor or body condition that prohibits a treatment from being administered; administration of the treatment would, in fact, make the factor or body condition

TABLE 3-1 Cautionary Sites

Site	Structures Involved	Appropriate Technique Approach
Area inferior to the ear	Facial nerve, styloid process, external carotid artery	Use lighter pressure
Anterior neck (defined by sternocleidomastoid, the sternal notch)	External carotid artery, jugular vein, vagus nerve, larynx, thyroid gland	Avoid the area
Vertebral column	Spinous processes	Avoid the area
Shoulder girdle	Spine of the scapula; clavicle	Use lighter pressure
Thoracic cage	Xiphoid process; lateral surfaces of the rib cage	Use lighter pressure
Axilla	Brachial artery, axillary artery, and vein; cephalic vein and brachial nerve plexus	Use lighter pressure or avoid the area
Medial upper arm (between biceps brachii and triceps brachii)	Brachial vein, musculocutaneous nerve	Use lighter pressure
Elbow		
Anterior elbow (antecubital region)	Brachial artery, median cubital vein, median nerve	Use lighter pressure
Posterior elbow (olecranon process)	Ulnar nerve	Use lighter pressure
Popliteal fossa	Popliteal artery and vein, tibial nerve	Use lighter pressure
Kidney area (on either side of the spine between the levels of L-3 and T-12)	The kidneys are loosely suspended in fat and connective tissue	Use lighter pressure; heavy percussion is contraindicated
Areas where the client has a great deal of sensitivity or pain		Use lighter pressure or avoid the area, depending on the client's tolerance
Bruises, open wounds, recent surgery (surgical incisions that have not yet healed)	The tissue is healing and therefore fragile. Massage over these areas will damage the tissue further, and can be painful. As part of the healing process, these areas contain blood clots that may dislodge under the pressure of massage technique application and travel throughout the body. There is also an increased chance of infection with open wounds.	Avoid the area
Areas of infection and inflammation	The tissue is healing and therefore fragile. Massage over these areas will damage the tissue further, possibly spread the infection or inflammation, and can be painful.	Avoid the area

worse. In this case, the factor is the amount of tissue protection. (On the other hand, an **indication** is a reason to perform a treatment. In other words, there is some factor or body condition that would be relieved by the application of a particular technique. An example is tight muscles being an indication for the technique of kneading.)

Location of Cautionary Sites

Many, but not all, of the cautionary sites of the body are joints. (The lesser tissue protection in joints is what allows for greater freedom of movement.) Other areas include bony projections and the kidney region. Cautionary sites also include any areas in which the client has a great deal of sensitivity or pain, bruises, open wounds or recent surgery (surgical incisions that have not yet healed), and areas of infection and inflammation. Table 3-1 shows the cautionary sites and the appropriate technique approach. Cautionary sites are also shown on Figure 3-25. Practitioners should note the popliteal fossa, which is not a concern for seated massage. However, Chapter 5, "Additional Techniques and Adaptations," explains how to transition the client to the massage table or futon to receive additional techniques, during which the popliteal fossa would be a cautionary site.

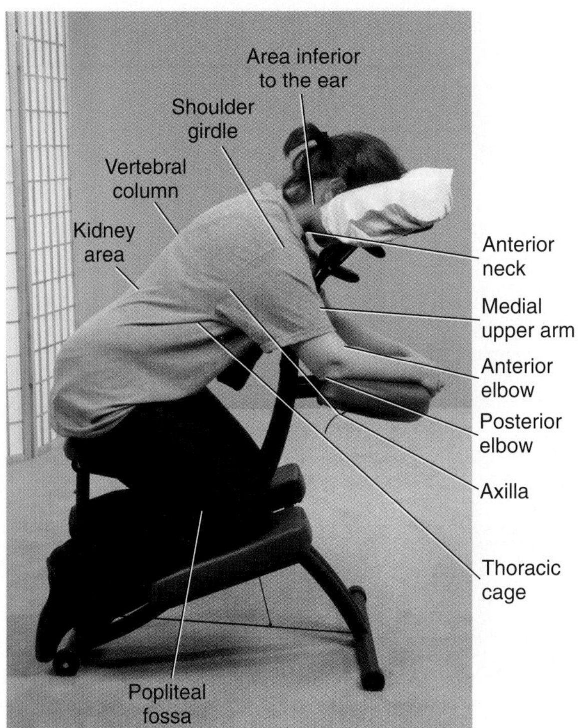

FIGURE 3-25 Cautionary sites on the anterior and posterior body.

BEFORE THE TREATMENT BEGINS

Considerations for Working on the Clothed Client

Chair massage practitioners must be able to work with many types of clothing and accessories that clients will be wearing. It is most important for the practitioner to make sure the client's tissues are engaged when working through clothing so that when pressure is applied, the fabric is not just moved around. Otherwise, the treatment can be abrasive to the client's skin and the practitioner's fingers. For example, blouses and shirts made of silky fabrics tend to be slippery, so it will be paramount that the practitioner be mindful of fully engaging with the client's tissues under the fabric. Otherwise, the work can be so abrasive it can actually cause a fabric burn on the client's skin.

Some fabrics, such as silk, linen, and ramie, wrinkle easily. If a client is wearing clothes made of these fabrics, the practitioner should let the client know that there will be some slight wrinkles in the outfit from leaning forward onto the sternum pad, from kneeling on the chair, and possibly from the techniques applied by the practitioner. The client could then choose whether or not to receive the treatment.

Sometimes practitioners may need to ask clients to remove certain items of clothing or other accessories if they interfere with providing an effective treatment. Examples would be thick wool sweaters, suit jackets, wide belts, and large jewelry (Figure 3-26). There is the possibility that clients may not be able to remove some of the clothing, such as when wearing a thick sweater without a shirt underneath. Therefore, the practitioner may want to consider bringing T-shirts that clients can change into if need be (as mentioned in the deluxe kit described in Chapter 2). Clients who are wearing ties should remove them and loosen the top two or three buttons of their shirts.

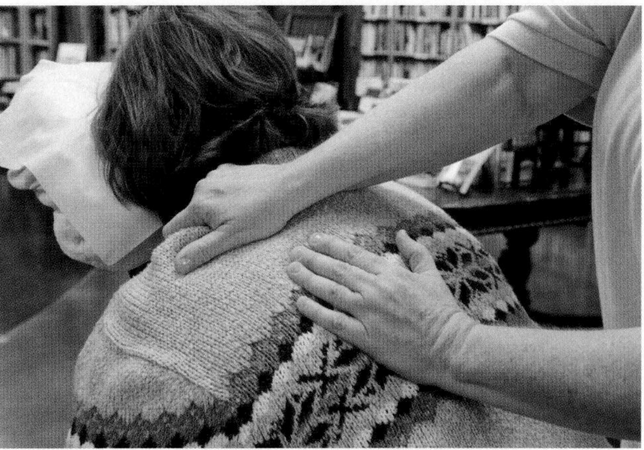

FIGURE 3-26 Client wearing a thick sweater.

Other items that clients should remove are eyeglasses, pens or other items in shirt pockets, and keys, coins, wallets, cell phones, and so forth from pants pockets. Practitioners can bring a small basket in which these items can be placed during the treatment (also mentioned in the deluxe kit in Chapter 2); practitioners should remind clients to pick these up after the treatment ends.

When asking clients to remove certain pieces of clothing and other items, the practitioner should explain why the request is being made. Some clients, though, may not be comfortable or may be unable to comply with the request. In this case, the practitioner must be flexible and adapt the treatment to the circumstances. For example, if it is not practical for clients who are wearing thick sweaters to change into a T-shirt or if clients are wearing jeans or bras with thick straps, then the practitioner may need to apply more pressure and check in more often with the client to see how it feels. The center of the horizontal strap of a bra may need to be avoided so as to not press the bra hooks into the client's skin. The practitioner may need to let the client wearing a thick sweater know that kneading techniques may not be therapeutically successful because of the inability to grasp the tissues through the clothing.

Practitioners should also remember that people have an energetic component to their physical body. Even if it seems that the techniques are not as effective through thick clothing, the practitioner is still affecting the client's energy (qi) by connecting with it and supporting it, even when the practitioner cannot address muscle and soft tissue fully and completely.

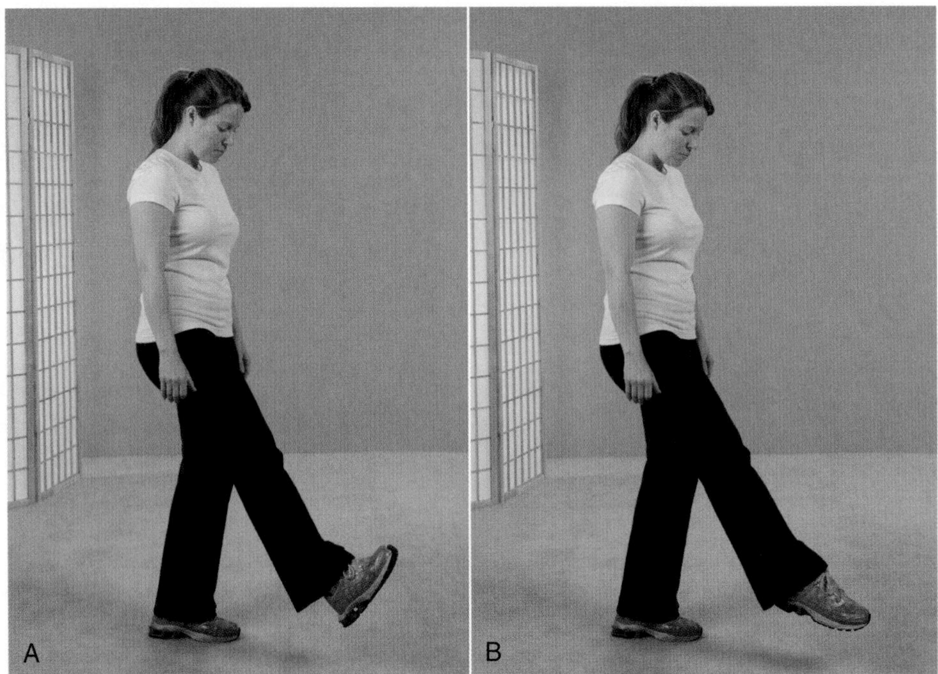

FIGURE 3-27 **A,** Ankle dorsiflexion. **B,** Plantarflexion.

Stretches and Warm-ups

Like all forms of bodywork, performing chair massage is a physical activity. Therefore, before setting up the massage chair and before working on the first client, practitioners should do some stretches and warm-ups. These will warm up their muscles and joints and will decrease fatigue and the chance of injury while working, maintaining, or improving balance and maintaining or improving flexibility. Stretches and warm-ups also increase the practitioner's flow of qi, which increases stamina and increases the practitioner's ability to connect with the client's qi to help support it.

The following are some basic stretches and warm-ups. They take only a few minutes to do and, done regularly, can become one of the practitioner's methods of health maintenance.

Ankle and Leg

While standing on one foot, lift the other foot off the floor in front of you. Plantarflex then dorsiflex your ankle several times (Figure 3-27). Repeat with the other foot.

While standing on one foot, lift the other foot off the floor in front of you. Circle your foot clockwise several times, then counterclockwise several times (Figure 3-28). Repeat with your other foot.

With your knees either together or shoulder width apart, slightly flex your knees, hold for several seconds, then extend them (Figure 3-29). Repeat several times.

With your knees together, move your knees clockwise several times, then counterclockwise several times (Figure 3-30).

Vertebral Column

Keeping your back straight, flex your vertebral column forward as far as is comfortable for you, hanging your arms forward or, if possible, placing your hands on the floor (Figure 3-31 A). Hold for several seconds. Keeping your back straight, extend your vertebral column as far back as is comfortable for you (Figure 3-31 B). *Do not force the extension.* This could result in injury to your back. Hold for several seconds, then release.

Keeping your back straight, circle your trunk clockwise several times, then counterclockwise several times (Figure 3-32). *Do not force your trunk into a wider circle than is comfortable for you.* This could result in injury to your back.

Shoulders and Arms

Shrug your shoulders as high as is comfortable for you (Figure 3-33 A). Hold for several seconds, then drop your shoulders (Figure 3-33 B). Repeat several times.

In as wide a movement as is comfortable for you, circle one arm forward several times, then circle it backward several times (Figure 3-34). Repeat with your other arm.

Extend one arm out in front, at, or just below shoulder height. With your other hand, grasp the fingers on the extended arm. Pull the hand to extend the wrist and stretch your forearm flexors (Figure 3-35 A). Hold for several seconds, then release. Flex the elbow of the extended arm. With your other hand, grasp the hand on the extended arm. Gently push the hand to flex the wrist and stretch your forearm extensors. The stretch can be intensified by pushing to curl the fingers under (Figure 3-35 B). Hold for several seconds, then release.

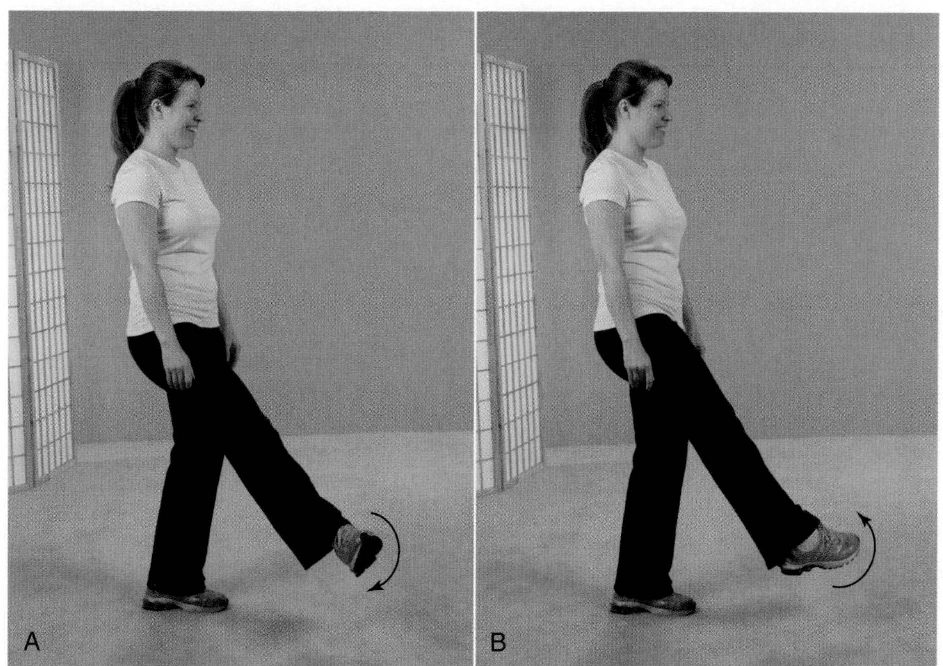

FIGURE 3-28 **A,** Ankle circles clockwise. **B,** Ankle circles counterclockwise.

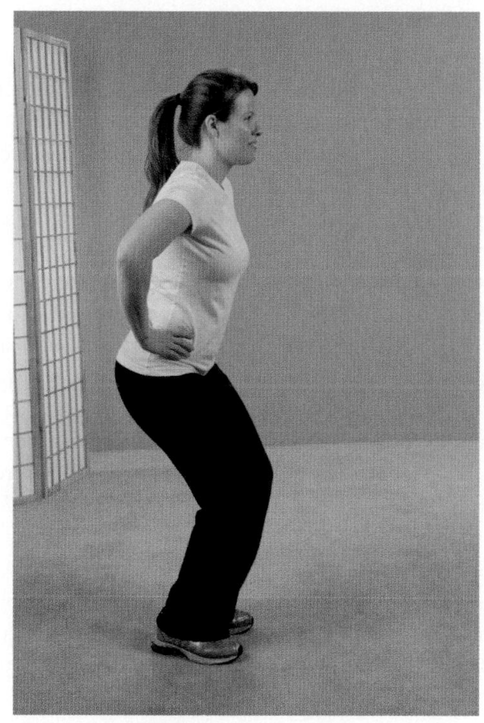

FIGURE 3-29 Knee flexion.

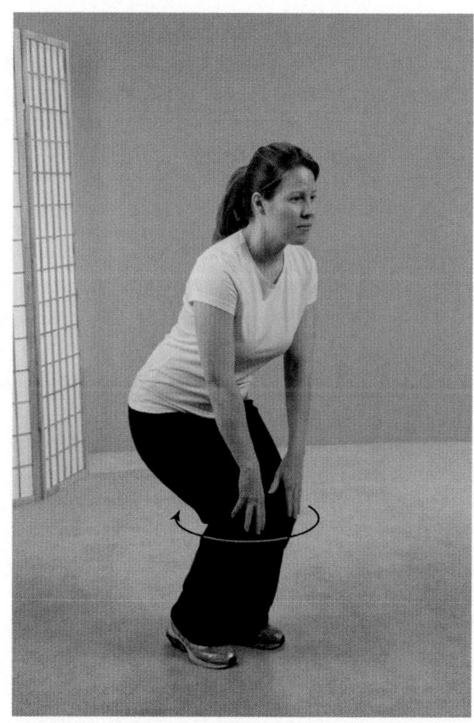

FIGURE 3-30 Knee circles, clockwise and counterclockwise.

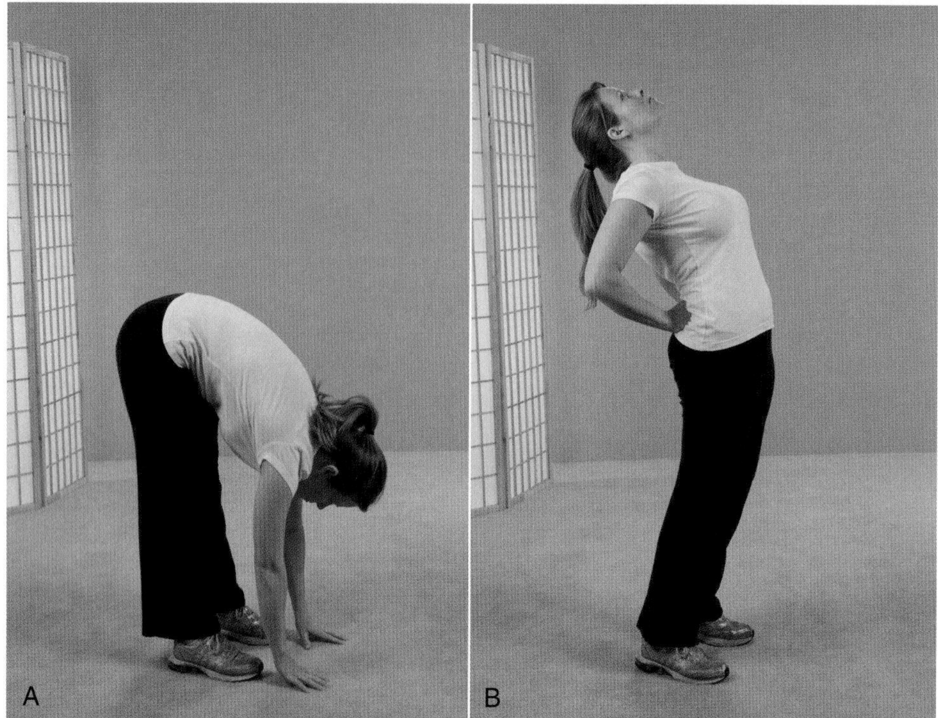

FIGURE 3-31 **A,** Vertebral column flexion. **B,** Vertebral column extension.

Place your fingertips together in a tentlike position. Gently push your hands together until you feel a stretch in your fingers (Figure 3-36). Hold for several seconds, then release.

Neck

Flex your neck forward as far as is comfortable for you to stretch your posterior neck muscles (Figure 3-37 A). You can intensify the stretch by interlacing your fingers, placing them on the back of your head, and gently pulling your head down. Hold for several seconds, then release. Flex your neck backward until your face is toward the ceiling (Figure 3-37 B). Gently stretch your anterior neck muscles for several seconds, then release.

Laterally flex your neck as far as is comfortable for you (Figure 3-38 A). This stretch can be intensified by placing your hand from the same side on top of your head and gently pulling down. Hold for several seconds, then release. Bring your head to center, then laterally flex your neck to the other side as far as is comfortable for you (Figure 3-38 B).

Circle your neck clockwise several times, then counterclockwise several times (Figure 3-39). *Do not force your neck into a wider circle than is comfortable for you.* This could result in injury to your neck.

Pretreatment Interview

Before performing chair massage, it is best to conduct a pretreatment interview, even a brief one. The practitioner can find out the following:

- The client's health history
- Whether or not the client has received any type of bodywork before, including chair massage
- If the client is experiencing any areas of pain, discomfort, or muscle tightness, and if so, where
- The goals for the treatment (e.g., pain relief, relaxation, rejuvenation)
- What the client will be doing after the treatment (for example, if the client is giving a big presentation, then scalp massage may be out of the question because it can mess up the hair; also, the client may not want to feel drowsy and relaxed afterward, and an invigorating treatment may be in order; the same is true for clients who have to go back to work; seeing their employees in a sedated state from the treatments most likely will not sit well with supervisors)

Some practitioners have clients fill out simple intake forms (discussed in more detail in Chapter 6, "The Business of Chair Massage") with health history questions, and they use this as well as a verbal interview to determine how to tailor the treatment to the client's needs.

Sample Script for the Practitioner to Say to a First-Time Chair Massage Client

The following is a sample script practitioners can use to talk with clients who are receiving their first chair massage. Practitioners are encouraged to develop their own styles of talking with clients, and this is intended for practitioners to use as a starting point.

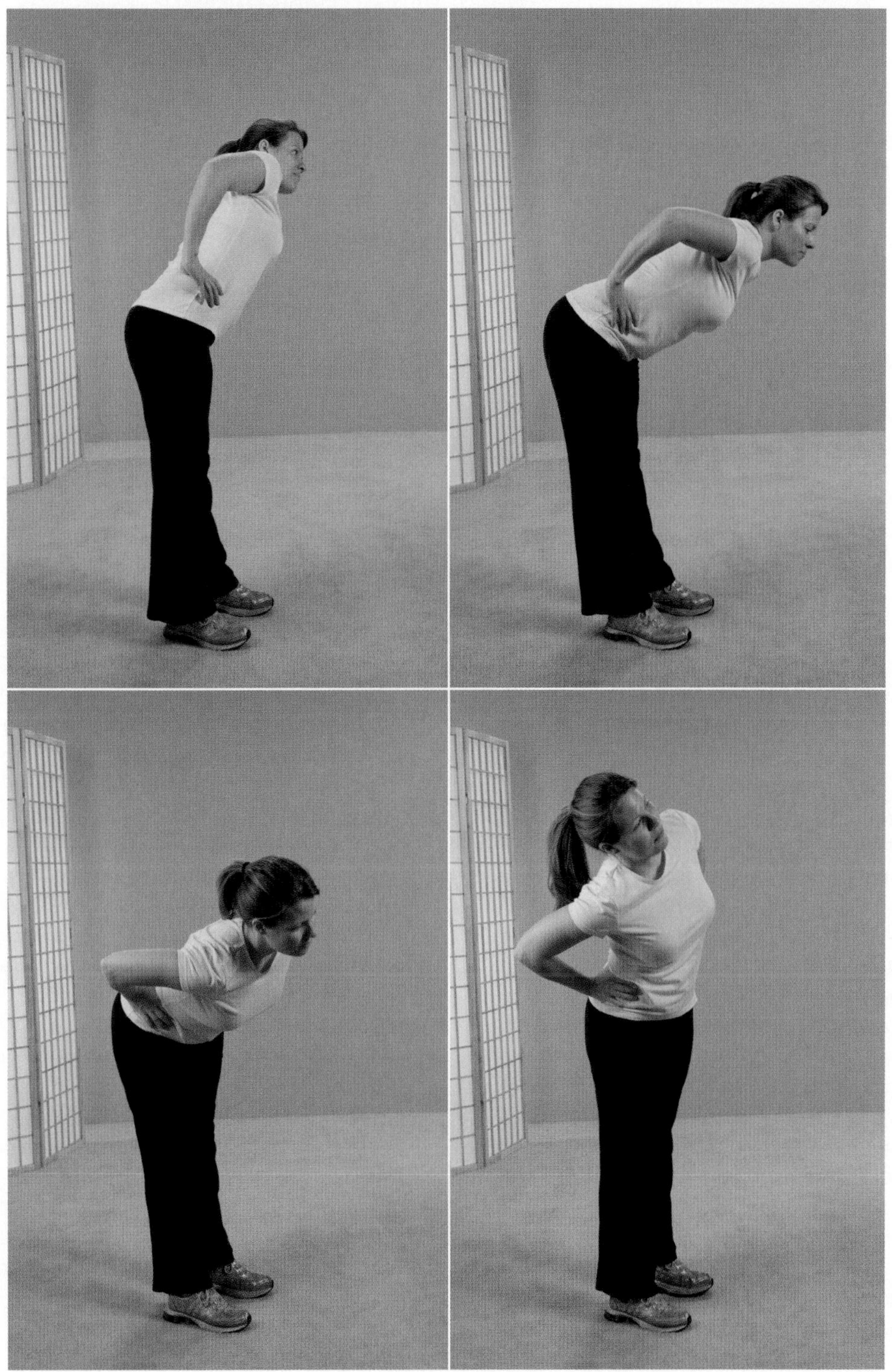

FIGURE 3-32 Trunk circles clockwise and counterclockwise.

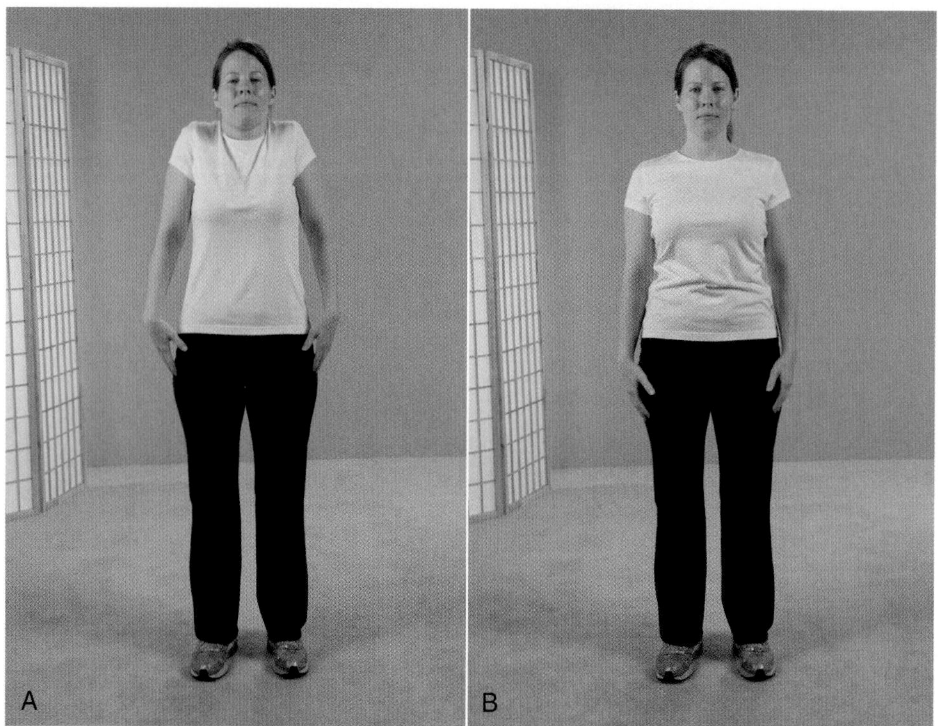

FIGURE 3-33 **A,** Shoulder shrugs up. **B,** Shoulder shrugs down.

"Hi. My name is Patricia, and I will be working with you today." (Reach out your hand to shake the client's hand firmly.)

"Since you have not received a chair massage before, there are a few things I want to share with you to help you get the most out of your treatment. The chair is ergonomically designed to totally support you so that you can relax and not have to do any work to hold yourself up. I'm going to show you how to sit in the chair and then how to get off the chair." (Demonstrate by getting into the chair, putting your face in the face cradle, and placing your arms on the armrest. Then demonstrate getting off the chair by sitting up straight, placing both feet firmly on the ground, standing up, and backing off from the chair.)

"Your treatment will consist of me softly kneading the tissue of your neck, shoulders, back, arms, and hands." (Point to these areas on yourself or on the client, depending on your preference.) "Have you had any recent accidents or injuries in these areas, or any other areas? Have you had any recent surgeries? Do you have any areas of infection or inflammation? Do you have any arthritis in your hands or fingers? There will also be some stretches at the end for the chest and the neck. Are you okay with being stretched in those areas? What will you be doing after the treatment today?"

"While I am working, please do not hesitate to tell me if you feel discomfort of any kind, if the pressure is too deep, not deep enough, or anything else that would be helpful for me to know to make sure you are enjoying the treatment. If you feel light-headed at any time during the treatment, just go ahead and sit up straight." (This sometimes happens if people have not eaten much during the day or have not had enough water. It can also happen due to vasovagal syncope, discussed in the "Vasovagal Syncope" section.")

"Before we get started, I am going put a clean face cloth here on the face cradle for sanitation purposes." (Take off the face cloth that you had placed your face on and replace it with a clean face cloth.) "Have a seat, and I will adjust the chair to match your size. What you should be looking for is a comfortable alignment of your back, shoulders, and neck as you lean forward. You should be able to breathe easily and not feel hunched at the shoulders or that your chin is pressing against anything uncomfortable." (Make the proper adjustments.) "How does that feel? Great. Now take a deep breath and exhale." (Begin the treatment.)

BASIC SEQUENCE

One of the challenges a practitioner experiences when first learning chair massage is the concept of reducing a 60-minute therapeutic session into one that is 15 minutes long. This is actually two challenges in one. First, the practitioner needs to reframe the idea that therapeutic bodywork can only be accomplished in a 50- or 60-minute,

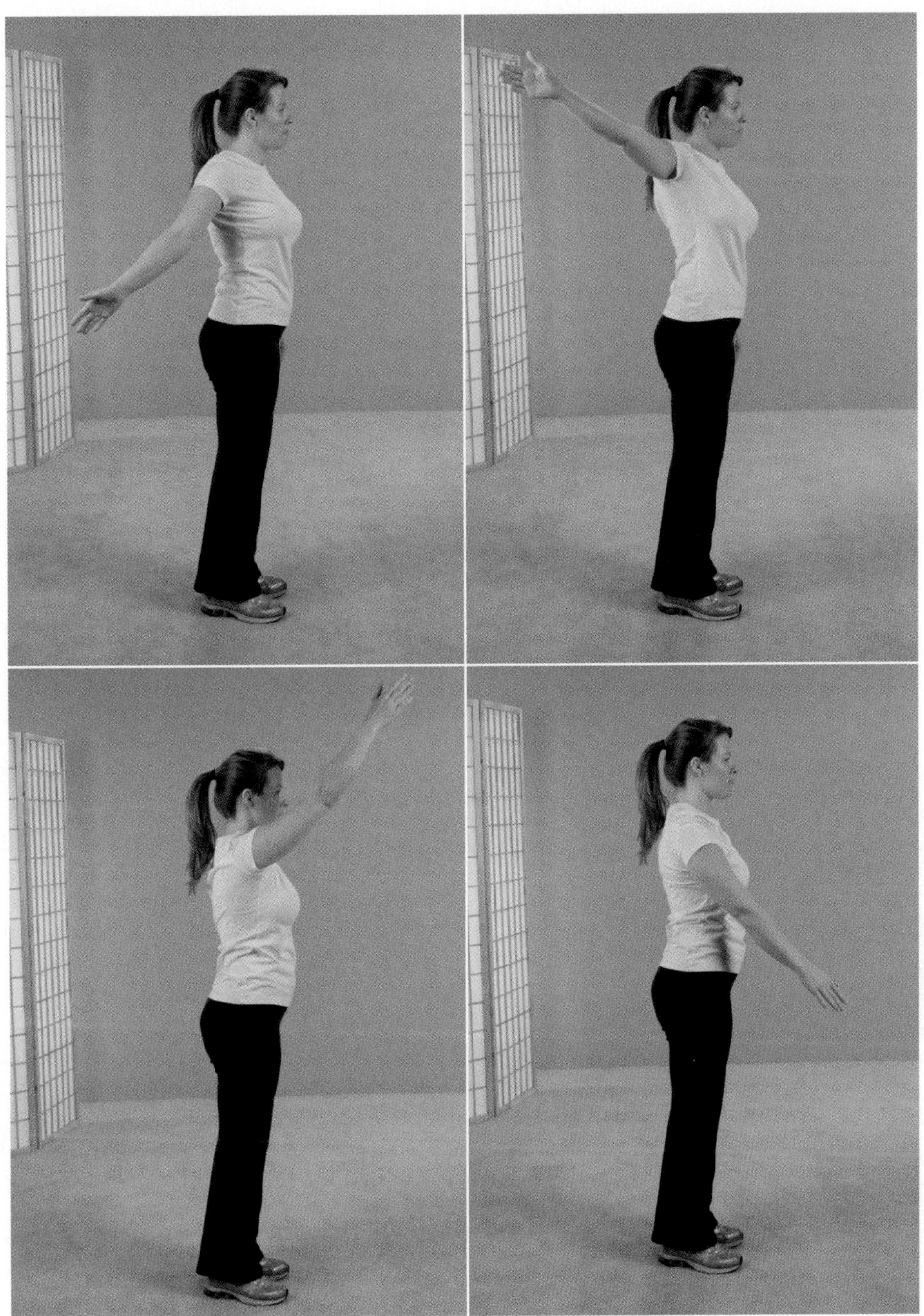

FIGURE 3-34 Large shoulder circles, forward and backward.

full-body treatment. The term *therapeutic* refers to any change in physical or emotional structure that assists a client in feeling better than before the session began. Therefore, it is important to not limit the concept of therapeutic effectiveness to a modality that addresses only the full body or one that occurs only within a specific time frame.

Second, practitioners may be overwhelmed by the thought of needing to cover the upper portion of a client's body in a certain time frame. They may think that they have to move on to another region even if they discern that the area they are working on needs more time. Although there can be opportunities for the practitioner to stay focused on a tense muscle until it releases, it is not the only way to help clients reduce stress. The ability to efficiently address several regions of the body, thereby releasing general physical tension, is a sign of skill, flexibility, and the ability to create a client-centered treatment.

A method that is helpful when learning to give an effective chair massage is to start with a **basic sequence** on the posterior body. A basic sequence provides a focus for

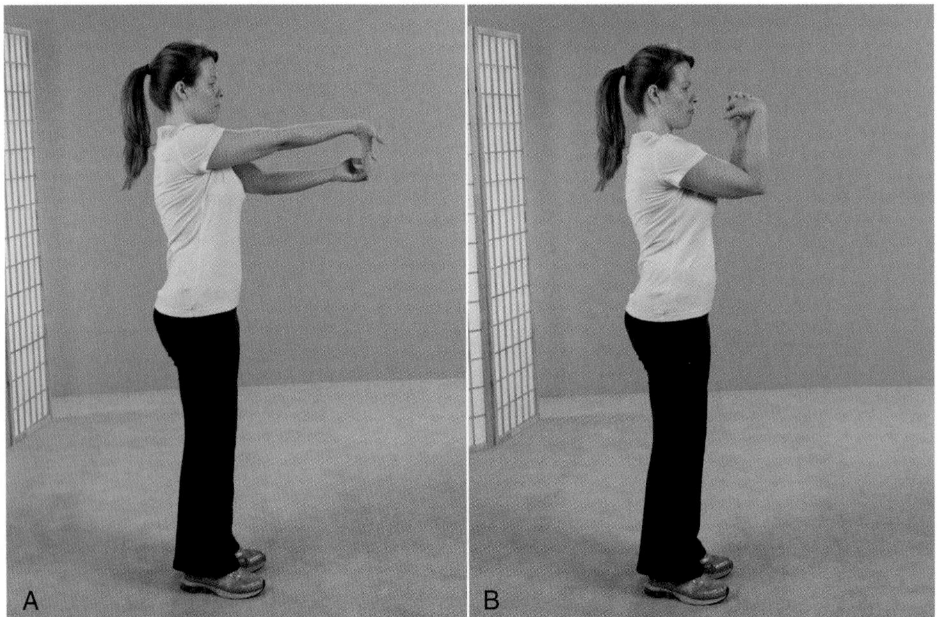

FIGURE 3-35 **A,** Forearm flexor stretch. **B,** Forearm extensor stretch.

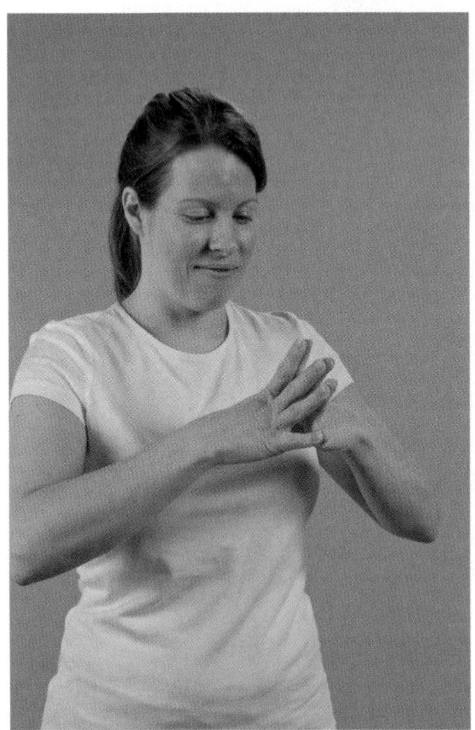
FIGURE 3-36 Finger stretch.

practice and a tool to make the techniques and movements of chair massage automatic. It is the equivalent of practicing scales when learning how to play the clarinet, or practicing free throws in basketball over and over until it becomes second nature. Having a specific sequence in the initial learning process can establish a sense of security for practitioners as well as a clearer understanding of how to begin the work of chair massage. It helps practitioners have organized treatments, which, through practice, they can execute in a fluid manner.

Once practitioners no longer need to concentrate consciously on body mechanics and techniques, treatments will feel more natural, smooth, and flowing. Practitioners will then move to a higher level of understanding the benefits of the treatments and how their touch affects clients. Practitioners may also then gain confidence in creating their own treatment protocols for individual clients and making their treatments client centered, which can lead to consistently high-quality treatments and greater client satisfaction.

Five Regions

The sequence starts by imagining the posterior torso, head, and neck divided into five regions as you face the back of the client (Figure 3-40):

- Upper right—upper trapezius, levator scapula, shoulder girdle muscles, arm, and hand
- Upper left—upper trapezius, levator scapula, shoulder girdle muscles, arm, and hand
- Lower right—the region from the level of the sixth thoracic vertebra inferior to the gluteals, including the mid and lower trapezius, rhomboids, erector spinae, and quadratus lumborum
- Lower left—the region from the level of the sixth thoracic vertebra inferior to the gluteals, including the mid and lower trapezius, rhomboids, erector spinae, and quadratus lumborum
- Posterior neck and head

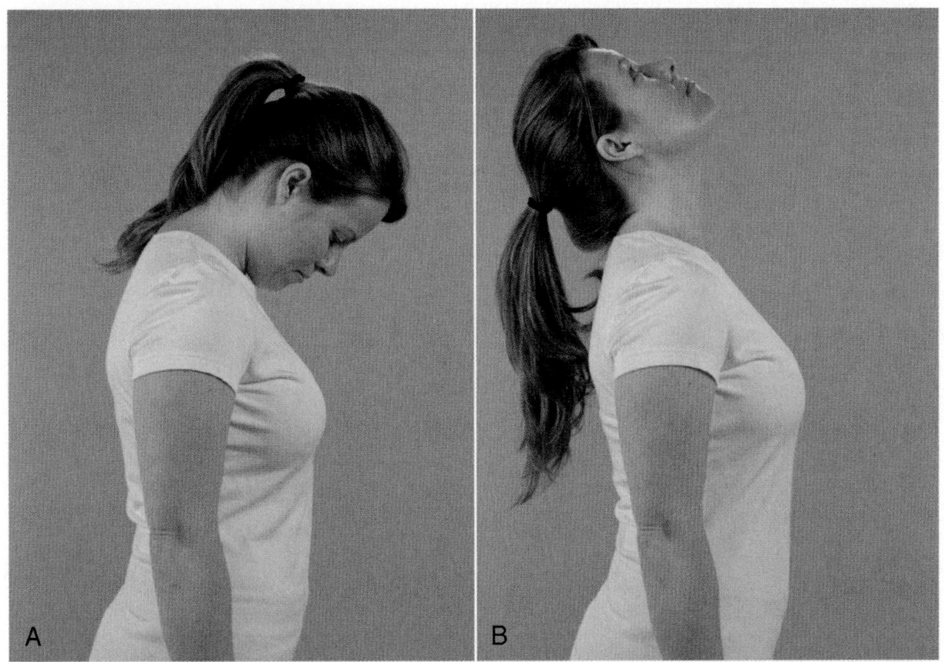

FIGURE 3-37 **A,** Neck forward flexion. **B,** Neck backward flexion.

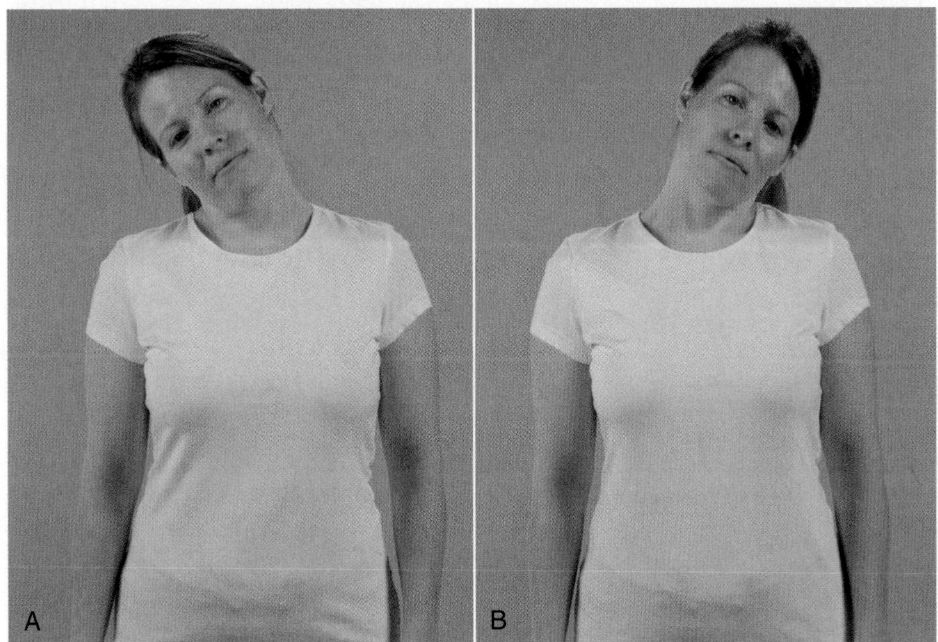

FIGURE 3-38 **A,** Neck lateral flexion to the left. **B,** Neck lateral flexion to the right.

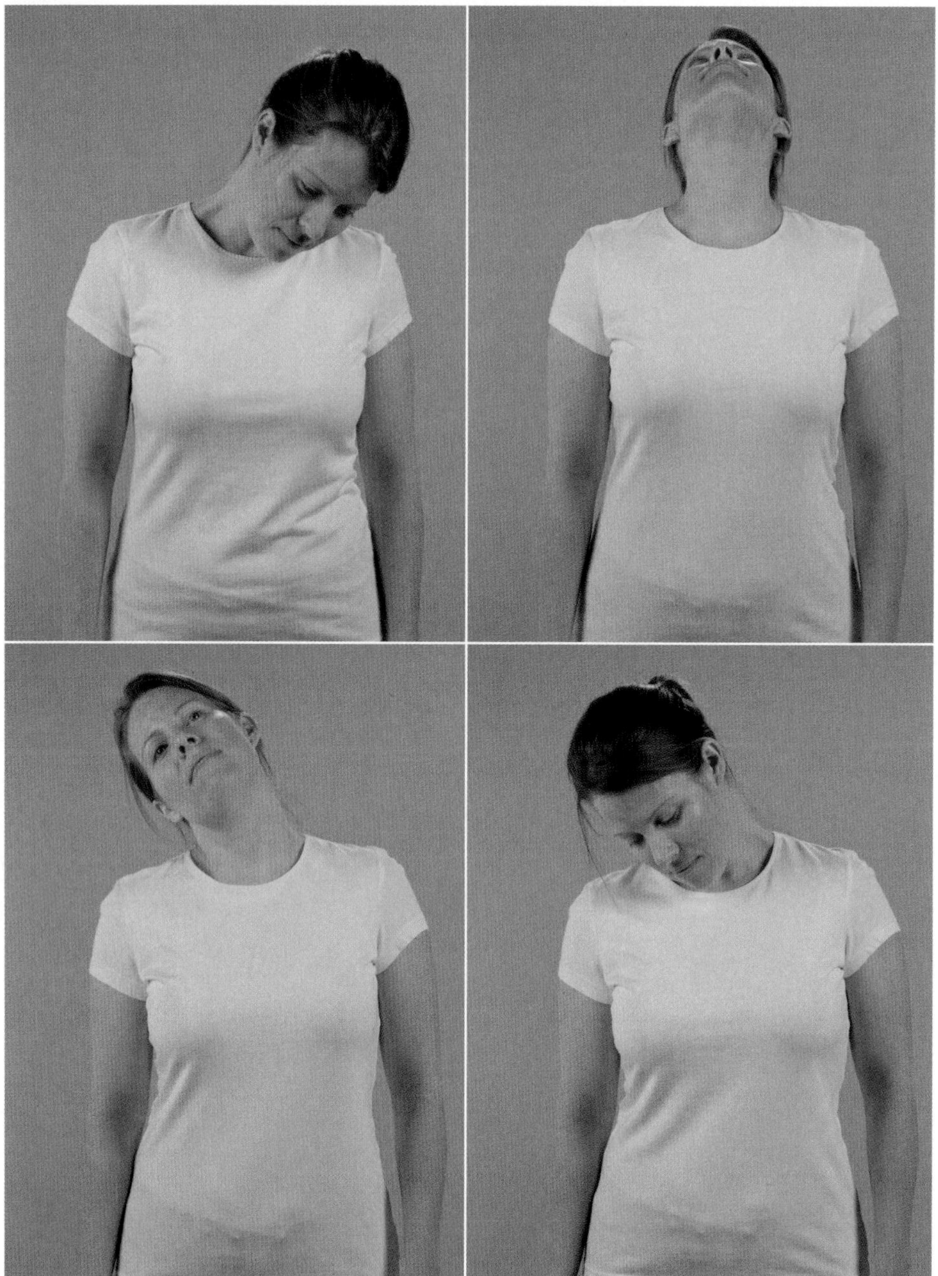

FIGURE 3-39 Neck circles, clockwise and counterclockwise.

Overview of Bony Landmarks and Muscles

Before starting to work on the client's back, it is helpful to palpate the bony landmarks of the regions and the muscles the practitioner will be working on. By palpating, the practitioner will know the location of the bony prominences of each region, joint structures, and muscles.

Figure 3-41 shows the bony landmarks of the back, posterior neck and skull, and the shoulder girdle, arm, and hand. Using this as a guide, practitioners should palpate the following on their clients:

- Occiput
- Spinous processes of the vertebrae
- Inferior rib cage
- Posterior iliac crests
- Sacrum
- Scapulae—medial border, lateral border, superior and inferior angles, spine, acromion process
- Glenohumeral joint
- Humerus—shaft, medial and lateral epicondyles, olecranon process
- Humeroulnar joint
- Radius—medial and lateral borders

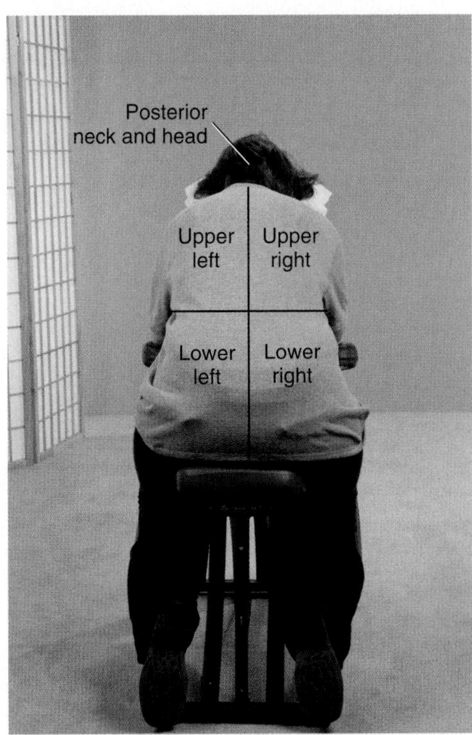

FIGURE 3-40 Posterior torso divided into five regions.

- Ulna—medial and lateral borders
- Carpals
- Metacarpals
- Phalanges

Figure 3-42 shows the muscles of the back and posterior shoulder girdle region. Figure 3-43 shows an anterior view of the posterior shoulder girdle region. This view shows the anterior trapezius, anterior deltoid, biceps brachii, and part of the triceps brachii. Figure 3-44 shows the erector spinae group and quadratus lumborum, which are deep to the muscles in Figures 3-41 and 3-42. Figure 3-45 and Figure 3-46 show the muscles of the upper arm, and Figure 3-47 and Figure 3-48 show the muscles of the forearm. Using this information as a guide, practitioners should palpate each muscle.

Helpful Treatment Reminders

Before performing the basic sequence, it is important to keep in mind that the client's body is three dimensional, not just a flat surface sitting on the chair. Make sure to address the many sides of the client's body by moving around the chair. For example, the upper trapezius and posterior neck can be grasped and lifted while standing behind, to the side of, and in front of the client. The shoulders and arms can be rolled and lifted as well.

Intention is important, and a good treatment can only be performed if the practitioner's mind is on the client and on the treatment. The practitioner should always be present to the client's needs and respond accordingly such as by adjusting pressure according to the client's request. The practitioner should lean into the client's body and wait for the body to respond. This can be thought of as listening to the body while applying techniques. Also, as practitioners release the pressure they are using, they should not break contact when moving around the body. Maintaining contact at all times makes the treatment flow better and makes the client feel more connected.

Practitioners should remember that neither they nor the client should hold their breath anytime during the treatment. They may need to gently remind clients to breathe, and ask about the quality of the pressure being applied and their comfort.

Most important, though, practitioners should relax and allow the sequence to flow. Enjoy the interaction and the exchange with the client. After some practice, practitioners may find that the sequence flows so well it is almost like doing no work at all, yet both they and their clients are deriving great benefit from it.

The Sequence

A recommended time frame for a 15-minute session is to do a brief opening by compressing the entire back, then allow three minutes for each upper region, two minutes for each lower region, three minutes for the posterior neck and head, and two minutes to close the session with brush strokes and percussion (Figure 3-49).

Opening: Compress the Entire Back

1. Standing behind the client in a lunge position, place both palms on the client's back on the erector spinae group on either side of the spine at approximately the level of T-1.
2. Lean forward, transferring your weight to your front leg as you exhale and apply pressure, then shift your weight to your back leg as you inhale and release the pressure. Continue to apply compressions rhythmically, working your way inferiorly to the level of T-6 (Figure 3-50 A).
3. At the level of T-6, curl your hands into soft fists and use the back of your hands to apply pressure (Figure 3-50 B). Continue compressing inferiorly until you reach the iliac crest. Compress superiorly back up to the top of the back.
4. Repeat two more times, ending with your hands on the left and right upper trapezius.

> **Tip** You may also instruct your client to inhale as you apply pressure and exhale as the pressure is released as a means for the client to relax into the treatment.

Knead the Left and Right Upper Trapezius

5. Still in a lunge stance, using both hands simultaneously, knead the upper trapezius bilaterally (Figure 3-51).

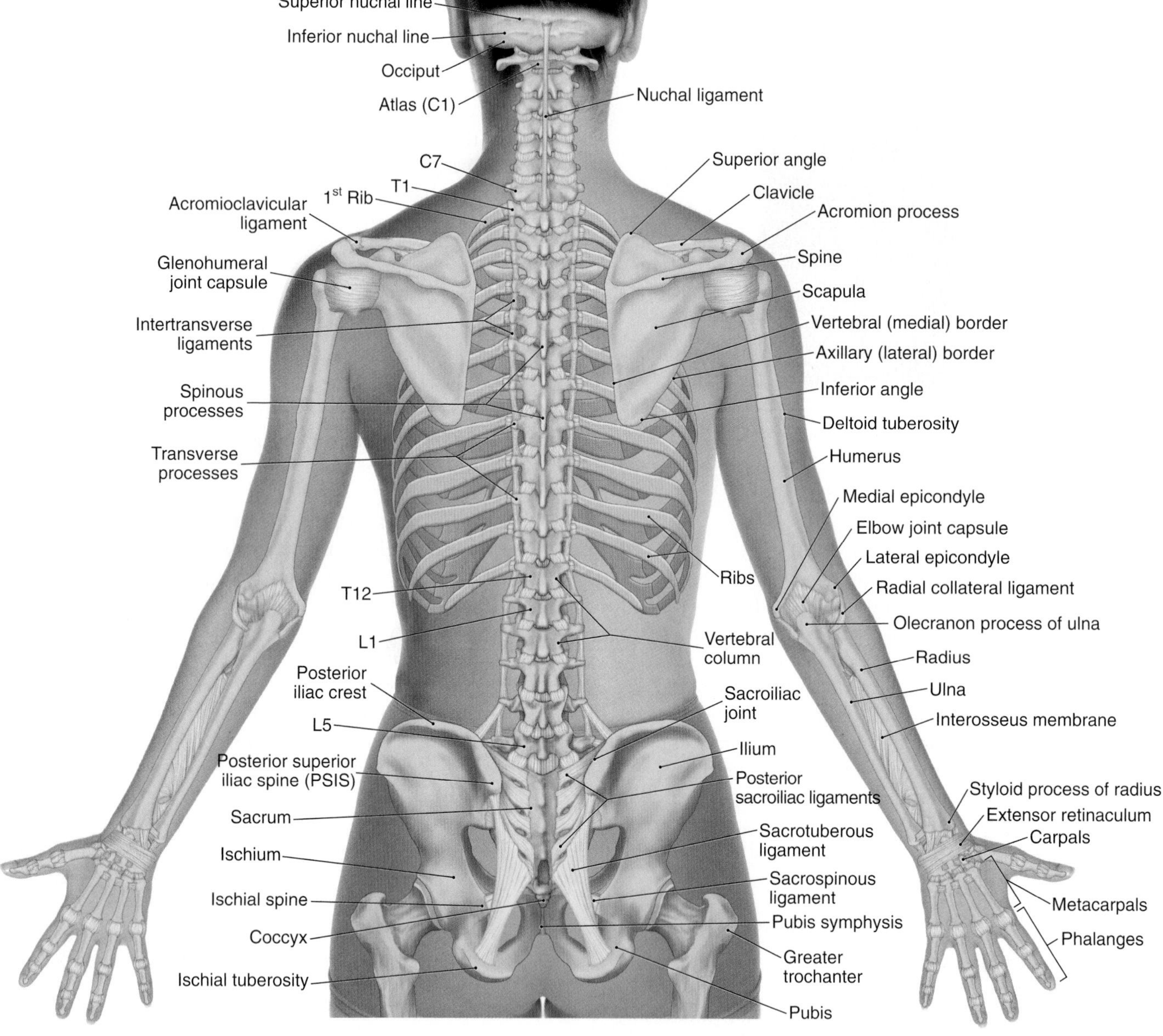

FIGURE 3-41 Bony landmarks of the posterior torso, neck, head, shoulder, arm, and hand. (Adapted from Muscolino JE: *The muscle and bone palpation manual with trigger points, referral patterns, and stretching.* St. Louis, 2009, Mosby.)

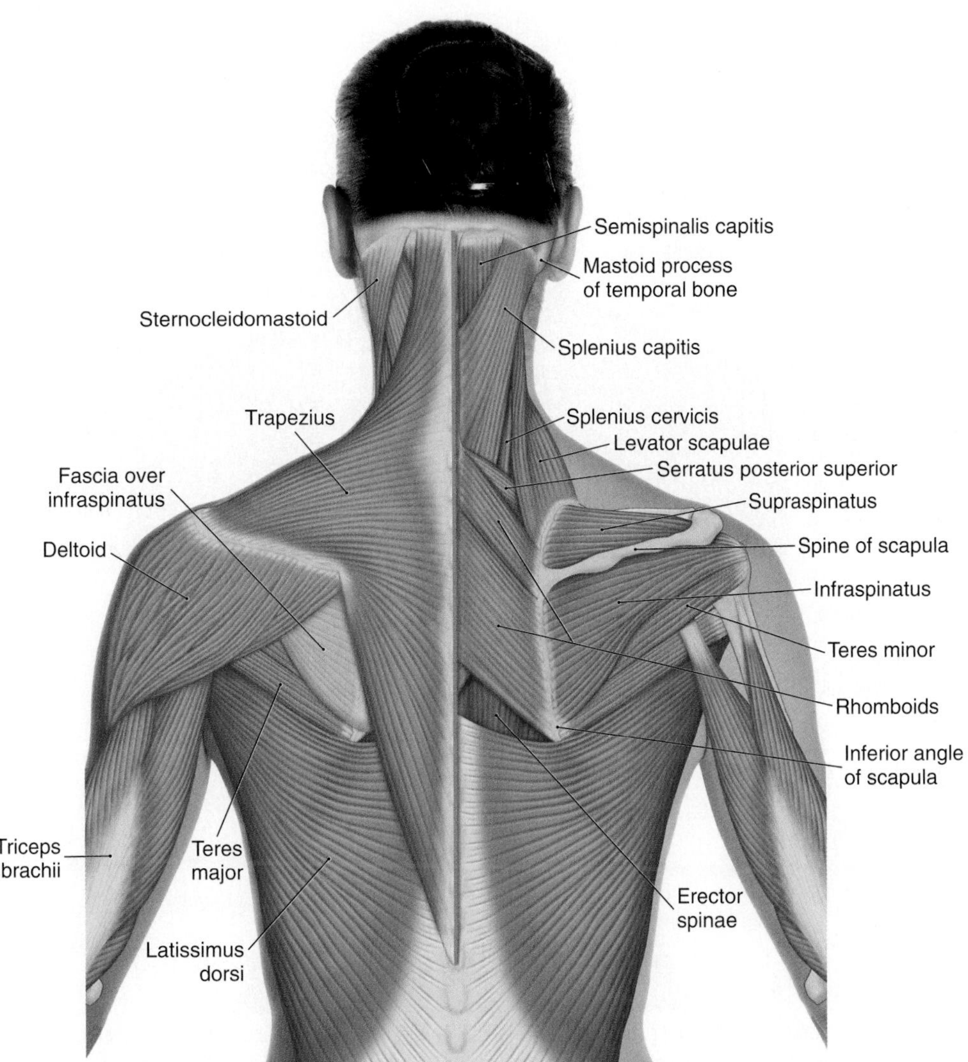

FIGURE 3-42 Muscles of the back and posterior shoulder girdle region. The left side is superficial; the right side is deep (the deltoid, trapezius, sternocleidomastoid, and infraspinatus fascia are removed). (Adapted from Muscolino JE: *The muscle and bone palpation manual, with trigger points, referral patterns, and stretching.* St. Louis, 2009, Mosby.)

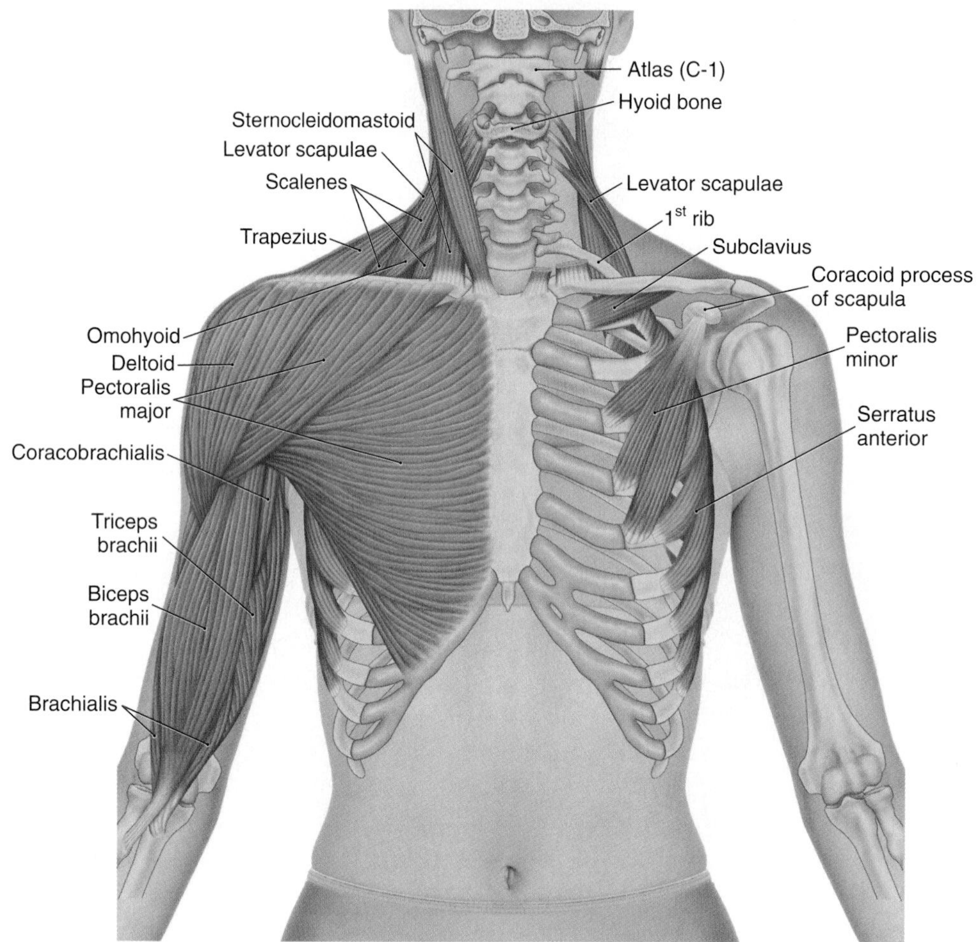

FIGURE 3-43 Muscles of an anterior view of the posterior shoulder girdle region. This view shows the anterior trapezius, anterior deltoid, biceps brachii, and part of the triceps brachii. (From Muscolino JE: *The muscle and bone palpation manual, with trigger points, referral patterns, and stretching.* St. Louis, 2009, Mosby.)

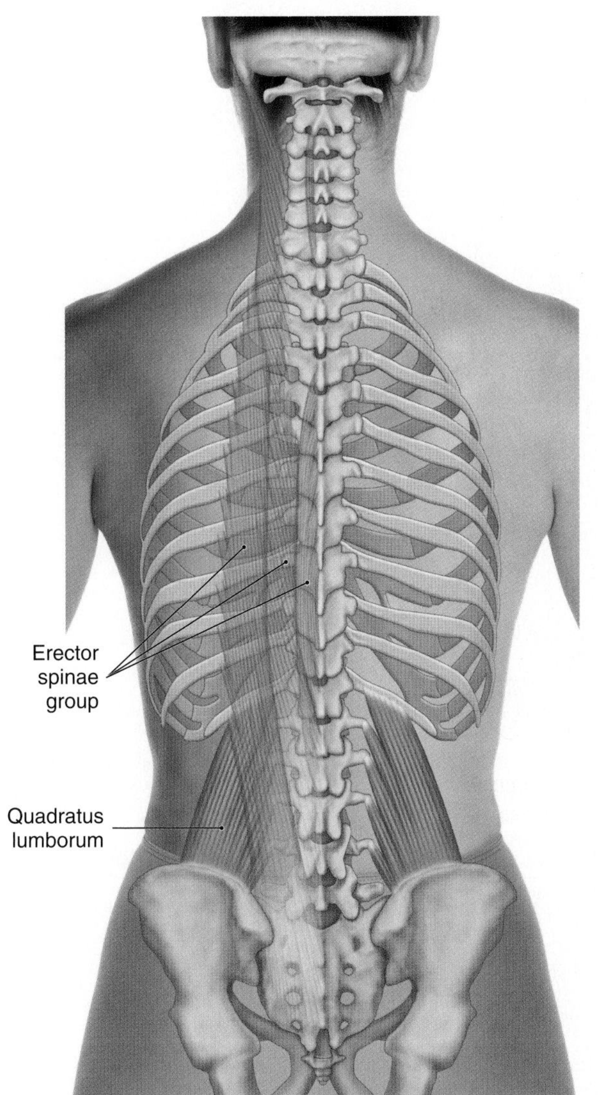

FIGURE 3-44 Erector spinae group and quadratus lumborum. (From Muscolino JE: *The muscle and bone palpation manual, with trigger points, referral patterns, and stretching.* St. Louis, 2009, Mosby.)

Forearm Press of the Left Upper Region at the Upper Trapezius

6. Move to the front of the chair and face your client in a lunge position, your right leg forward and your left leg back. Place your left hand on your client's right shoulder to stabilize the area. Place your right forearm on the upper trapezius just lateral to C-7. Press downward with your forearm in rhythmic compressions while flexing your knees and rocking forward and backward. You can also use your client's upper shoulder as a fulcrum and rock back and forth to create movement in the tissue. With each downward compression stroke, move your forearm slightly lateral until you reach the glenohumeral joint (Figure 3-52).
7. Work your way back to the starting point.
8. Repeat two more times.

> **Tip** The focus of this stroke is to address the soft muscle tissue of the upper trapezius. You do not want to press on any bones with your forearm.

Forearm Compression of the Entire Upper Left Region of the Back

9. Move to the right side of your client and resume a lunge position, this time with your left leg forward and right leg back. With your left hand, grasp the client's right deltoid to stabilize the arm. Use your right forearm to compress downward and in a circular motion on the rhomboids, supraspinatus, infraspinatus, and middle trapezius. Stay in a lunge position while rocking back and forth as you perform the technique (Figure 3-53).

This technique can also be done as a sweeping motion with your right forearm moving back and forth along the area, mimicking the motion of the windshield wipers on a car (Figure 3-54).

Deep Specific and Circular Friction on the Left Scapula

10. Move back to the right side of the client and change to a straight stance. Place one hand on top of the other with straight fingers and slightly cupped palms. With your fingertips, focus your touch downward, and use a circular motion while applying specific friction to all the posterior muscles that attach to the scapula (Figure 3-55). You can also use your thumb pads in a circular or linear direction to address the muscles in this area.

Elbow Compressions in the Rhomboids and Upper Trapezius

11. Move behind to the right side of your client, and resume the lunge stance with your left leg forward and your right leg back. To outline the rhomboids, position your left hand so that the web portion between your thumb and index finger is at the level of the inferior angle of the left scapula; your thumb touches the spinous processes of the vertebral column, and your index finger is on the medial border of the scapula (Figure 3-56 A). Using this as a guide, place your flexed right elbow in the rhomboids at the level of the inferior angle of the scapula (Figure 3-56 B). Slightly extend your elbow into the tissue as you lean forward. Continue this motion superiorly until you reach the level of the superior angle of the scapula.
12. Work your way inferiorly back down to the level of the inferior angle of the scapula.
13. Repeat two more times, then work your way back up, ending with your elbow placed at the levator scapula attachment at the superior angle of the scapula (Figure 3-56 C).

Text continued on page 90.

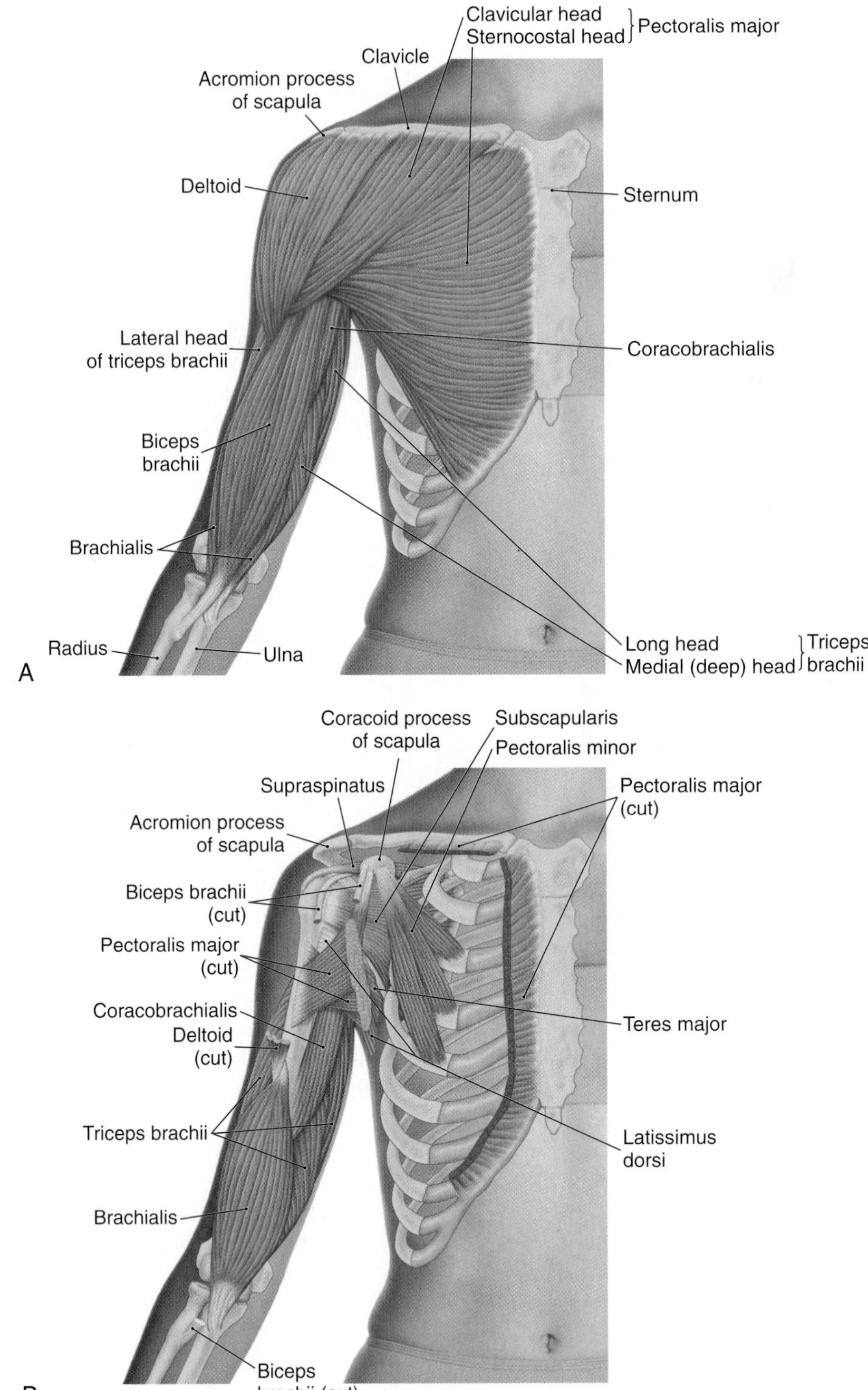

FIGURE 3-45 A, Muscles of the anterior upper arm. **B,** Muscles of the anterior upper arm with pectoralis major and deltoid cut. (From Muscolino JE: *The muscle and bone palpation manual, with trigger points, referral patterns, and stretching.* St. Louis, 2009, Mosby.)

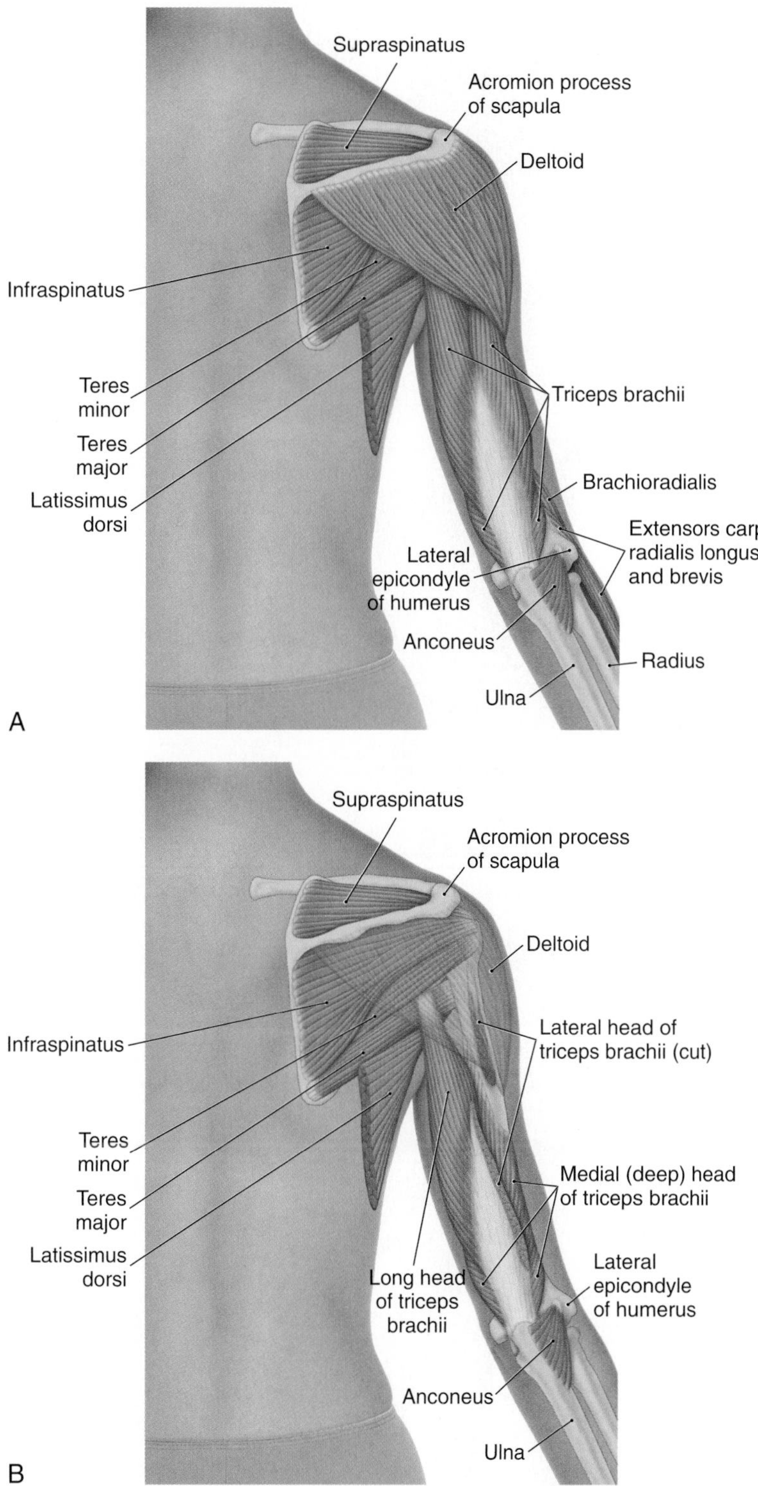

FIGURE 3-46 A, Muscles of the posterior upper arm. **B,** Muscles of the posterior upper arm with deltoid cut. (From Muscolino JE: *The muscle and bone palpation manual, with trigger points, referral patterns, and stretching.* St. Louis, 2009, Mosby.)

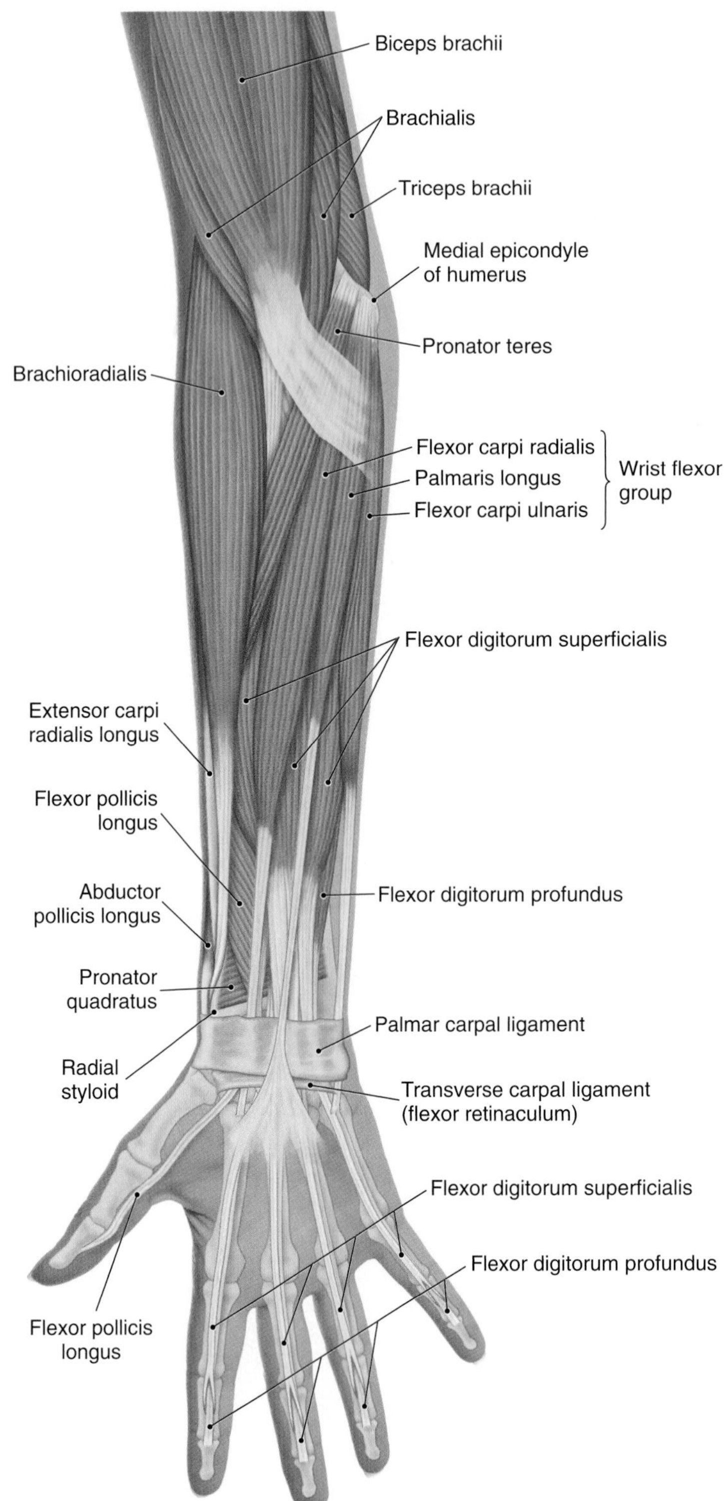

FIGURE 3-47 Muscles of the anterior forearm. (From Muscolino JE: *The muscle and bone palpation manual, with trigger points, referral patterns, and stretching*. St. Louis, 2009, Mosby.)

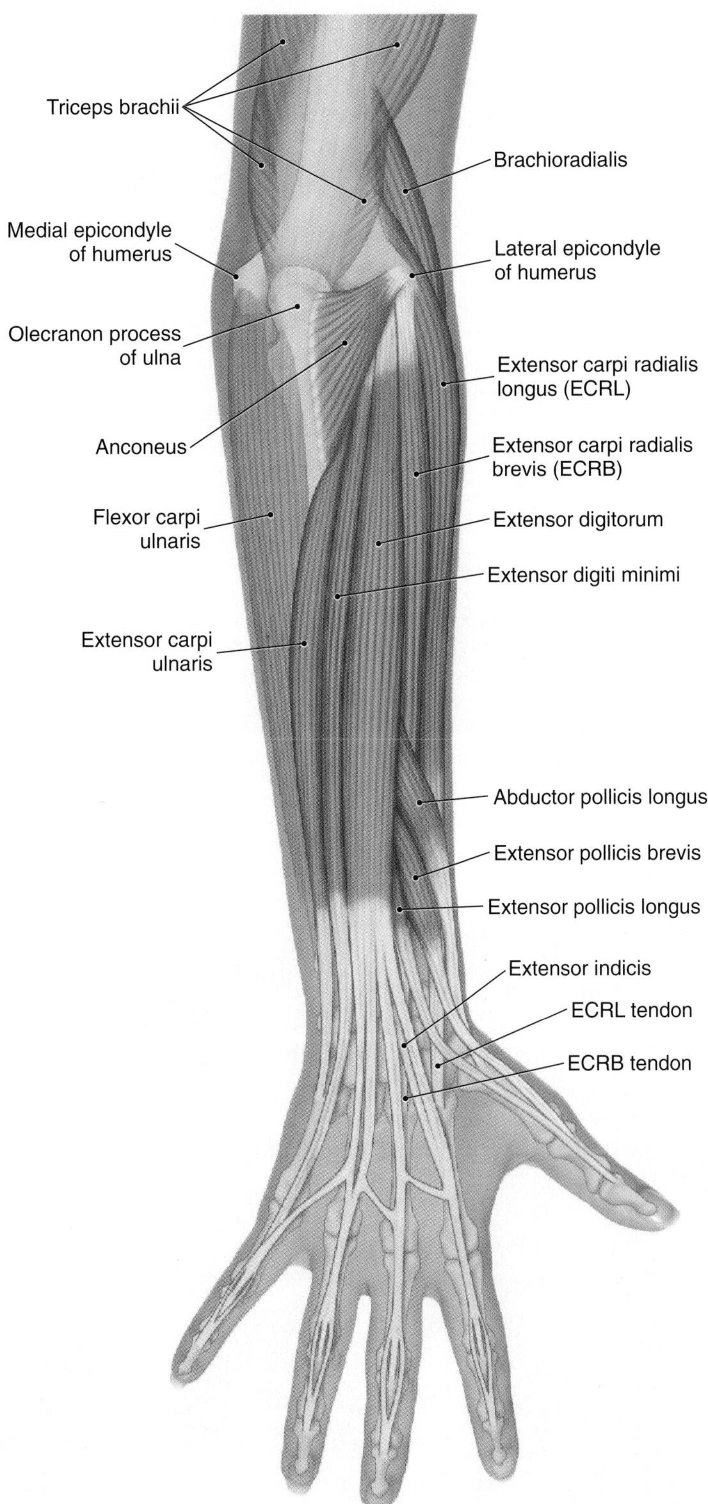

FIGURE 3-48 Muscles of the posterior forearm. (From Muscolino JE: *The muscle and bone palpation manual, with trigger points, referral patterns, and stretching.* St. Louis, 2009, Mosby.)

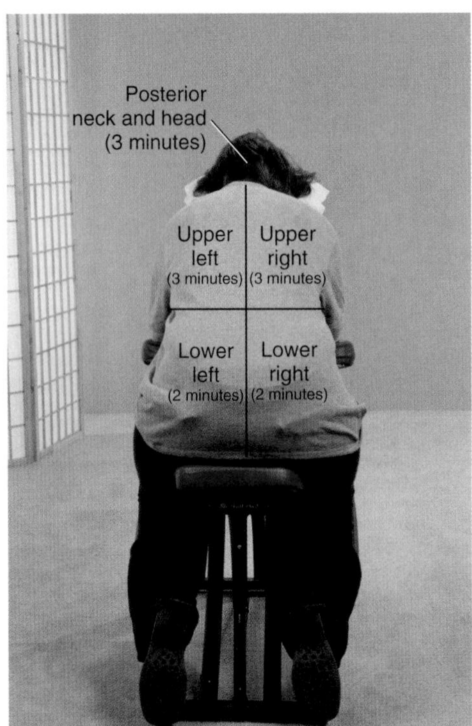

FIGURE 3-49 Posterior torso head and neck divided into five regions.

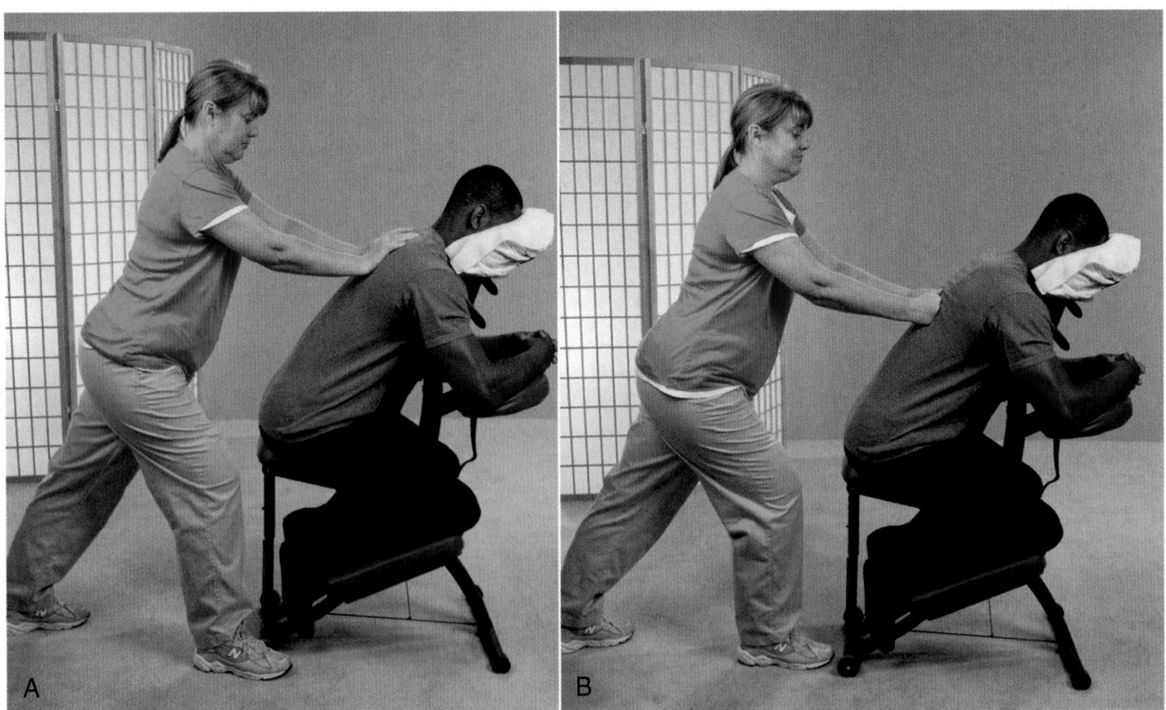

FIGURE 3-50 **A,** Apply compressions down the erector spinae starting at T-1. **B,** At T-6, apply compressions with the backs of the hands in soft fists.

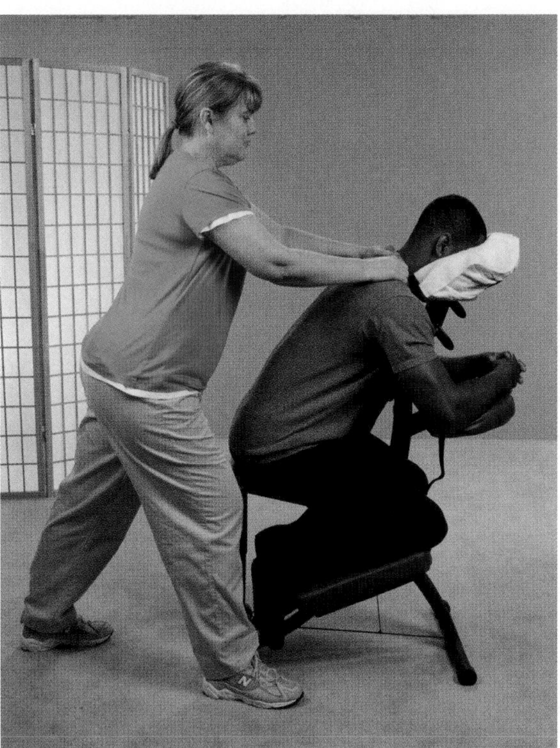

FIGURE 3-51 Knead both upper trapezius muscles simultaneously.

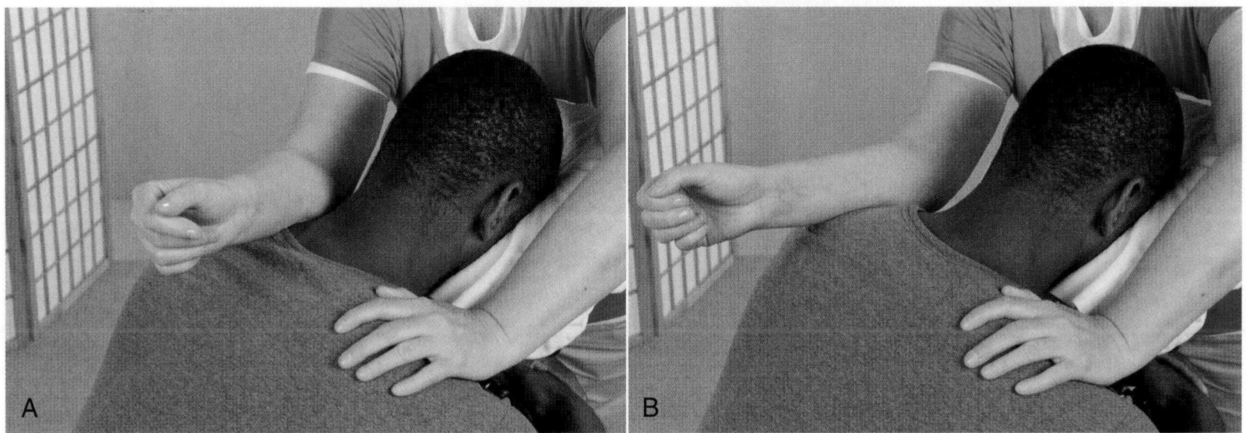

FIGURE 3-52 Forearm press on the upper trapezius starting just lateral to C-7 **(A)** and just medial to the glenohumeral joint **(B).**

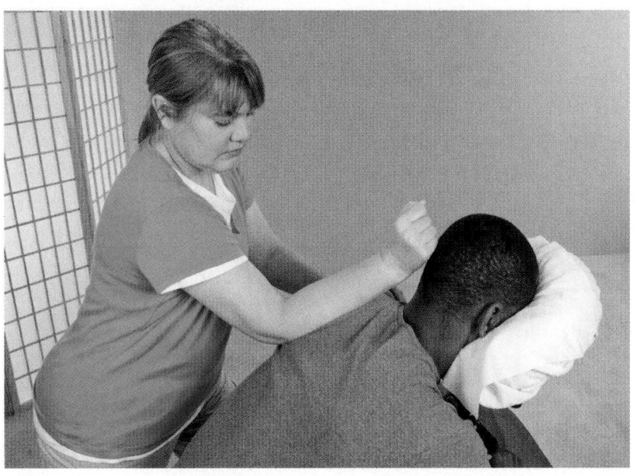

FIGURE 3-53 Forearm compression downward and in a circular motion on the rhomboids and infraspinatus.

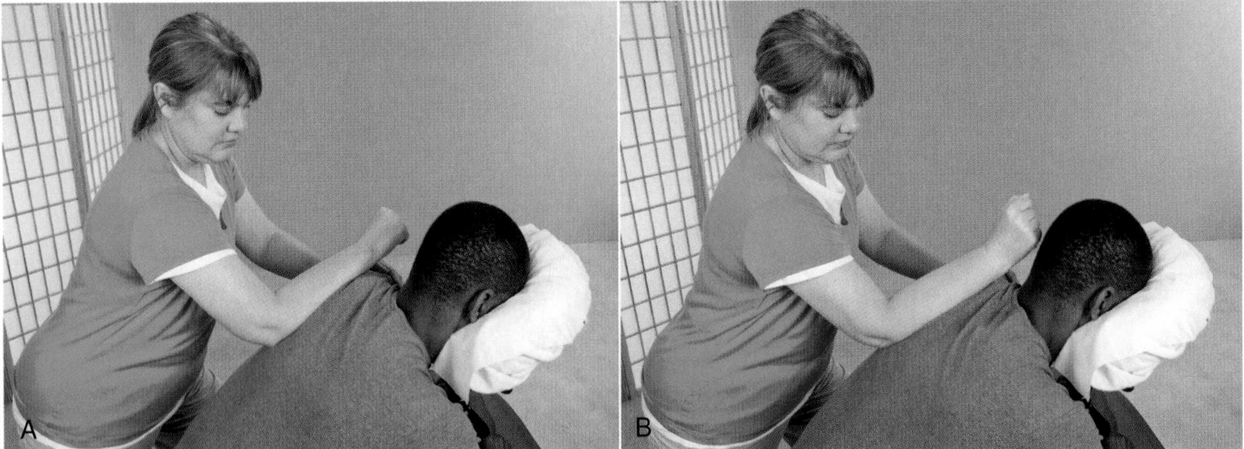

FIGURE 3-54 Sweeping motion of the forearm back **(A)** and forth **(B)** on the area.

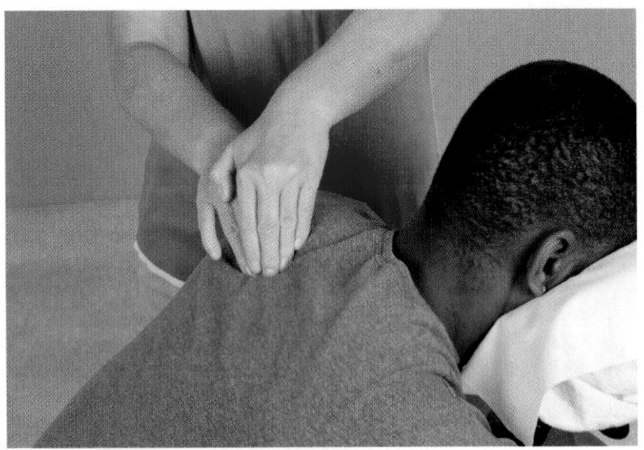
FIGURE 3-55 Deep specific and circular friction with the fingertips on posterior muscles that attach to the scapula.

14. Use your elbow on the upper trapezius by keeping your elbow flexed and compressing downward into the tissue. Move laterally, then back medially, working the entire width of the upper trapezius (Figure 3-57).
15. Repeat two more times.

> **Tip** Pressure from this stroke can be increased by placing more of your weight on the front foot as you lean forward. The heel of your back foot will lift up when the lunge is complete (Figure 3-58). You can modify the elbow work by adding a small circular movement with the elbow as the pressure is applied.

16. Apply elbow pressure and circles into the infraspinatus (Figure 3-59).
17. Once the elbow work has been completed, use kneading and compression on the area to close.

Working the Arm and Hand

17. Move to the left front of your client, and resume a lunge position with your left leg forward and your right leg back. Pick up your client's arm from the armrest so that the elbow is extended with fingers pointing to the ground. Grasp the upper arm with both of your hands just below the axillary fold (Figure 3-60). Pull the arm slightly laterally (so that the client's hand does not hit the knee pads of the massage chair), and gently vibrate the arm by rolling the upper arm between both of your hands (Figure 3-61).
18. After a few rolls, bring both of your hands back to the starting position. Place your thumbs side by side as you use both hands to do compressions from the deltoid to the wrist (Figure 3-62 A). It may be easier to kneel on your right knee for this technique (Figure 3-62 B).
19. Repeat two more times.
20. If you are kneeling on your right knee, stand up while holding the client's hand. Resume the lunge position with your left leg forward and your right leg back as you turn the client's hand palm side down. Grasp it with both of your hands, and apply pressure downward and outward to spread the metacarpals apart (Figure 3-63).
21. Repeat two more times.
22. Hold your client's hand with your left hand. Starting with your client's thumb, use the thumb and index finger of your right hand and knead the length of each digit, ending each one with a small shake (Figure 3-64).
23. Turn the client's hand so it is palm up. Use both of your thumb pads to glide over the entire surface of the palm with a slight downward pressure (Figure 3-65).
24. Shake the arm again with the same rolling motion as in Step 17, then place it back on the armrest. Stand behind your client and simultaneously knead the left and the right upper trapezius bilaterally.

Working the Client's Right Upper Region and Arm

25. Move to the client's right side, and repeat Steps 6 through 24.

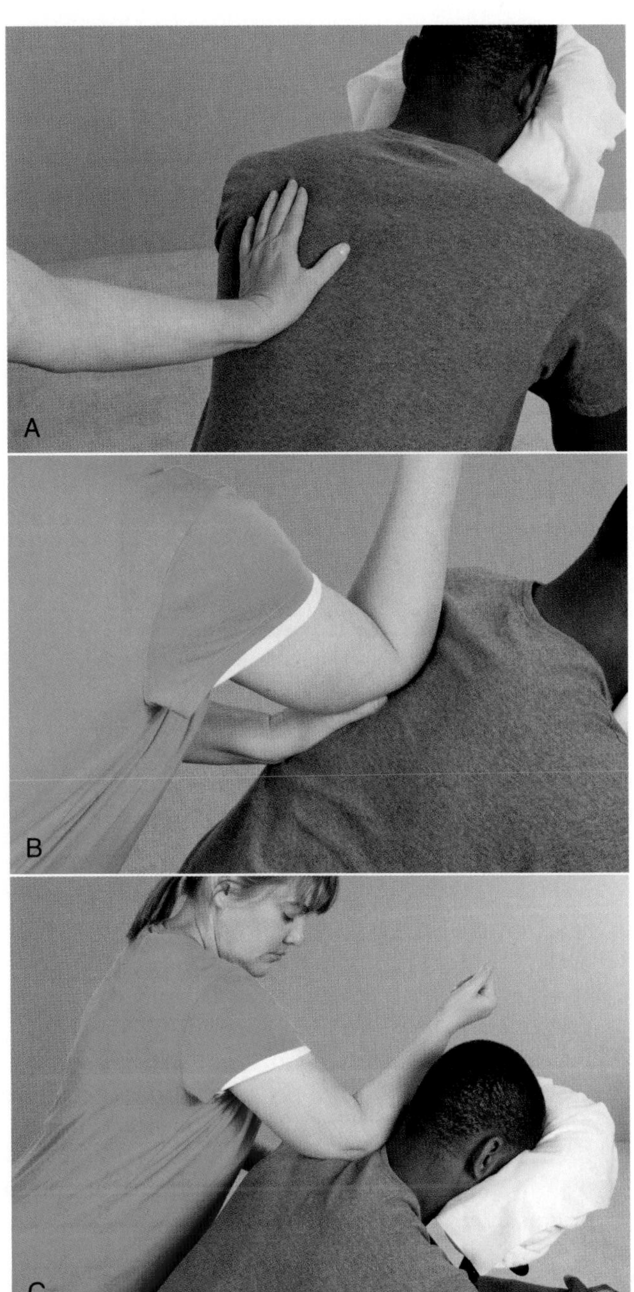

FIGURE 3-56 **A,** Positioning of left hand on the inferior angle of the scapula. **B,** Using this as a guide, place your flexed right elbow in the rhomboids at the level of the inferior angle of the scapula. **C,** Elbow placed at the levator scapula attachment at the superior angle of the scapula.

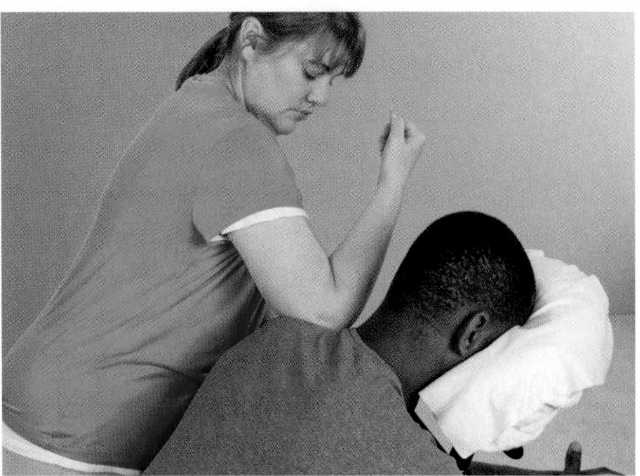

FIGURE 3-57 Using elbow on the upper trapezius starting medially.

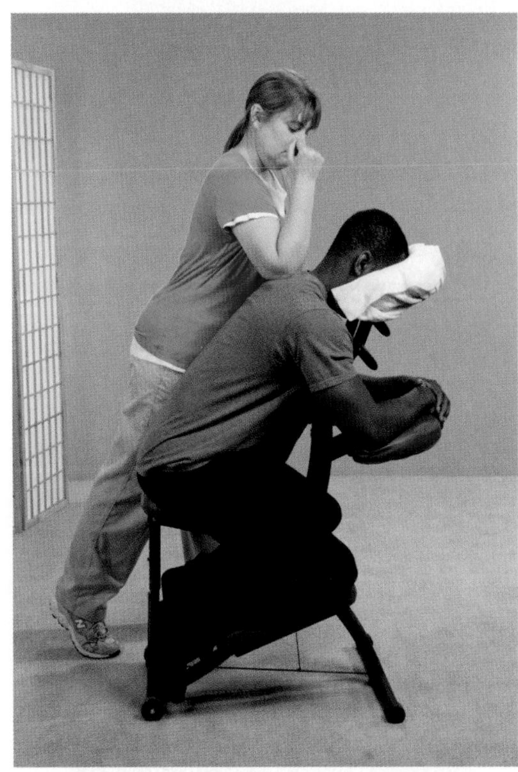

FIGURE 3-58 Increasing pressure by leaning forward onto the front foot.

Compressions of the Lower Regions

26. Stand behind your client in a lunge position with your left leg forward and your right leg back. With your hands in soft fists, thumbs on top of the fists, place each hand on the erector spinae group on either side of the spine just below the level of T-6 (Figure 3-66). Lean forward and, with neutral wrists, apply compressions on the erector spinae muscle group, remembering to use your body weight, rocking back and forth, and coordinating your breath. Continue compressing inferiorly until you reach the iliac crest. Compress superiorly back up to the level of T-6.
27. Repeat two more times.

Working the Client's Right Lower Region

28. Move slightly to the client's right, still in a lunge. Place one hand on top of the other, keeping your fingers braced and slightly curved. Use deep gliding strokes

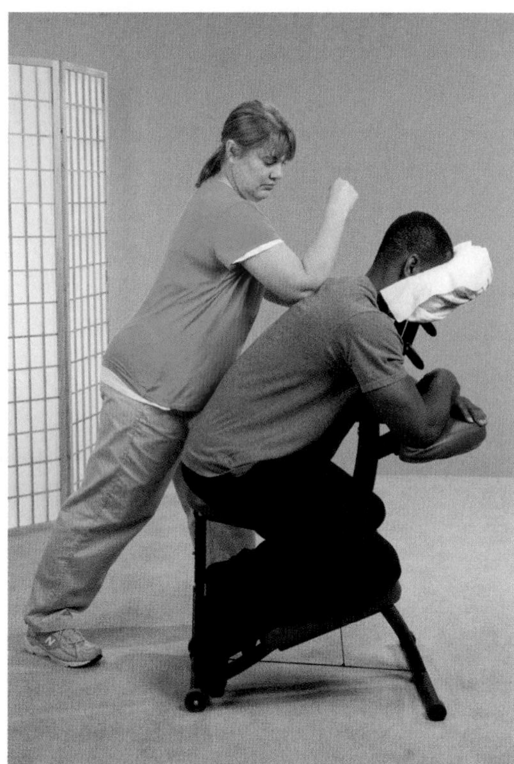

FIGURE 3-59 Apply elbow pressure and circles into the infraspinatus.

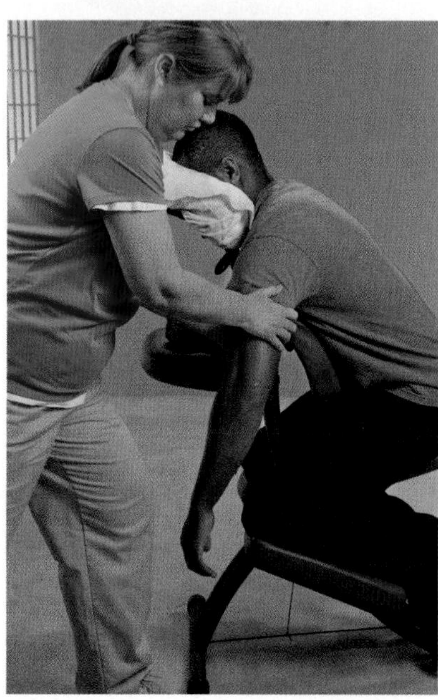

FIGURE 3-60 Grasp the upper arm with both hands.

with your fingertips, placing one hand on top of the other if needing to apply more pressure, to work the right erector spinae group from the level of T-6 down to the iliac crest (Figure 3-67). Follow this movement with circular friction on the erector spinae from the level of T-6 down to the iliac crest (Figure 3-68). Remember to keep your back straight, using the large

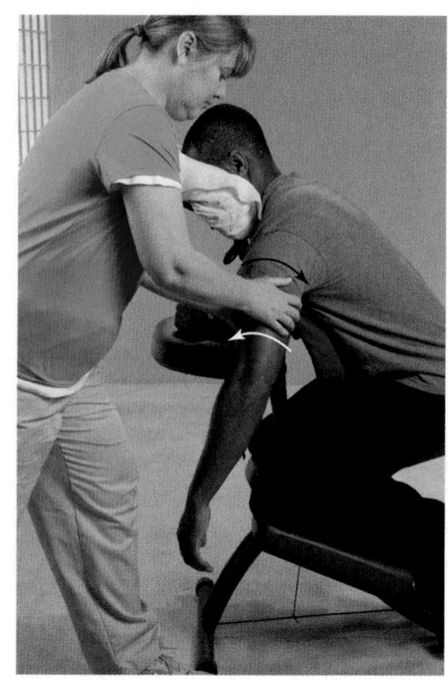

FIGURE 3-61 Roll the humerus between both hands.

muscles of your legs as you rise, and sink down while your hands move along the erector spinae group.

29. Repeat two more times.
30. When you reach the iliac crest for the third time, make both of your hands into soft fists. Knead the muscle attachments along the iliac crest laterally toward the greater trochanter, then back medially (Figure 3-69).
31. Repeat two more times.
32. Continue kneading into the gluteal region (Figure 3-70). Keep the pace rhythmic and consistent.
33. Complete the region by returning back up to the level of T-6 and bilaterally compress both erector spinae groups inferiorly to the iliac crests.

Working the Client's Left Lower Region

34. Repeat Steps 26 through 33 on the client's left side.

Brush Strokes for Connection

35. Once you have finished all four regions of the back, use a series of brush strokes to provide a sense of connection for the entire back. Start superiorly and continue inferiorly until you have brushed the entire back (Figure 3-71).

Neck and Scalp

36. Move to a straight stance at the left of the client, and use both hands to knead the posterior neck muscles (Figure 3-72). Use your right thumb to perform friction along the occipital ridge. Start laterally at the mastoid process and move medially to the center of the neck (Figure 3-73).

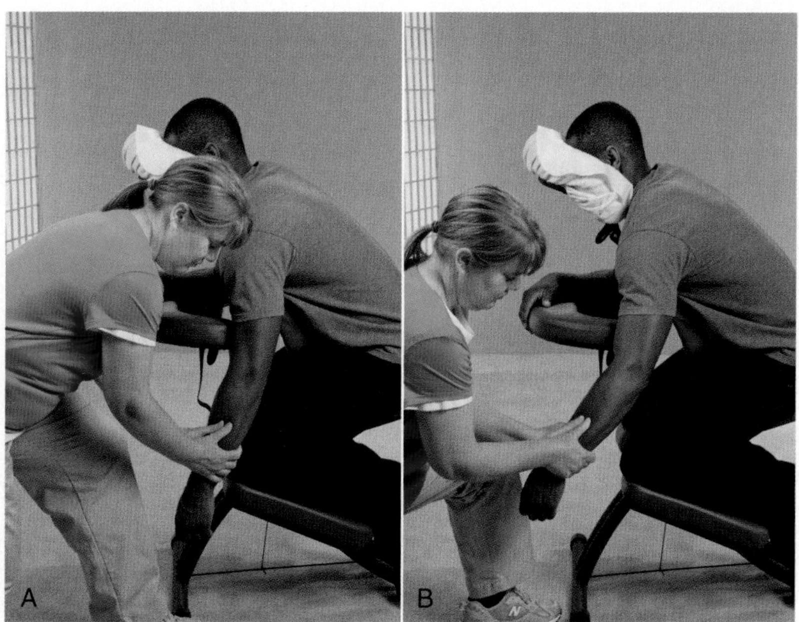

FIGURE 3-62 **A,** Thumbs side by side to do compressions from the deltoid to the wrist. **B,** Kneeling position while doing compressions down the arm.

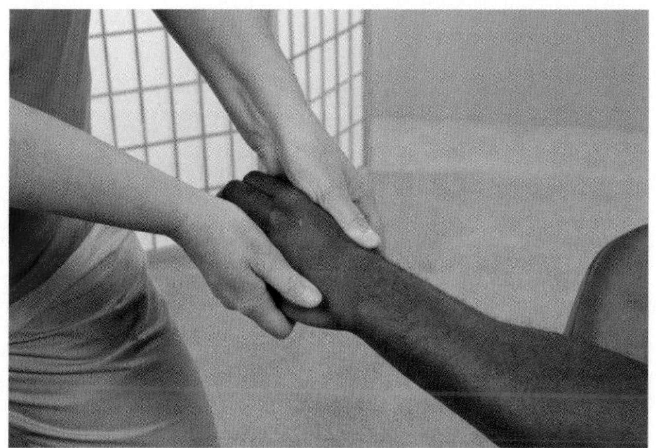

FIGURE 3-63 Spreading the metacarpals.

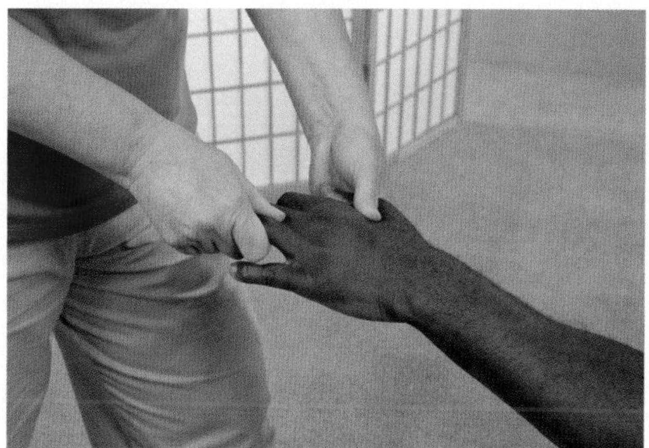

FIGURE 3-64 Knead each of the fingers.

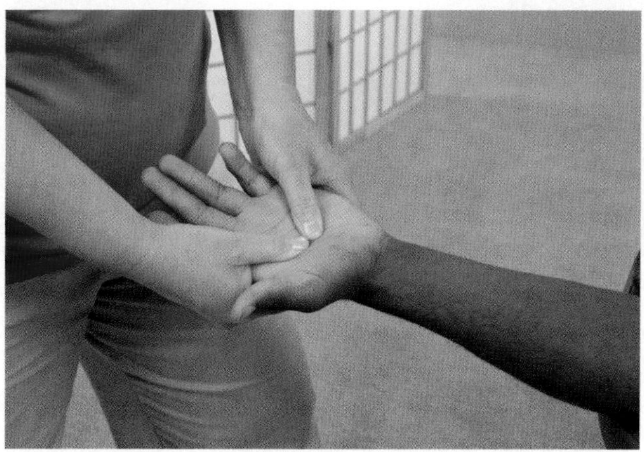

FIGURE 3-65 Thumb pad glides over the entire surface of the palm.

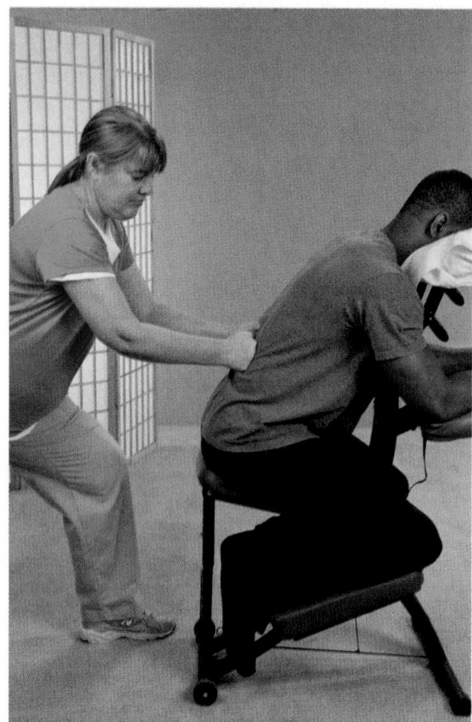

FIGURE 3-66 Compress the erector spinae from T-6 down to the iliac crest.

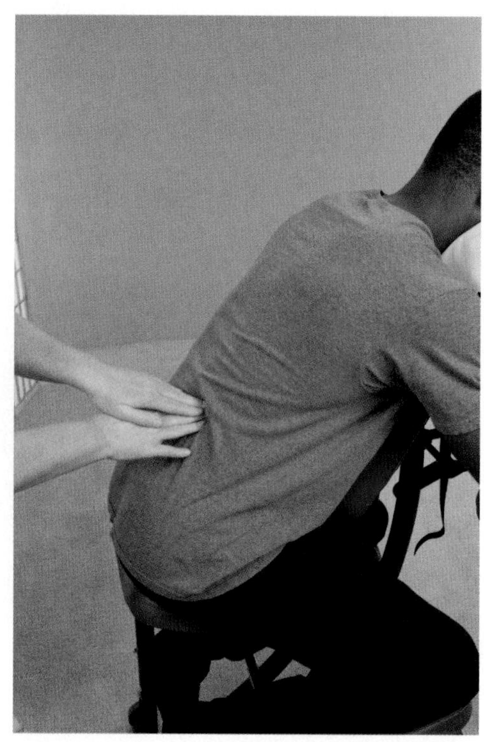

FIGURE 3-67 Deep gliding strokes with one hand on top of the other.

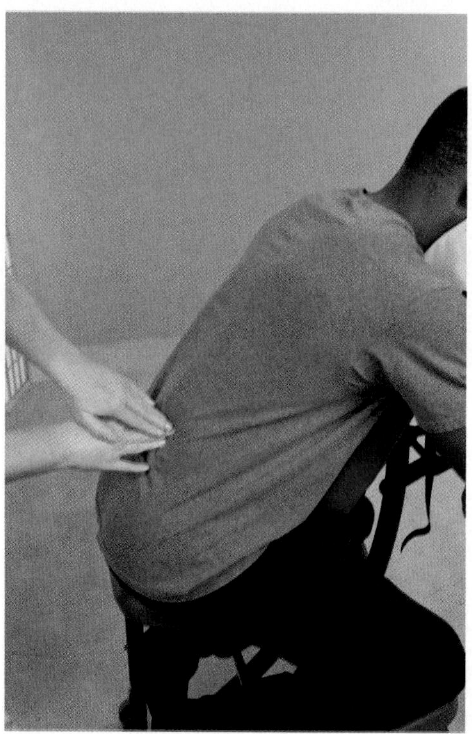

FIGURE 3-68 Circular friction.

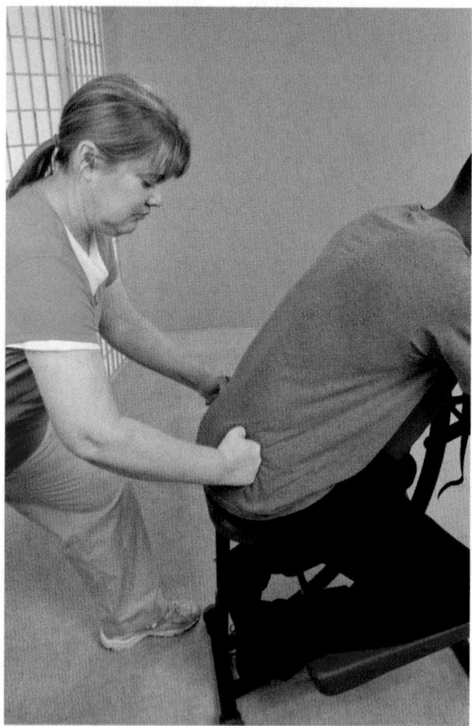

FIGURE 3-69 Knead the muscle attachments along the crest starting at the sacrum and moving laterally.

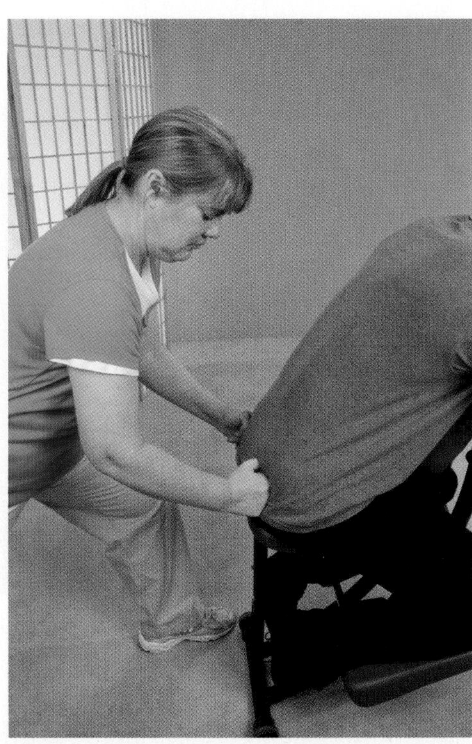

FIGURE 3-70 Continue the kneading strokes into the gluteal region.

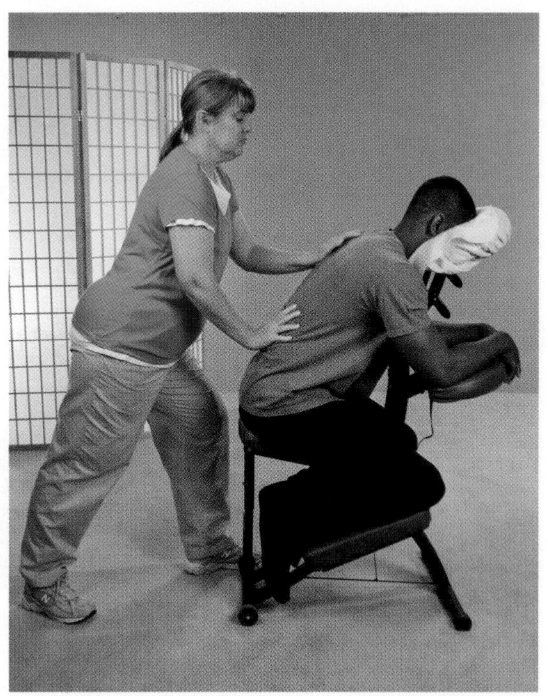

FIGURE 3-71 Brush strokes starting superiorly and continuing inferiorly to connect the entire back.

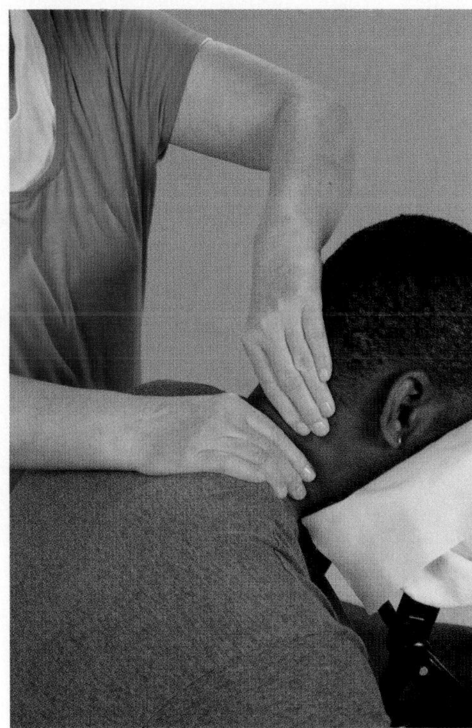

FIGURE 3-72 Knead the posterior neck muscles.

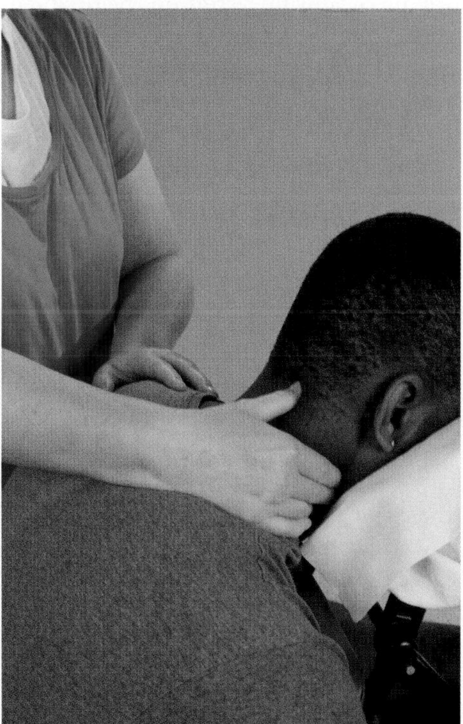

FIGURE 3-73 Circular friction on the suboccipitals.

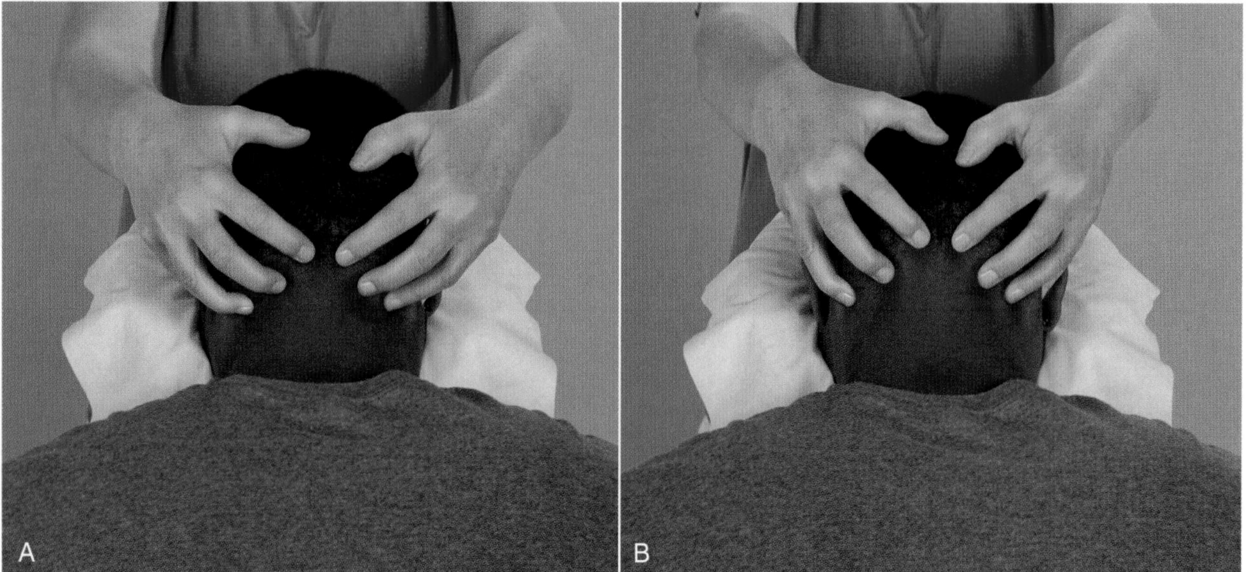

FIGURE 3-74 Fingertips at the occipital ridge and small circular friction along the entire occipital ridge **(A)** and followed by a slight lift upward to stretch the neck **(B).**

37. Move to the right side of the client and repeat Step 36, using your left hand to provide the strokes.
38. Move to front of the chair and face your client in a straight stance. With the fingers of both your hands cupped, place your fingertips on the occipital ridge of the client's skull where the muscles attach. Provide small circular friction along the entire occipital ridge (Figure 3-74 A). Follow this with a slight lift upward to stretch the posterior neck (Figure 3-74 B).
39. Continue by massaging the client's entire scalp (with client consent, of course), using circular motions with your fingertips. Make sure to not pull on the hair.

Closing the Treatment

40. Move back behind the chair, and stand in a lunge with your left leg forward and right leg back. Perform brush strokes followed by percussion on the client's entire back (Figure 3-75).

Assisting the Client off the Chair

41. Ask the client to sit up straight; be sure to hold on to the face cradle cover so that it does not stick to the client's face (Figure 3-76). Check to see if the client is feeling dizzy or light-headed. If so, have the client sit for a moment until it passes.
42. When the client is ready, have the client place both feet on the floor. Place your left hand on the chair to prevent it from falling over, and with your right hand placed gently on the client's back, guide him or her out of the chair (Figure 3-77).
43. Once the client is off the chair, conduct a brief post-treatment feedback session, offer water (if available), and thank the client for the opportunity to work together.

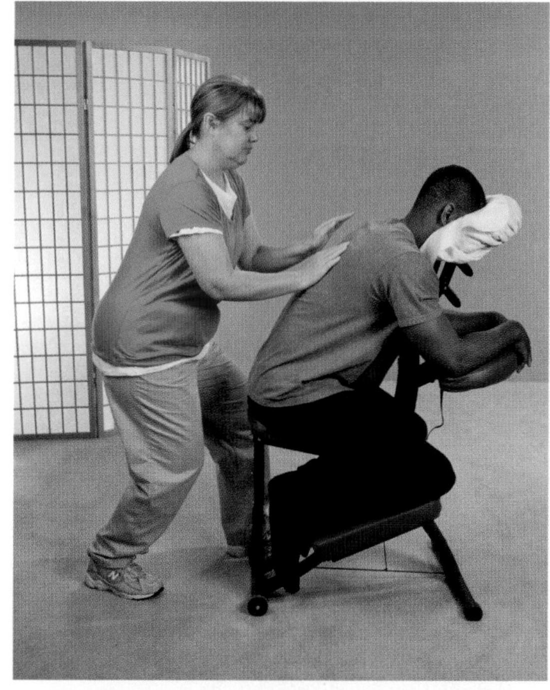

FIGURE 3-75 Percussion strokes on the back.

VASOVAGAL SYNCOPE

As mentioned at the end of the basic sequence, clients may feel some dizziness or light-headedness at the end of a treatment. This can happen if clients have not had much to eat or have not drunk enough water before receiving the treatment. The most common reason is decreased blood flow to the brain. The client may have become so relaxed that his

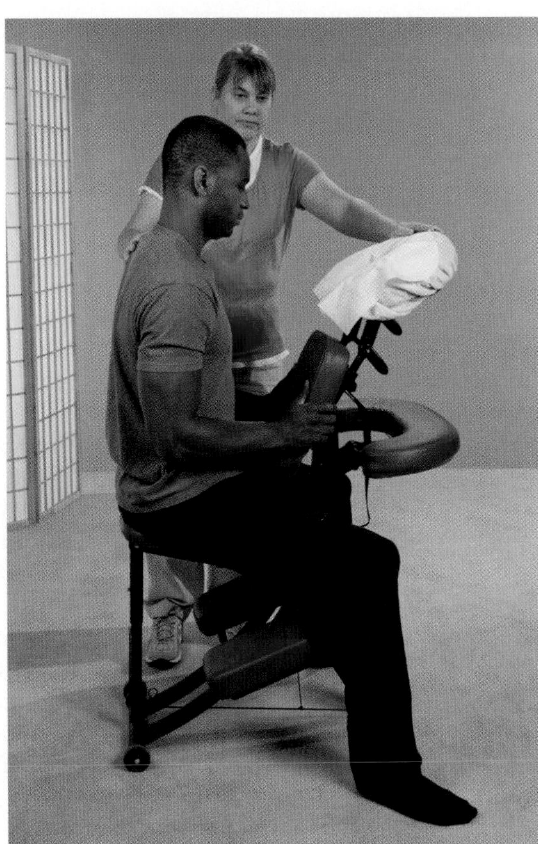

FIGURE 3-76 Holding onto the face cradle cover so that it does not stick to the client's face.

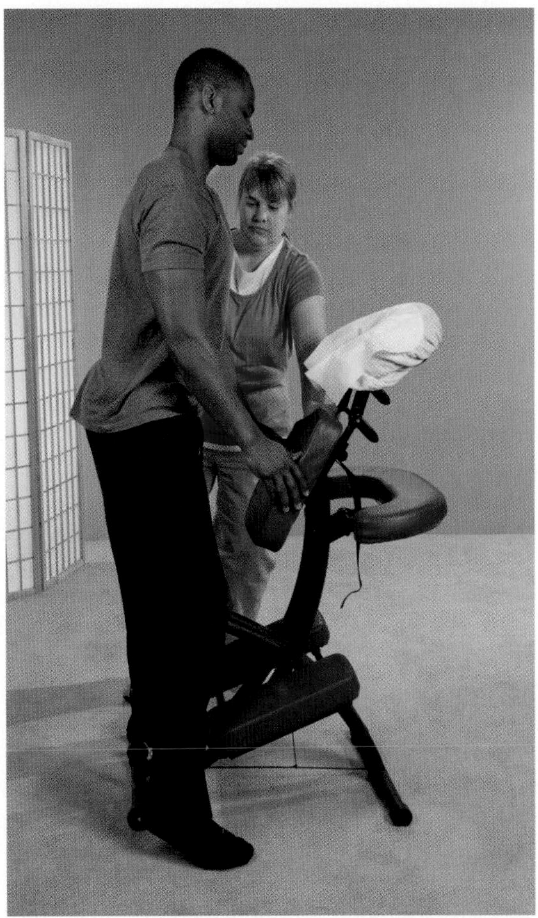

FIGURE 3-77 Placing one hand on the chair to prevent it from falling over while placing the other hand on the client's back to guide him or her out of the chair.

or her heart rate slowed down, resulting in decreased pressure of the blood flowing to the client's brain. It may take a few moments for the dizziness to pass. If the client is dehydrated, his or her blood volume could be lowered, which can also lead to a decrease in blood pressure to the brain. This is one of the reasons why it is helpful to offer clients water after the treatment.

Some chair massage clients, though, may experience a condition more serious than slight dizziness, called syncope. **Syncope**, or fainting, is defined as a sudden, temporary loss of consciousness (not the result of head trauma), followed by spontaneous recovery. It is most commonly caused by a lack of sufficient blood flow to the brain. **Vasovagal syncope** is a more descriptive term for this event, because the vagus nerve is involved ("vagal") and so is blood in blood vessels ("vaso").

The vagus nerve is the major parasympathetic nerve in the body, innervating 70% to 80% of the internal organs, including the heart. Nerve impulses from the vagus nerve keep the heart rate slowed to whatever a person's resting heart rate is. With increased activity, the nerve impulses along the vagus nerve are inhibited, and heart rate increases. An example of this occurs when a person stands up from sitting or lying down. When standing up, heart rate increases slightly to increase blood pressure to the brain (and to the rest of the body) in response to increased activity.

Sometimes, though, the impulses along the vagus nerve are not inhibited quickly enough, and the heart does not increase its rate, resulting in an excessive decrease in blood pressure to the brain. Or if the knees have been locked, such as in the kneeling required for sitting on a massage chair, blood flow back to the heart can slow. Then, upon standing up, less blood volume is available than is needed to be pumped by the heart to the brain. This also results in decreased blood pressure to the brain. The outcome is a feeling of light-headedness (sometimes known as a "head rush") or fainting.

Before losing consciousness, the person may experience the following:

- Light-headedness
- Nausea, sometimes to the point of vomiting
- Sweating
- Ringing in the ears
- An uncomfortable feeling in the heart
- Weakness
- Visual disturbances

These symptoms may last for at least a few seconds before consciousness is lost. If the client displays any of these symptoms, the practitioner should remain calm and professional. If the client was standing, the practitioner should make sure the client does not fall and become injured. The practitioner should help the client sit or lie down, if it is safe to do so. The client's feet should be raised if at all possible. By lying down or sitting with the feet raised, the client's effective blood flow to the brain will be restored, and, if the client has passed out, he or she should wake up in a few moments. After waking, is likely that the client will be nauseated, pale, and sweaty for a while longer. If the client tries to sit or stand up too soon, the symptoms may recur, and the client may even pass out again.

The client may require medical attention, so practitioners should be prepared to contact the business's medical services (if available) or call 9-1-1 if necessary. If providing seated massage treatments at an athletic event, practitioners should make sure they are aware of where the first-aid area is located before setting up their treatment space in case they need to direct a client there for help. Ideally, the practitioner should also have a contact phone number for first-aid staff in case someone needs to come to the treatment area to assist a client.

The clients most susceptible to vasovagal syncope are the elderly, those with heart conditions, frail clients, and prenatal clients. The elderly are more likely to have heart conditions or low blood pressure and are at an increased risk for dehydration. Frail clients may also have low blood pressure to begin with, or they may have other conditions that make them subject to low blood pressure. Prenatal clients have an increased blood volume, which is needed to nourish the developing infant. This increased blood volume can tax the heart, making the client more susceptible to a vasovagal episode.

SUMMARY

The application of seated massage techniques needs to be accompanied by efficient practitioner postures and stances—in short, proper body mechanics. These reduce the possibility of injury to the practitioner and to the client, as well as increase the effectiveness of the techniques. The three key elements to appropriate body mechanics are keeping the back straight, using larger muscles to do the work, and remembering to breathe.

The stances used to perform seated massage include lunge, straight, and kneeling. Practitioners may also choose to use a stool while working. The basic techniques used are compressions, palming, thumb and finger pressure, deep gliding, kneading, friction, forearm work, elbow work, vibration, brush strokes, and percussion. Practitioners also need to be aware of cautionary sites on the body that may require changes in treatment approach or avoidance all together.

There are several considerations for working on clothed clients that practitioners need to keep in mind, such as the fabric of the client's clothing and accessories and items the clients may have in their pockets. The practitioner may need to ask the client to remove certain pieces of clothing and items; if the client is unwilling or unable to do so, the practitioner may have to adapt the treatment to the circumstances.

Because performing seated massage is a physical activity, practitioners need to do warm-ups and stretches for their ankles, legs, back, shoulders, arms, and neck. Practitioners should also conduct a pretreatment interview with the client that includes the client's health history; whether or not the client has received any type of bodywork before, including chair massage; if the client is experiencing any areas of pain, discomfort, or muscle tightness; the goals for the treatment; and what the client will be doing after the treatment.

To assist practitioners in making the techniques and movements of chair massage automatic, a basic sequence is provided as a focus for practice. The sequence involves dividing the client's body into five regions and spending specified amounts of time performing certain techniques in each region. Practitioners are encouraged to practice this sequence until they feel comfortable that doing it is second nature.

Some clients experience vasovagal syncope at the end of a seated massage treatment. Practitioners should watch for signs of light-headedness, nausea (sometimes to the point of vomiting), sweating, ringing in the ears, an uncomfortable feeling in the heart, weakness, and visual disturbances. If these occur, the practitioner should remain calm and make sure the client sits until the symptoms pass. If the client has stood up, then the practitioner should have the client lie down and raise his or her feet. The practitioner should also be prepared to call for medical attention if necessary.

STUDY QUESTIONS

Answers to Study Questions are located on page 227.

Multiple Choice

1. In what type of stance is one foot in front of the other, with the toes of both feet facing forward, and the hips facing the same direction as the feet?
   a. Straight
   b. Lunge
   c. Kneeling
   d. Horse

2. Where is the practitioner's source of strength in the lunge stance?
   a. Shoulder muscles
   b. Locked elbows
   c. Rear leg
   d. Flexed knee

3. What is it called when the ulnar sides of both hands strike alternately up and down on the client's body?
   a. Hacking
   b. Vibration
   c. Palming
   d. Friction

4. Which of the following is an appropriate question for the practitioner to ask the client in the pretreatment interview?
   a. Do you have a history of any medical conditions?
   b. Have you received chair massage before?
   c. Where are your areas of pain and discomfort?
   d. All of the above

5. Which of the following is a cautionary site on the body?
   a. Deltoid muscles
   b. Kidney area
   c. Quadriceps femoris muscles
   d. Mid-back area

Fill in the Blank

1. The three most important components of proper body mechanics for performing chair massage are to keep the back ____________________, use ____________________ muscles to do the work, and remember to ____________________.

2. Because pressure should be applied in a way to minimize the compressive force on the shoulder and arm joints, it should pass ____________________ ____________________ the joint, not at a(n) ____________________.

3. The compression stroke is performed by placing one or both palms of the hand on the soft muscle tissue and pumping at a(n) ____________________ angle into the tissue.

4. The two types of friction are ____________________ and ____.

5. Areas of the body in which there is little tissue protection of nerves, blood vessels, and body projections, making them subject to damage and pain when massage techniques are applied, are called ____.

Short Answer

1. Compare and contrast the proper body mechanics for chair massage and table massage.

____

____

____

____

____

STUDY QUESTIONS

2. Explain the palpation considerations for working on a clothed client.

3. Describe the ways vibration can be used during a chair massage treatment.

4. List and describe cautionary sites on the body and the appropriate technique approach to each of these areas.

5. Explain the causes, symptoms, and appropriate practitioner response to a client who is experiencing vasovagal syncope.

ACTIVITIES

1. Have someone, such as another student of chair massage or a practitioner learning chair massage, put on a white T-shirt and sit in the massage chair. Palpate the bony landmarks that can be felt on the back and shoulders. Use a washable marker to draw the bony landmarks on the shirt. Use a different color of washable marker to draw the muscles in the basic sequence.

2. Write your own script for greeting a client who is new to seated massage and explaining the procedures.

3. Practice the basic routine on at least 10 people such as friends and family. Work on people with various body sizes and shapes. Keep track of the time to ensure that you spend the appropriate amount of time in each body section of the basic routine.

Enhancing Treatment Sessions

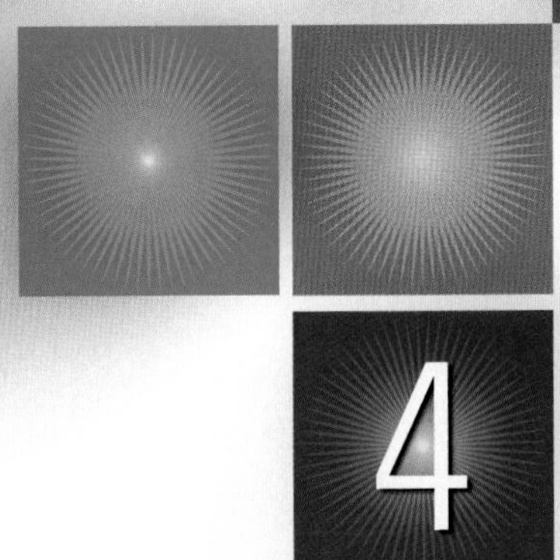

OBJECTIVES

Upon completion of this chapter, the reader will have the information necessary to do the following:

1. Define repetitive stress injuries (RSIs).
2. Describe the symptoms and causes of, and treatments and massage considerations for, adhesive capsulitis, carpal tunnel syndrome, disk herniation, tendinitis and tenosynovitis, lateral epicondylitis, medial epicondylitis, muscle strain, sprain, tension headache, and thoracic outlet syndrome.
3. Describe the location, attachment sites, and kinesiology of the muscles addressed in the upper region of the posterior body.
4. Perform techniques to address the upper region of the posterior body, including key tsubos.
5. Describe the location, attachment sites, and kinesiology of the muscles addressed in the mid- and low back.
6. Perform techniques to address the mid- and low back, including key tsubos.
7. Describe the location, attachment sites, and kinesiology of the muscles addressed in the head and neck.
8. Perform techniques to address the head and neck, including key tsubos.
9. Describe the location, attachment sites, and kinesiology of the muscles addressed in the arm and hand.
10. Perform techniques to address the arm and hand, including key tsubos.
11. Explain how to close the treatment session with the client.

KEY TERMS

Adhesive capsulitis	Overuse injuries
Analgesic	Repetitive stress injuries (RSIs)
Carpal tunnel syndrome	Sprain
Disk herniation (slipped disk)	Tendinitis
Lateral epicondylitis (tennis elbow)	Tenosynovitis
Medial epicondylitis (golfer's or pitcher's elbow)	Tension headache
Muscle strain	Thoracic outlet syndrome
Noodling	Torticollis (wry neck)
	Tsubo

When performing chair massage, practitioners are likely to encounter a wide variety of conditions and complaints. These can be anything from general muscle tightness and fatigue—such as tight necks, shoulders, arms, and low back—to **repetitive stress injuries (RSIs)**, or **overuse injuries**. These are injuries that result from constant and repeated stress placed on bones, joints, or soft tissues; from a joint being forced into an extreme range of motion; or from prolonged strenuous activity. Some examples of RSIs include tendinitis, carpal tunnel syndrome, and thoracic outlet syndrome.

This chapter covers specific techniques for the neck, shoulders, arms and hands, and the low back, including the gluteals, and are designed to address the most common conditions and complaints chair massage clients have in each of these regions. (Chapter 5 contains additional techniques that can be useful for these conditions and complaints as well.) Along with more specific massage techniques, this chapter includes **tsubos** that would be helpful to press for each condition/area of the body. As practitioners of shiatsu know, a tsubo is a point that is an opening or gateway into one of the channels of energy (qi) in the body and is a direct link between the channel and the outside world. It is a place where qi can be changed, dispersed, or supported through thumb or finger pressure. See Appendix A for an overview and description of each of the traditional Chinese medicine organ channels.

OVERVIEW OF MUSCLES

The following figures are taken from *The Muscle and Bone Palpation Manual* by Joseph Muscolino. They are intended to provide an overview of the areas of focus in this chapter.

Figure 4-1 A shows the muscles of the back and posterior shoulder girdle region, as well as some of the posterior neck muscle. Figure 4-1 B shows the anterior view of the posterior shoulder girdle and neck regions. This view shows the anterior trapezius, anterior deltoid, biceps brachii, and part of the triceps brachii.

Figure 4-2 shows the quadratus lumborum.

Figure 4-3 shows the gluteus medius and maximus.

Figure 4-4 shows the scalenes and the suboccipitals.

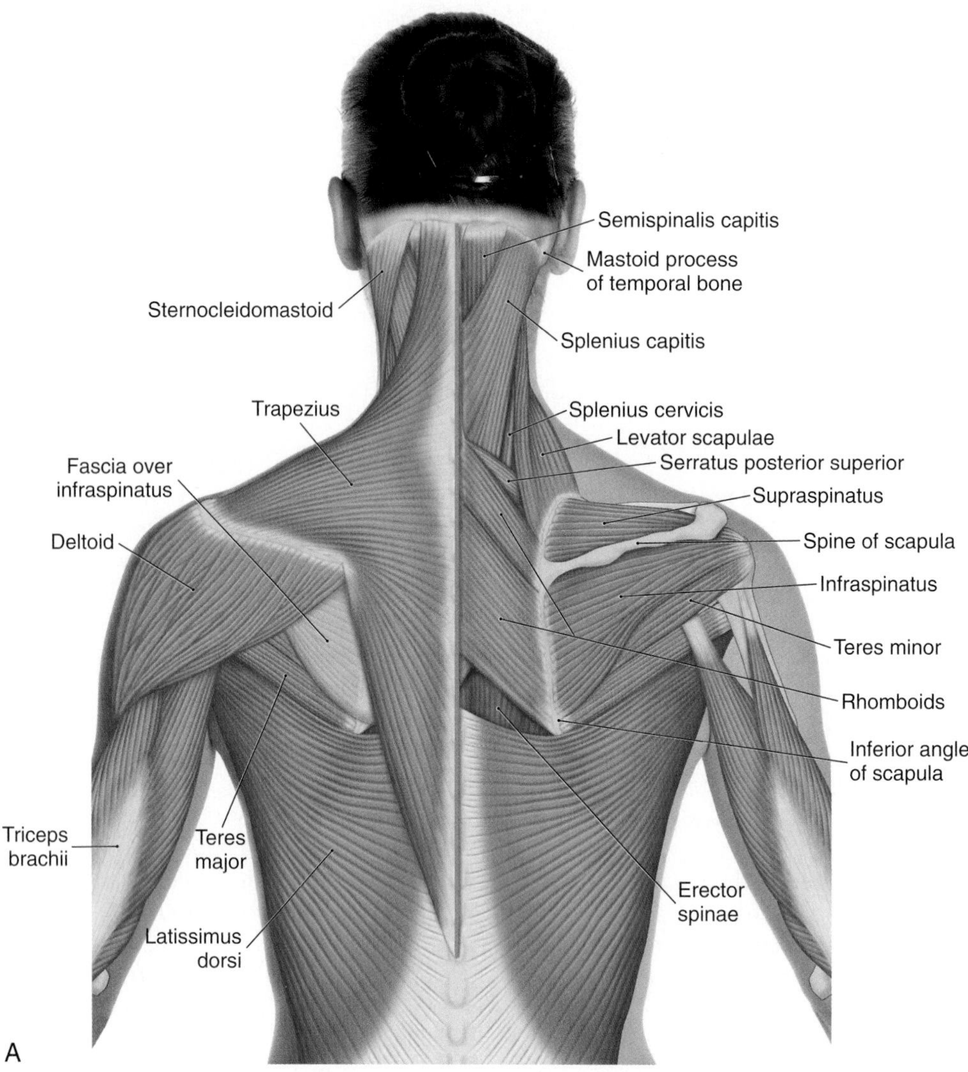

FIGURE 4-1 A, Muscles of the back and posterior shoulder girdle region. The left side is superficial; the right side is deep (the deltoid, trapezius, sternocleidomastoid, and infraspinatus fascia are removed). (From Muscolino JE: *The muscle and bone palpation manual, with trigger points, referral patterns, and stretching.* St. Louis, 2009, Mosby.)

Figure 4-5 A shows the anterior view of the upper arm muscles, and Figure 4-5 B shows the posterior view of the upper arm muscles. Figure 4-6 A shows the forearm flexors, and Figure 4-6 B shows the forearm extensors.

Before performing more specific treatment techniques on a particular region of the client's body, palpate each muscle and its attachments. For a more detailed review of the specific muscles discussed in each region of the body, see Appendix B, "Anatomy and Kinesiology Review."

UPPER REGION OF THE POSTERIOR BODY

Many seated massage clients have muscle tension and tightness in the shoulders and upper back. Mental or emotional stress can cause the muscle tension and even result in muscle pain. It can also be caused by long hours sitting at desks, working at a computer, and talking on the telephone. Jobs that require lifting and reaching above the head, such as working on overhead machinery or on automobiles that have been lifted by hydraulic hoists, can lead to tight upper back and shoulder muscles as well. However, practitioners should not assume the source of any client's muscle tension and pain. Instead, the pretreatment interview should be used as a tool to determine the focus of the treatment.

The muscles addressed in the upper region of the posterior body are trapezius, the rotator cuff muscles (supraspinatus, infraspinatus, teres minor, and subscapularis), teres major, and rhomboids. See Appendix B for the specific attachments and actions of these muscles.

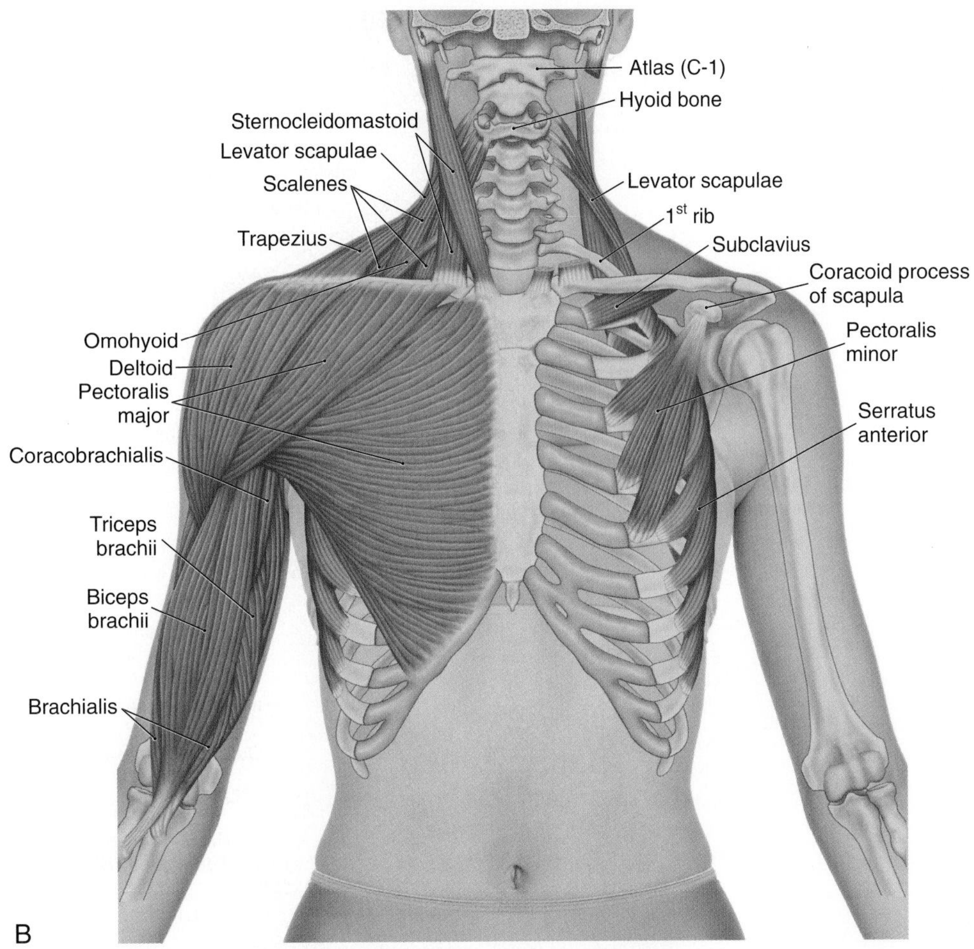

FIGURE 4-1, cont'd B, Muscles of the anterior view of the posterior shoulder girdle region. This view shows the anterior trapezius, anterior deltoid, biceps brachii, and part of the triceps brachii. (From Muscolino JE: *The muscle and bone palpation manual, with trigger points, referral patterns, and stretching.* St. Louis, 2009, Mosby.)

Shoulder Conditions

Besides general muscle tension and tightness in the shoulders and upper back, adhesive capsulitis is a shoulder disorder that practitioners may encounter in chair massage clients.

Adhesive Capsulitis (Frozen Shoulder)

Definition: **Adhesive capsulitis** is the restricted range of motion of the glenohumeral joint resulting from inflammation and stiffening of the surrounding connective tissue and adhesions. It can last from approximately five months to three years or more and may resolve, at least partially, spontaneously. It usually occurs in people 50 to 70 years of age.

Symptoms: In addition to severely restricted range of motion, there is also chronic pain, characterized as diffuse, dull, and aching, in the shoulder. Certain movements can cause sudden onset of pain and muscle cramping that can last several minutes.

Causes: The exact cause is unknown. It may be caused by injury or trauma to the shoulder area. It may also be an autoimmune disorder in which the body's immune system attacks healthy tissue in the shoulder. The shoulder joint loses movement because of chronic inflammation, the formation of adhesions, and a decrease of synovial fluid.

Treatments: Treatment can be painful. It consists of physical therapy, various pain relief and anti-inflammatory medications, massage therapy, and, in severe cases, surgery.

Chair massage considerations: Practitioners should ask clients if they are taking any **analgesics** (pain relievers) or anti-inflammatory medications, even over-the-counter ones. Clients who are taking an analgesic have altered pain perception and may not be able to give accurate feedback about pressure of the techniques being applied during the treatment. For this reason, practitioners should ask clients when they took their most recent dose, and if it is on the same day as the chair massage treatment, practitioners

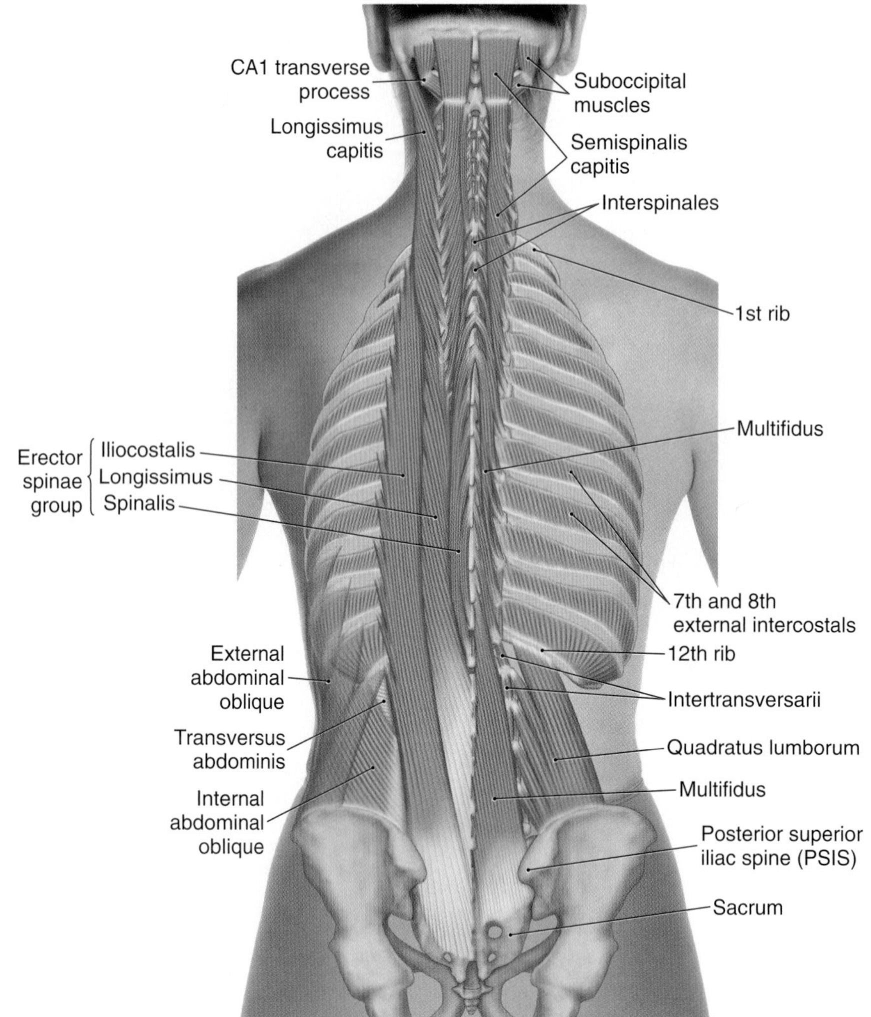

FIGURE 4-2 Quadratus lumborum. (From Muscolino JE: *The muscle and bone palpation manual, with trigger points, referral patterns, and stretching.* St. Louis, 2009, Mosby.)

should use lighter pressure to avoid the risk of damaging tissues. Practitioners should ask clients who are taking an anti-inflammatory medication how long they have been taking it and when they took their most recent dose. Anti-inflammatory medications can alter pain perception, and long-term use can also compromise the integrity of the tissues. If the client has been taking an anti-inflammatory medication for a short time and the most recent dose is taken the same day as the chair massage treatment, or if the client has been taking an anti-inflammatory medication for a long time (three or more months), practitioners should apply lighter pressure to avoid the risk of damaging tissues. Shoulder girdle muscles can be addressed, including the rotator cuff muscles, biceps brachii, triceps brachii, and deltoid. Because sudden movements of the shoulder joint can result in severe pain and muscle cramping that can last for several minutes, the shoulder should be moved slowly and with caution. The practitioner should consider alerting the client before moving the shoulder, indicate that the movement will be slow, and ask that the client immediately report if any movement causes pain.

Treatment Protocol

1. Begin the treatment by warming up the area with palm-press compressions. Stand behind the client in a lunge position, place both hands on each side of the spine, and lean forward to apply pressure from the level of C-7 inferiorly to the level of T-6. (Remember to inhale deeply as you lean forward and exhale as you release the compression.) When you reach T-6, retrace superiorly to C-7. Repeat two more times,

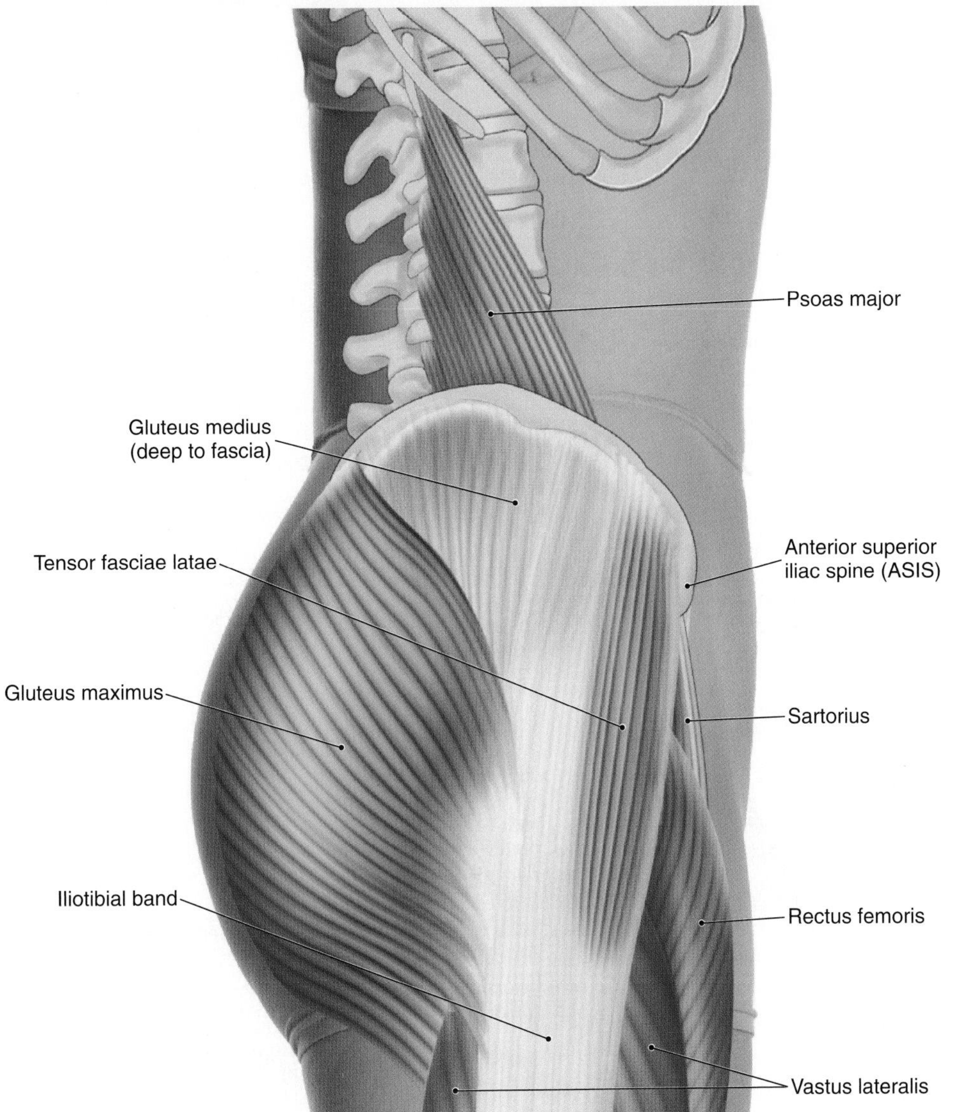

FIGURE 4-3 Gluteus maximus and medius. (From Muscolino JE: *The muscle and bone palpation manual, with trigger points, referral patterns, and stretching.* St. Louis, 2009, Mosby.)

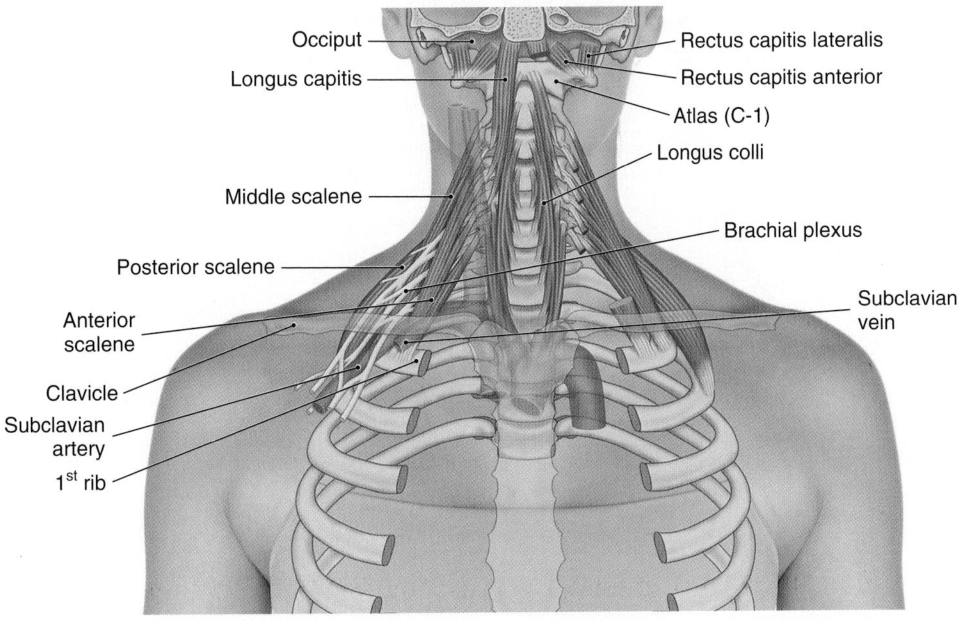

FIGURE 4-4 Scalenes and suboccipitals. (From Muscolino JE: *The muscle and bone palpation manual, with trigger points, referral patterns, and stretching.* St. Louis, 2009, Mosby.)

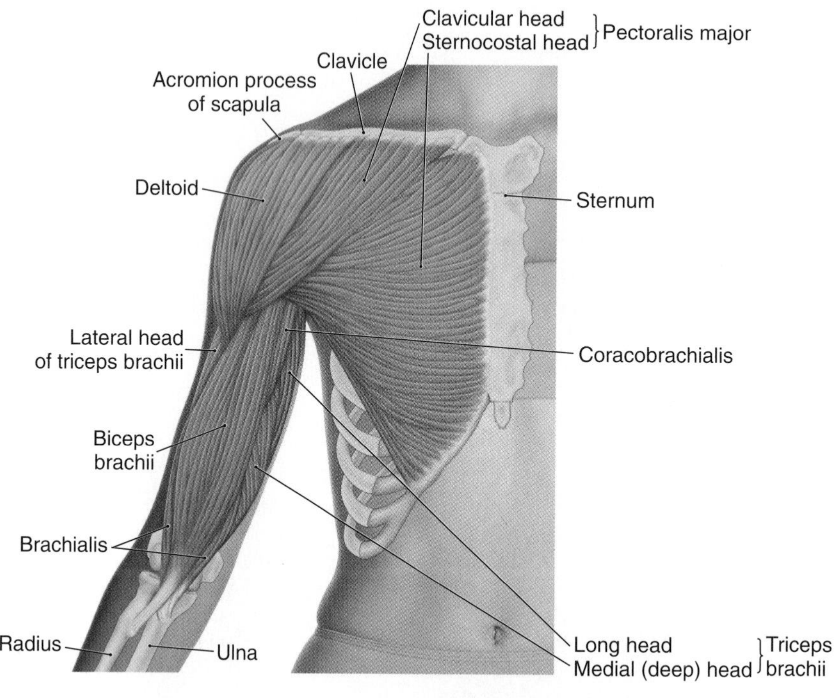

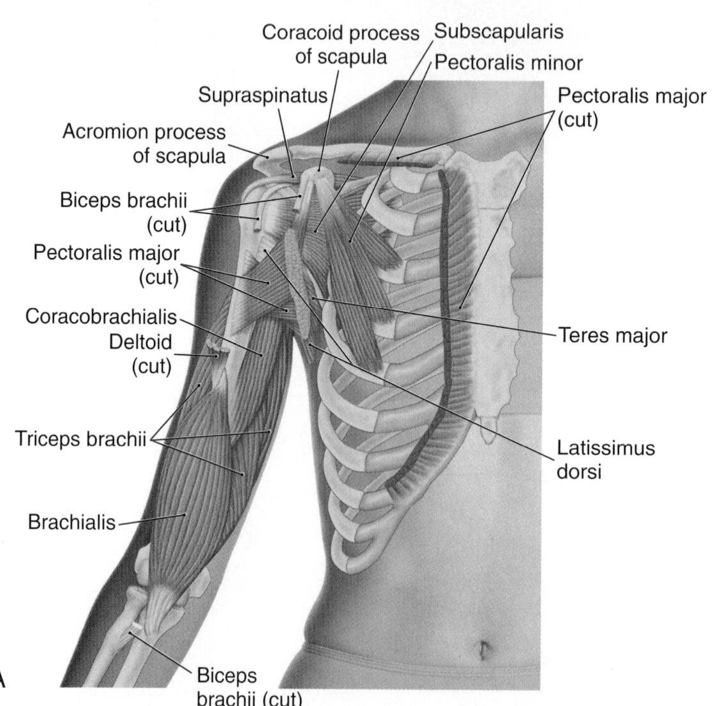

FIGURE 4-5 A, Anterior view of the upper arm muscles. (From Muscolino JE: *The muscle and bone palpation manual, with trigger points, referral patterns, and stretching.* St. Louis, 2009, Mosby.)

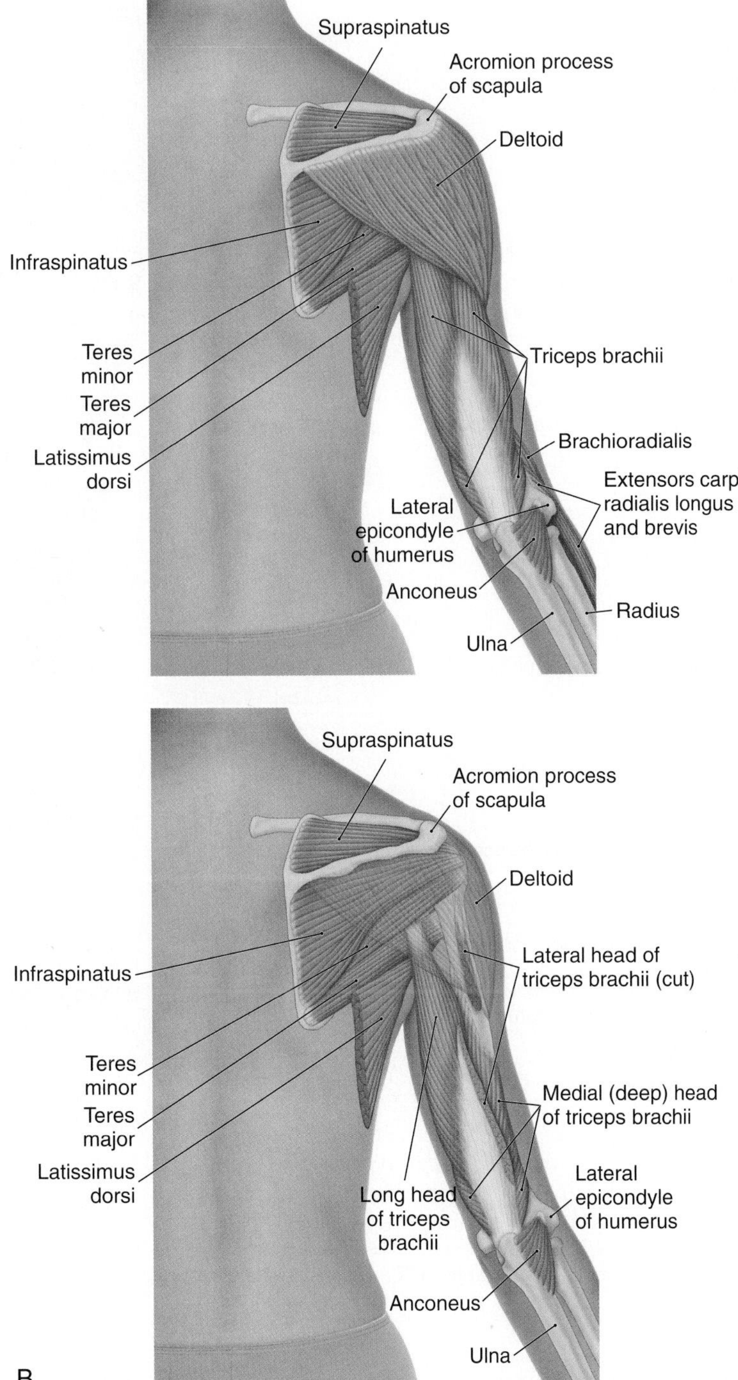

FIGURE 4-5, cont'd B, Posterior view of the upper arm muscles. (From Muscolino JE: *The muscle and bone palpation manual, with trigger points, referral patterns, and stretching.* St. Louis, 2009, Mosby.)

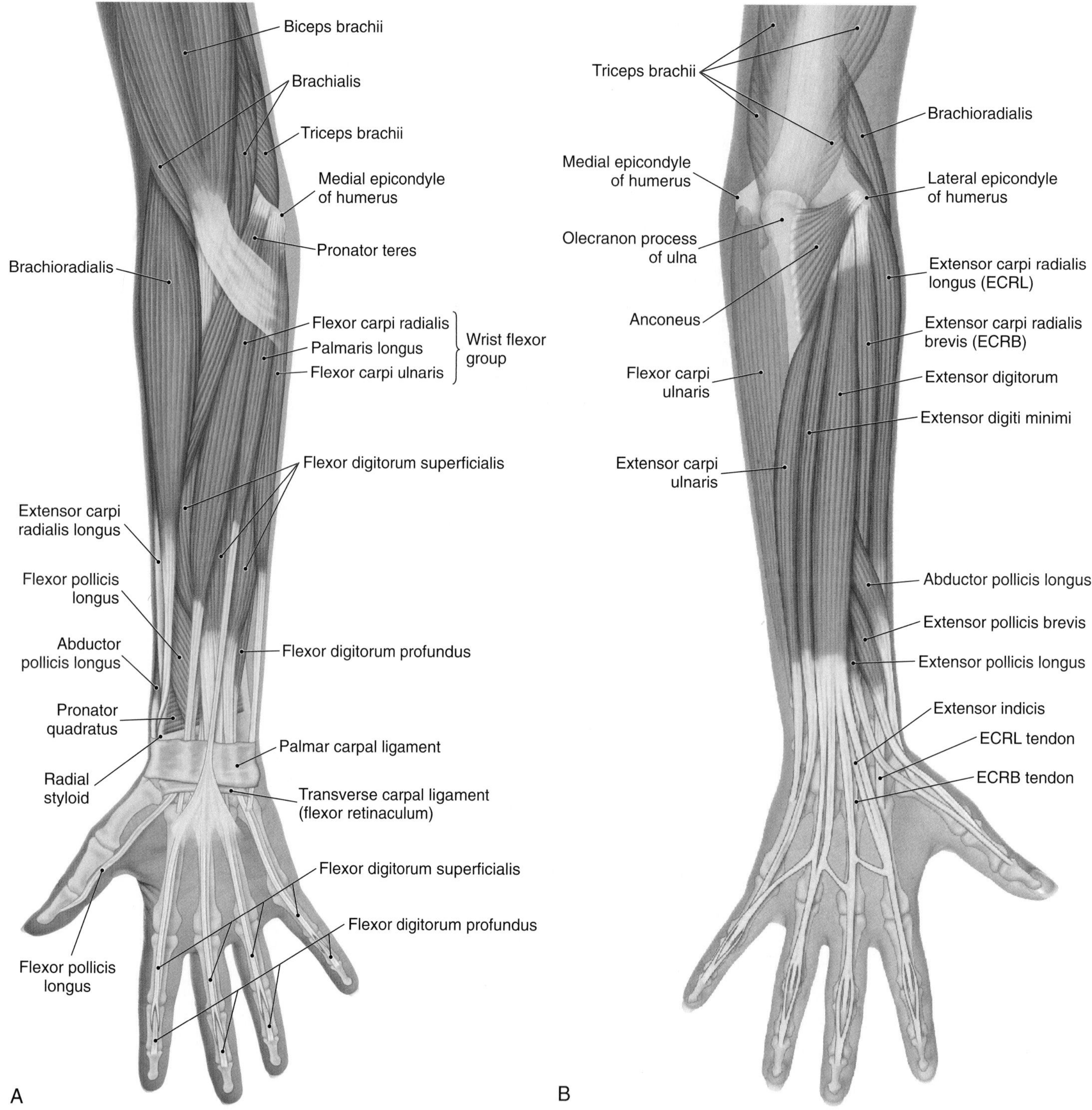

FIGURE 4-6 A, Forearm flexors. **B,** Forearm extensors. (From Muscolino JE: *The muscle and bone palpation manual, with trigger points, referral patterns, and stretching.* St. Louis, 2009, Mosby.)

ending with your hands on the client's upper trapezius (Figure 4-7).

2. Knead the upper trapezius muscles bilaterally until you feel the tissue softening (Figure 4-8).
3. Standing in a lunge position, place your left forearm on the client's right upper trapezius at the level of C-7, and place your left hand on the client's right upper arm to stabilize the region while pressure is applied. Depress your forearm into the tissue by bending the knees and leaning downward into the tissue. With each downward motion, move your forearm laterally toward the lateral shoulder, being sure to not press down on the acromion process. When the edge of the shoulder is reached, retrace your movements back toward the neck (Figure 4-9). Repeat two more times.

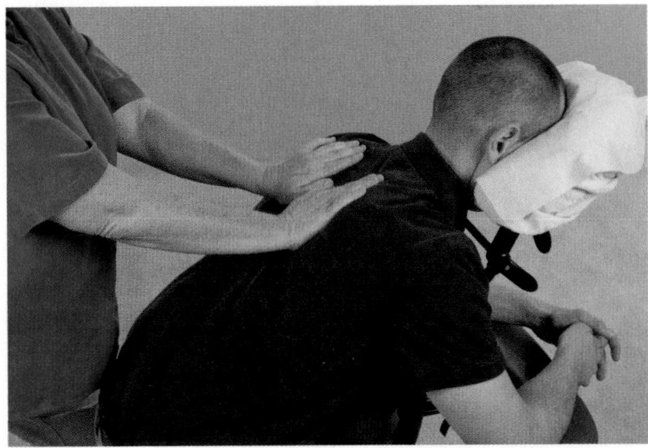

FIGURE 4-7 Compressions down the erector spinae from C-7 to T-6.

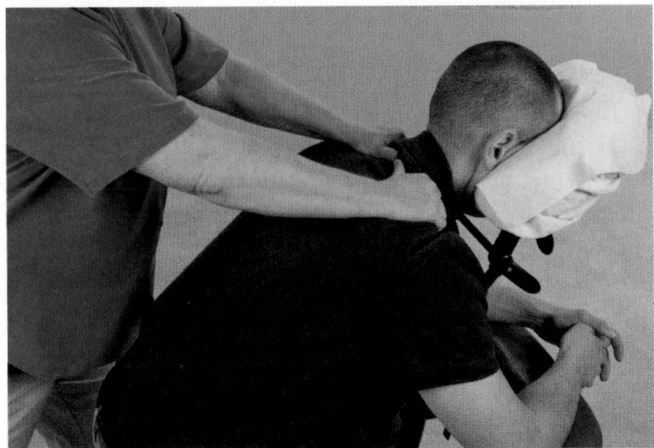

FIGURE 4-8 Kneading the upper trapezius bilaterally.

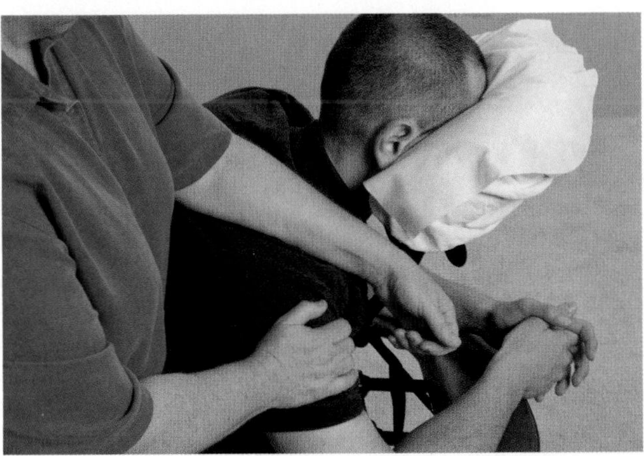

FIGURE 4-9 Pressing the forearm into the upper trapezius.

4. With your thumb and finger pads, apply circular motions along the supraspinatus and infraspinatus muscles from medial to lateral and back again (Figure 4-10). Do this several times until the tissue softens.
5. Place your left hand on the client's right upper arm again to stabilize, and use your left forearm to make broad circular motions along the rhomboid and shoulder girdle area (Figure 4-11).

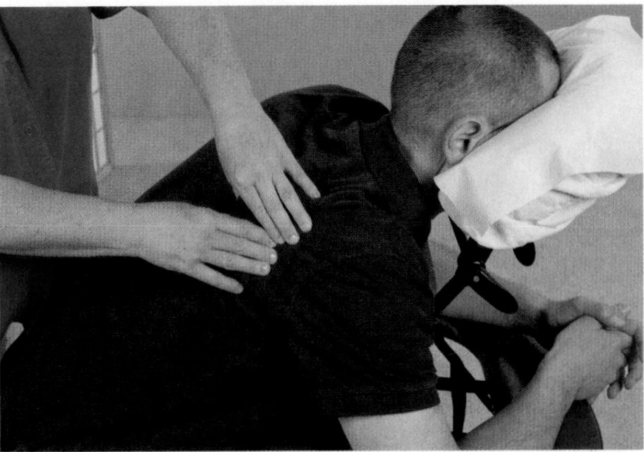

FIGURE 4-10 Circular friction applied with the thumb and finger pads along the supraspinatus and infraspinatus.

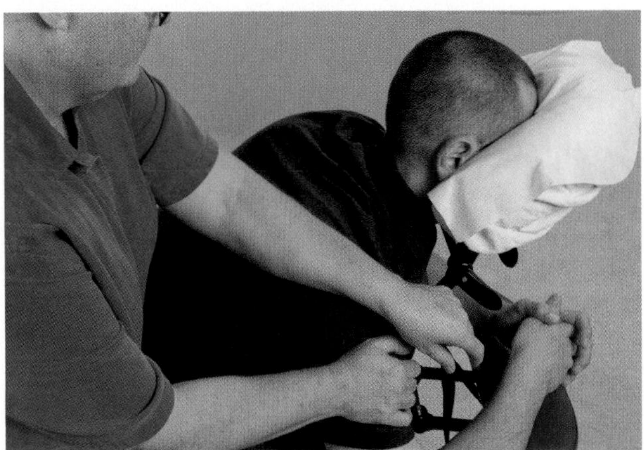

FIGURE 4-11 Make broad circular motions with the forearm along the rhomboid and shoulder girdle area.

6. Move to the left side of the client and, standing in a straight stance, place one hand on top of the other to brace the fingers. Use your fingertips to apply downward pressure as you glide deeply on the rhomboids from the vertebral column to the medial border of the scapula. Make sure to engage the entire muscle, lengthening the tissue (Figure 4-12 A). Make several passes of the area, then use thumb pressure to further soften the tissue along the medial border of the scapula (Figure 4-12 B).
7. Move to the right side of the client and stand in either a lunge position or straight stance. Place your right hand under the client's right arm, and cradle the shoulder joint. With your right hand, retract the shoulder joint posteriorly to wing the right scapula (Figure 4-13). Use the thumb or fingers of your left hand to apply pressure into the subscapularis attachments on the medial border of the scapula while moving the scapula posteriorly. This should be done in a fluid motion as

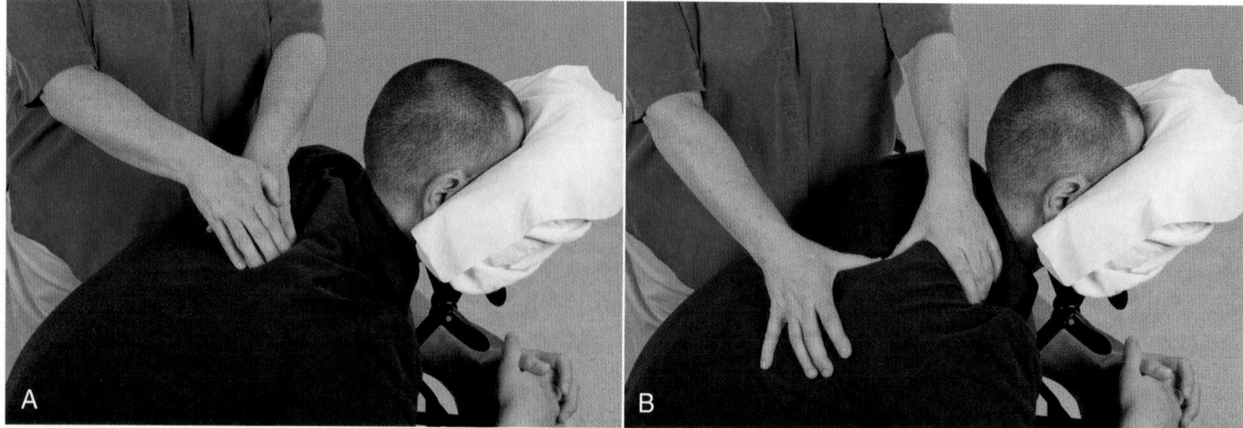

FIGURE 4-12 **A,** Deep fingertip gliding from the vertebral column to the medial border of the scapula. **B,** Using thumb pressure to further soften the tissue along the medial border of the scapula.

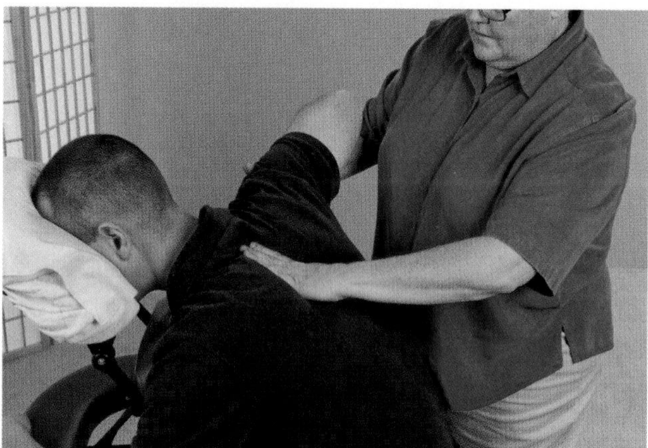

FIGURE 4-13 Winging the scapula.

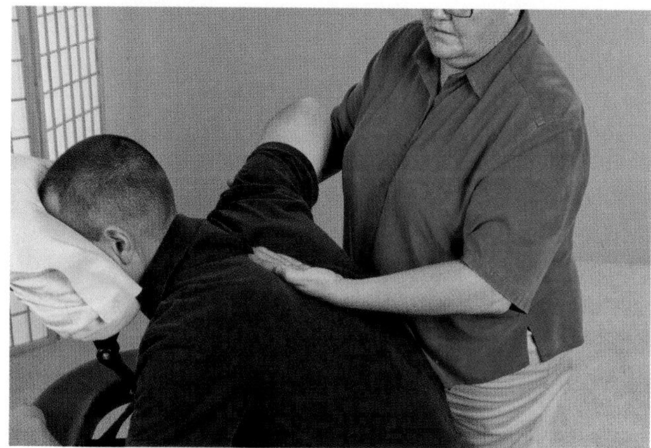

FIGURE 4-14 Working the fingers along the medial border of the scapula.

your thumb or fingers (whichever is most comfortable for you) work along the medial border of the scapula from the inferior angle to the superior angle and back again (Figure 4-14). The thumb or fingers act as pivot points while the posterior movement of the shoulder joint allows for the application of pressure from the digits into the subscapularis.

Repeat two more times. When finished, remove your left hand from under the client's arm and place it back on the armrest.

8. The area should now be warmed up for firmer pressure from the elbow. Palpate the region to locate the medial border of the scapula and the vertebral column. Move to a lunge position behind the client and slightly to the right. With your right hand holding the client's right shoulder area, place your flexed left elbow on the rhomboids at the inferior angle of the scapula. Apply pressure in a forward motion, slightly extending your elbow as you gently lunge forward, then release. Continue applying your elbow along the medial border of the scapula to the superior angle, retrace your movements back to the inferior angle, then back up to the superior angle (Figure 4-15). While at the superior angle of the scapula, use your flexed elbow to gently palpate for the levator scapula attachment; it should feel like a thick knot at the top of the scapula. Once located, soften your knees in the lunge stance to apply pressure directly downward at the attachment site. Make small circular motions with the elbow to fully address this area.
9. Using your left hand, gently knead the right upper trapezius to complete the deep work performed on this area.
10. Place the palm of your left hand on the rhomboids, lean into the area, and firmly move the tissue under the palm in a clockwise manner (envision the movement of opening a jar) (Figure 4-16). Perform this motion several times to complete the deep work performed on this area.
11. Standing behind your client in a straight stance, knead the upper trapezius muscles bilaterally.
12. Move to the client's left side and repeat Steps 1 through 11.

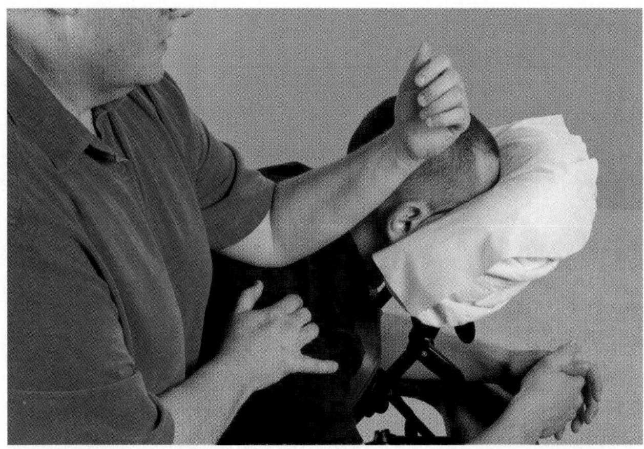

FIGURE 4-15 Applying pressure with flexed elbow along the medial border of the scapula.

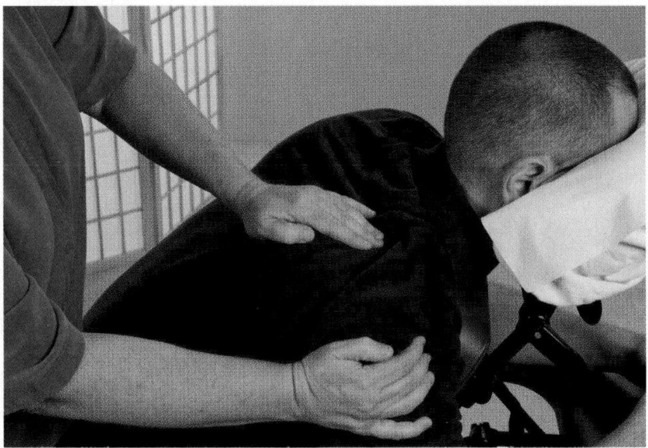

FIGURE 4-16 Using the palm to firmly move the tissue in a clockwise manner.

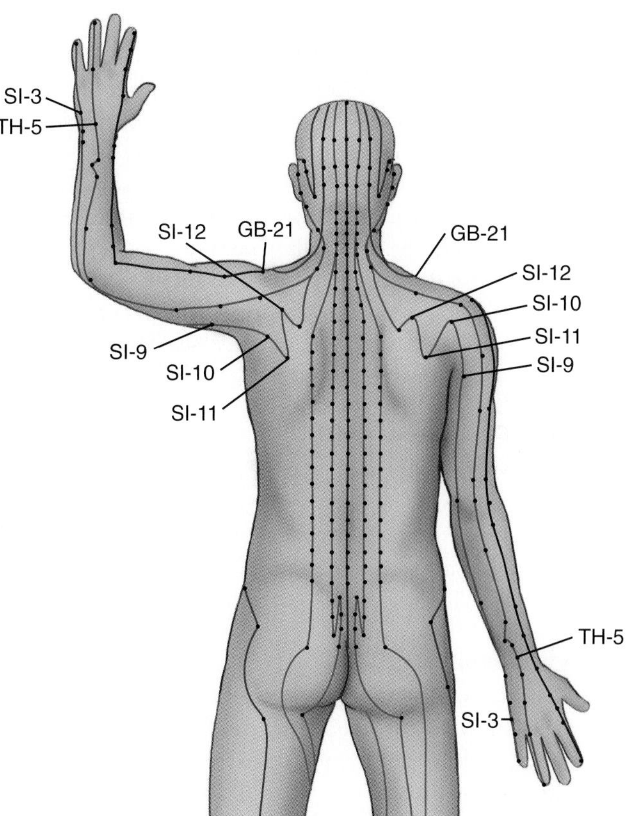

FIGURE 4-17 Tsubos to press to alleviate pain and discomfort in the shoulders and upper back. (Modified from Anderson SK: *The practice of shiatsu.* St. Louis, 2008, Mosby.)

Tsubos

There are several tsubos that practitioners may find helpful to press to alleviate pain and discomfort in the client's shoulders and upper back. These are all shown in Figure 4-17.

GB-21: "Shoulder Well," *Jianjing*

This point is located on the mound of the shoulder, halfway between the neck and the acromion process. It is helpful with relieving neck and shoulder stiffness. Because it creates a strong downward movement of qi, which may bring on labor prematurely, *this point is not to be used on a pregnant client.* If, however, the baby is overdue, it may be beneficial to press this point, with the mother's consent.

SI-3: "Back Ravine," *Houxi*

On a loose fist, this point is proximal to the head of the fifth metacarpal on the medial side of the hand. It supports the back and spine, and it relieves headache, stiff neck and shoulder, and tight muscles of the elbow, arm, and fingers.

SI-9: "Shoulder Integrity," *Jianzhen*

This point is located approximately one inch superior to the posterior axillary crease. It relieves pain in the scapular area, arm, and hand.

SI-10: "Scapula Hollow," *Naoshu*

This point is located in the depression just inferior and posterior to the acromion process of the scapula, directly superior to SI-9. It relieves pain and supports the qi in the shoulder and arm.

SI-11: "Celestial Gathering," *Tianzong*

This point is located in the center of the scapula. It is a key point to the back. It diffuses qi stagnation in the chest and ribcage.

SI-12: "Grasping the Wind," *Bingfeng*

This point is located in the suprascapular fossa directly superior to SI-11. It relieves pain and numbness in the shoulder, arm, and hand.

TH-5: "Outer Gate," *Weiguan*

This point is located 1.5 inches proximal to the wrist crease in between the radius and the ulna. It is helpful for headache and pain anywhere in the upper body.

MID- AND LOW BACK

Low back pain is the most common complaint in the United States. Sometimes the pain is relatively mild and simply from sitting for long periods of time. In this posture, the muscle fibers have shortened, and if the person does not periodically stand up and stretch, the muscle fibers can become *chronically* short, which generally causes pain. The muscles addressed in the mid and low back are the latissimus dorsi, the erector spinae group, quadratus lumborum, gluteus maximus, and gluteus medius. See Appendix B for the specific attachments and actions of these muscles.

Low Back Conditions

More severe pain can be due to muscle injury, injury to the ligaments of the joints between the vertebrae or between the sacrum and ilium, and issues with the intervertebral disks (such as malposition or herniation). The following are common low back issues that chair massage can help.

Muscle Strain (Pull)

Definition: **Muscle strain** refers to a stretch or tear in the muscle; it may also include the fascia surrounding the muscle. The strain can involve a few muscle fibers up to a large area of the muscle.

Symptoms: Pain, loss of muscle function.

Causes: Usually an abnormal muscle contraction during abrupt movement, such as improper lifting by using the small muscles of the back instead of the large muscles of the legs, and twisting while lifting.

Treatments: Analgesics, anti-inflammatory medications, rest, ice, compression.

Chair massage considerations: Massage is contraindicated until the inflammation has subsided or 72 hours after the initial injury, whichever comes first. Practitioners should ask clients if they are taking any analgesics or anti-inflammatory medications, even over-the-counter ones. Clients who are taking an analgesic have altered pain perception and may not be able to give accurate feedback about the pressure of the techniques being applied during the treatment. Therefore, practitioners should ask clients when they took their most recent dose, and if it is the same day as the chair massage treatment, practitioners should use lighter pressure to avoid the risk of damaging tissues.

Practitioners should ask clients who are taking an anti-inflammatory medication when they took their most recent dose. Anti-inflammatory medications can also alter pain perception, and if the most recent dose is taken the same day as the chair massage treatment, practitioners should apply lighter pressure to avoid the risk of damaging tissues. Light gliding strokes and light friction around the area can help to increase blood circulation and support healing. Once healing is fully completed and the client is no longer taking an analgesic or anti-inflammatory medication, deep friction in the area to loosen adhesions may be helpful.

Sprain

Definition: **Sprain** refers to a joint trauma that stretches or tears the ligaments of joint, but in which no bones are dislocated. A first-degree sprain involves stretching of the ligaments without tearing; a second-degree sprain involves partial tearing of the ligaments; a third-degree sprain involves complete tearing of the ligament. In the low back, sprains can occur in the intervertebral joints and the sacroiliac joint.

Symptoms: Pain, inflammation, skin discoloration.

Causes: Low back sprains are usually caused by lifting using the small muscles of the back instead of the large muscles of the legs and twisting the torso at the same time.

Treatments: Analgesics, anti-inflammatory medications, rest, ice, compression.

Chair massage considerations: Massage is contraindicated until the inflammation has subsided or 72 hours after the initial injury, whichever comes first. Practitioners should ask clients if they are taking any analgesics or anti-inflammatory medications, even over-the-counter ones. Clients who are taking an analgesic have altered pain perception and may not be able to give accurate feedback about the pressure of the techniques being applied during the treatment. For this reason, practitioners should ask clients when they took their most recent dose, and if it is on the same day as the chair massage treatment, practitioners should use lighter pressure to avoid the risk of damaging tissues.

Practitioners should ask clients who are taking an anti-inflammatory medication when they took their most recent dose. Anti-inflammatory medications can also alter pain perception, and if the most recent dose is taken the same day as the chair massage treatment, practitioners should apply lighter pressure to avoid the risk of damaging tissues. Light gliding strokes and light friction around the area can help to increase blood circulation and support healing. Once healing is fully completed and the client is no longer taking an analgesic or anti-inflammatory medication, deep friction in the area to loosen adhesions may be helpful.

Disk Herniation (Slipped Disk)

Definition: **Disk herniation** occurs when the fibrocartilage surrounding the intervertebral disk ruptures, releasing the nucleus pulposus. This condition most often occurs in the lumbar region, involving the L-4 or L-5 disks.

Symptoms: Resulting pressure on spinal nerve roots may cause pain and damage to surrounding nerves. Pain radiates from the gluteal area down the lateral or posterior thigh, through the calf, and sometimes into the foot. Sometimes there can be spasms in the surrounding muscles.

Causes: Intervertebral disks act as shock absorbers. Disk herniations can occur from general wear and tear, such as jobs that require constant sitting such as at a desk or driving a truck. Traumatic injury to lumbar disks commonly occurs through lifting using the small muscles of the back (trunk flexion) instead of lifting using the large muscles of the legs with a straight back. Minor back pain and chronic back

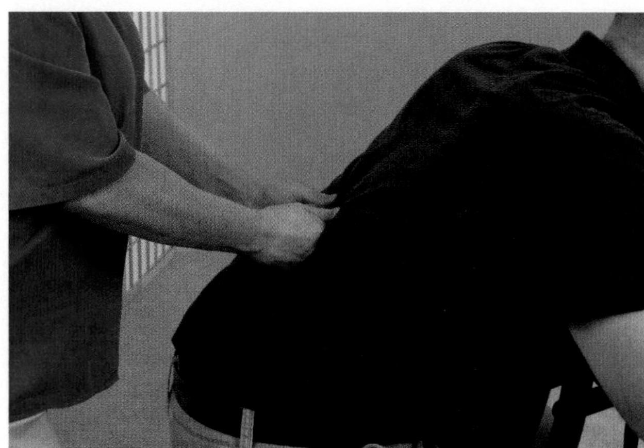

FIGURE 4-18 Soft fists on either side of the vertebral column on the erector spinae muscle group at the level of T-6.

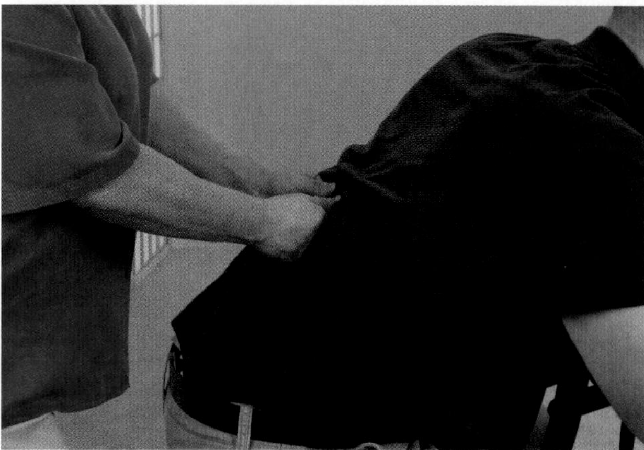

FIGURE 4-19 Applying pressure into the muscles, moving inferiorly to the iliac crest, superiorly back to T-6, and inferiorly to the iliac crest again.

fatigue are indicative of general wear and tear; these can make the person susceptible to a traumatic herniated disk from something as simple as bending to pick up a pen or a briefcase from the floor.

Treatments: Analgesics, bed rest, traction, physical therapy, and exercises.

Chair massage considerations: Practitioners should ask clients if they are taking any analgesics, even over-the-counter ones, or muscle relaxants. Clients who are taking these medications have altered pain perception and may not be able to give accurate feedback about the pressure of the techniques being applied during the treatment. For this reason, practitioners should ask clients when they took their most recent dose, and if it is on the same day as the chair massage treatment, practitioners should use lighter pressure to avoid the risk of damaging tissues. Massage on the muscles surrounding the area can help to reduce muscle spasms. Pressure should not be applied directly over the area of disk herniation.

Treatment Protocol

1. Stand behind the client in a lunge position. Make soft fists with both hands and, with thumbs pointing up, place them on either side of the vertebral column on the erector spinae muscle group at the level of T-6 (Figure 4-18). Apply pressure into the muscles, moving inferiorly to the iliac crest (Figure 4-19). At the iliac crest, retrace your movements superiorly to the level of T-6 and then inferiorly to the iliac crest again.
2. Trace your movements back up to the level of T-6, and add circular friction with your soft fists to slightly stretch the erector spinae muscle group attachment sites along the vertebral column. The circular motion can be either clockwise or counterclockwise (Figure 4-20). Repeat two more times.
3. Focusing on the lower right region of the back, place one of your hands on top of the other. With straight fingers, lean forward into the erector spinae group and glide upward to engage the tissue (Figure 4-21).

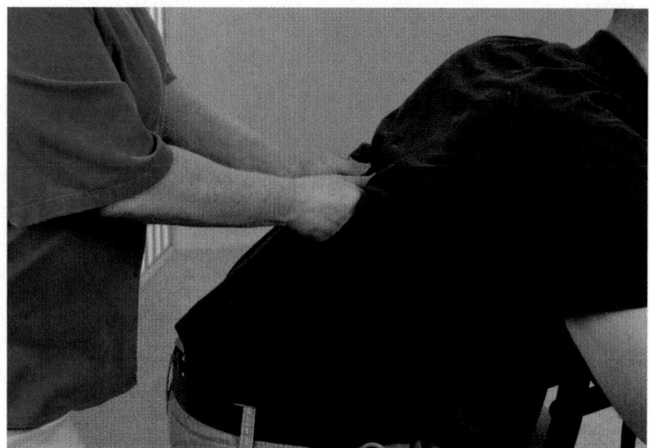

FIGURE 4-20 Circular friction with soft fists.

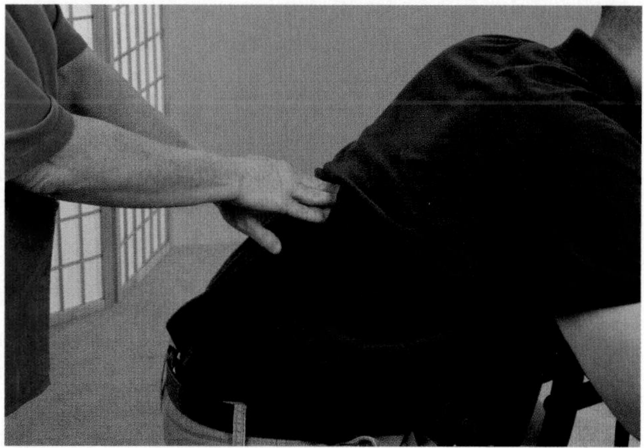

FIGURE 4-21 With one hand on top of the other, use straight fingers to lean forward into the erector spinae group and glide upward to engage the tissue.

Continue applying this combination of stretching and deep gliding into the tissue from the level of T-6 inferiorly to the iliac crest. At the iliac crest, retrace your movements superiorly to the level of T-6. Repeat one more time.

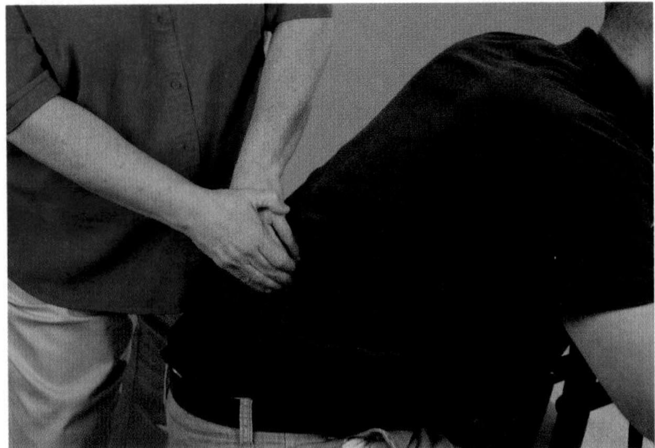

FIGURE 4-22 Apply circular friction with your fingertips on all three attachment sites for the quadratus lumborum.

4. With your fingertips, gently palpate the attachment sites for the quadratus lumborum (the 12th rib, the transverse processes of L-1 to L-4, and the posteriolateral iliac crest). Apply circular friction with your fingertips on all three attachment sites (Figure 4-22).
5. Standing on the right side of your client in a straight stance, place one hand on top of the other. With straight fingers, apply small circular motions to the lateral portion of the quadratus lumborum while gently directing your pressure medially (toward the lumbar attachment) (Figure 4-23 A). Depending on the length of the client's torso, you may be able to address several inches of the muscle's length, or even the entire length. Practitioners should take care to use gentle pressure, as this can be a sensitive area for many people. Continue the circular motion of your fingertips along the iliac crest to soften this attachment site (Figure 4-23 B).

> **Tip** Because the quadratus lumborum is a deep muscle, it is difficult to fully access it. Practitioners may find it helpful to visualize this aspect of the body in 3-D, then focus their touch deep to the erector spinae muscle group.

6. To finish working the quadratus lumborum, move to a straight stance on the client's left side and reach across to apply gentle kneading along the entire area (Figure 4-24).
7. Move to a half kneeling stance behind the client's right side. Use soft fists to knead the gluteus maximus (Figure 4-25).
8. Place your left forearm on the client's left gluteus medius, and place your right hand on the client's right greater trochanter of the femur to stabilize the hips. Use your forearm in a sweeping movement upward; be sure to fan out over the entire muscle (Figure 4-26). Once the area is softened with forearm work, place your left elbow along the client's right iliac crest and slowly lean in to provide deep specific pressure at the attachment sites (Figure 4-27). Finish by kneading the area.
9. With your hands in soft fists, place them on either side of the vertebral column on the erector spinae muscle group at the level of T-6, and apply deep circular friction inferiorly to the iliac crest. At the iliac crest, retrace your movements superiorly to the level of T-6.
10. Repeat Steps 3 through 9 on the client's left side.

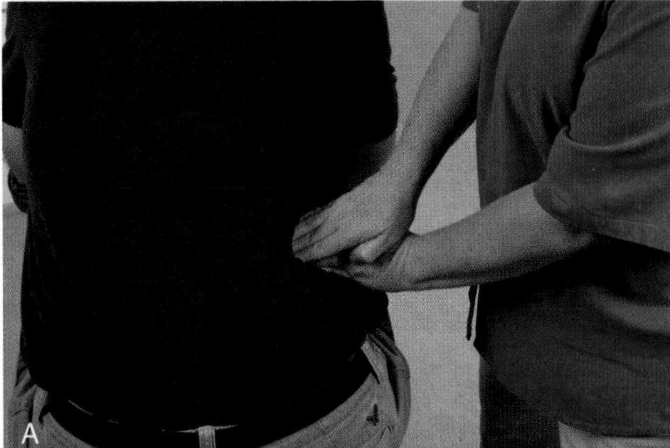

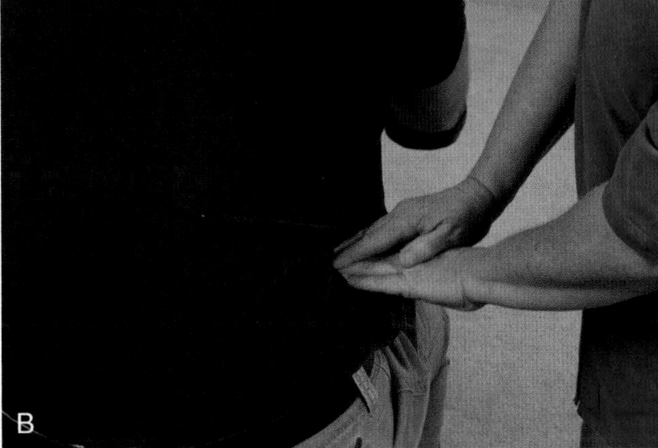

FIGURE 4-23 **A,** Applying small circular while gently directing pressure medially toward the lumbar attachment. **B,** Continuing circular motions of the fingertips along the iliac crest.

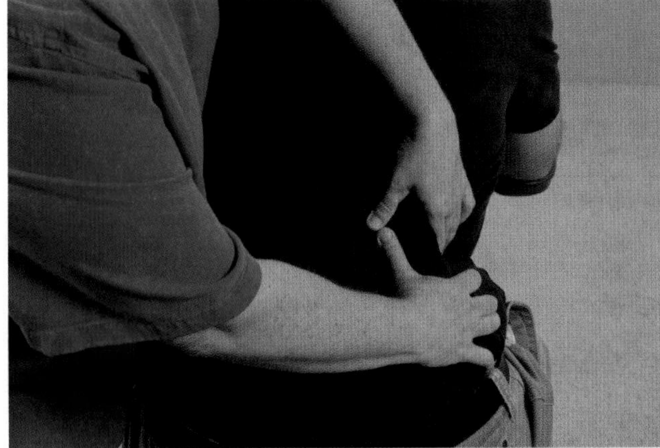

FIGURE 4-24 Standing on the client's left side and reaching across to apply gentle kneading along the entire quadratus lumborum area.

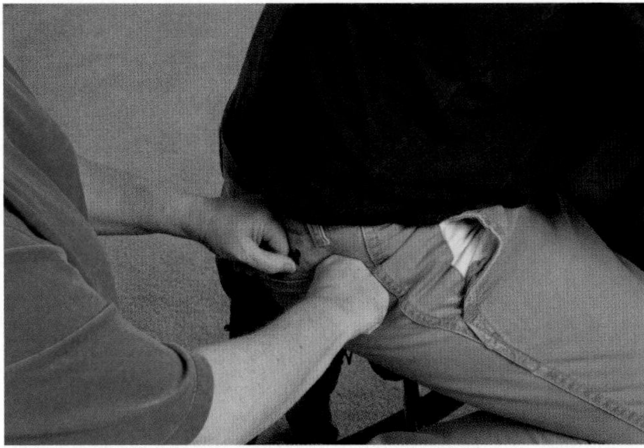

FIGURE 4-25 Half kneeling behind the client's right side and using soft fists to knead the gluteus maximus.

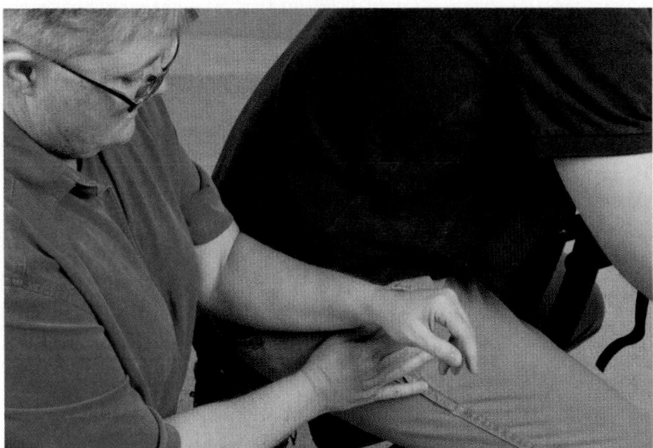

FIGURE 4-26 Using the forearm in a sweeping movement upward.

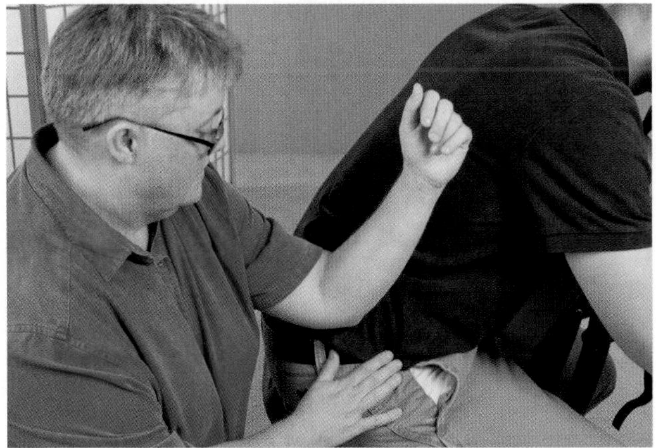

FIGURE 4-27 Providing deep, specific elbow pressure at the attachment sites.

Tsubos

There are several tsubos that practitioners may find helpful to press to alleviate pain and discomfort in the client's mid and low back. These are all shown in Figure 4-28.

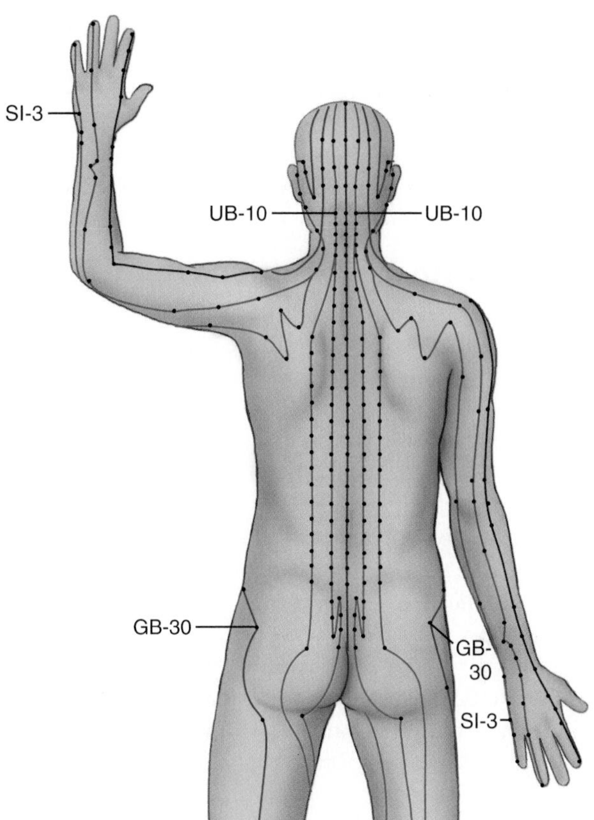

FIGURE 4-28 Tsubos to press to alleviate pain and discomfort in the mid and low back. (Modified from Anderson SK: *The practice of shiatsu.* St. Louis, 2008, Mosby.)

UB-10: "Celestial Pillar," *Tianzhu*

This point is located within the posterior hairline, along the suboccipital groove, approximately ¾ inch lateral to the midline of the posterior neck. Relieves lower back pain, stiff neck, and headache.

GB-30; "Jumping Circle," *Huantiao*

This point is located one third of the distance between the greater trochanter and the sacrum. It helps decrease pain in the hip and pelvis and helps relieve sciatic pain.

SI-3: "Back Ravine," *Houxi*

On a loose fist, this point is proximal to the head of the fifth metacarpal, on the medial side of the hand. It supports the back and spine, and it relieves headache, stiff neck and shoulder, and tight muscles of the elbow, arm, and fingers.

TECHNIQUES FOR THE NECK AND HEAD

The head on average weighs 12 to 15 pounds. The muscles responsible for keeping the head upright and for moving it into all the possible positions for the eyes to see have quite a bit of tension placed on them. These muscles are constantly making adjustments. Along with the stresses of everyday life, each different occupation puts various strains on the muscles of the neck and head depending on what is required of the person to do the work.

The muscles addressed in techniques for the neck and head are the upper trapezius, sternocleidomastoid (SCM), splenius capitis and cervicis, semispinalis capitis, scalenes, the suboccipital group, and levator scapula. See Appendix B for the specific attachments and actions of these muscles.

Neck and Head Conditions

In addition to general muscle tension and fatigue, there are specific neck and head conditions that chair massage clients are likely to present with.

Tension Headache

Definition: A **tension headache** refers to pain in the head from any cause.

Symptoms: The pain usually feels dull, persistent, and achy, and there can be a feeling of tightness around the head, temples, forehead, or occipital area.

Causes: Contracted muscles place pressure on the nerves and blood vessels in the area, causing pain. The contracted muscles can be due to mental or emotional stress, hours of looking at a computer screen, or any work in which the head is placed in a position so that the eyes are looking in one direction for prolonged periods of time such as looking downward at paperwork on a desk or looking upward at overhead machinery.

Treatments: Analgesics, rest, relaxation techniques.

Chair massage considerations: Practitioners should ask clients if they are taking any analgesics, even over-the-counter ones. Clients who are taking an analgesic have altered pain perception and may not be able to give accurate feedback about the pressure of the techniques being applied during the treatment. Therefore, practitioners should ask clients when they took their most recent dose, and if it is on the same day as the chair massage treatment, practitioners should use lighter pressure to avoid the risk of damaging tissues. Placing the face in the face cradle may cause the headache to worsen for some clients, so consider other massage positions to accommodate that possibility.

Thoracic Outlet Syndrome

Definition: **Thoracic outlet syndrome** refers to the compression or entrapment of one or more of the structures of the neurovascular bundle (brachial nerve plexus and associated blood vessels) located in the neck, upper chest, and axilla.

Symptoms: Shooting pain, weakness, and numbness in the shoulder and scapular regions and down the arm, and sometimes in the chest and neck.

Causes: Impingement caused by tight pectoralis minor or scalene muscles. This can be due to excessive arm movements or chronic tight scalene muscles such as from cradling a telephone receiver on the shoulder. Other causes include herniated cervical disks or cervical spondylosis.

Treatments: Postural changes, physiotherapy, massage therapy, chiropractic adjustments, or osteopathic manipulation.

Chair massage considerations: If the symptoms are due to tight muscles, massage can be performed to reduce muscle tension. If the symptoms are due to herniated cervical disks or spondylosis, massage will have little to no effect, and, for safety considerations, massage over the area should be performed with light pressure.

Torticollis (Wry Neck)

Definition: **Torticollis** is the condition in which the head is tilted toward one side and the chin is elevated and turned toward the opposite side.

Symptoms: Involves spasms of the sternocleidomastoid, although the scalenes, trapezius, and splenius capitis and cervicis can be involved as well.

Causes: Trauma to the neck, tumors of the base of the skull (compress the nerve supply to the neck), infections in the pharynx and the ear (can irritate the nerves supplying the neck muscles).

Treatments: Surgery if the cause is due to tumors; antibiotics if the cause is infection; physical therapy and massage therapy.

Chair massage considerations: The treatment should focus on relaxing the neck muscles, releasing trigger points, gently stretching the contracted muscles, and performing neck range of motion techniques. All of these techniques should be performed within the client's comfort; none should be forced.

Treatment Protocol

1. Standing behind your client in a lunge stance, knead the trapezius muscles bilaterally. Move to your client's left side and stand in a straight stance to knead the posterior neck muscles (Figure 4-29).
2. Once the area is warmed up, place your left hand on the client's left shoulder. Use your right thumb, index, and middle finger to gently lift the lateral portion of the neck muscles away from the nuchal ligament in a pincer grip (Figure 4-30).

   Gently hold the neck tissue in the pincer grip while kneading. The stroke is performed with the thumb, index, and middle finger briskly moving. Continue to use pincer-grip kneading along the entire length of the posterior neck.

> **Tip** The key to the effectiveness of this technique is to not be timid about pulling the muscle tissue away from the neck.

3. Address the left suboccipitals by using your right thumb pad to apply deep specific friction superiorly and inferiorly along the attachment sites on the occipital ridge of the skull (Figure 4-31).

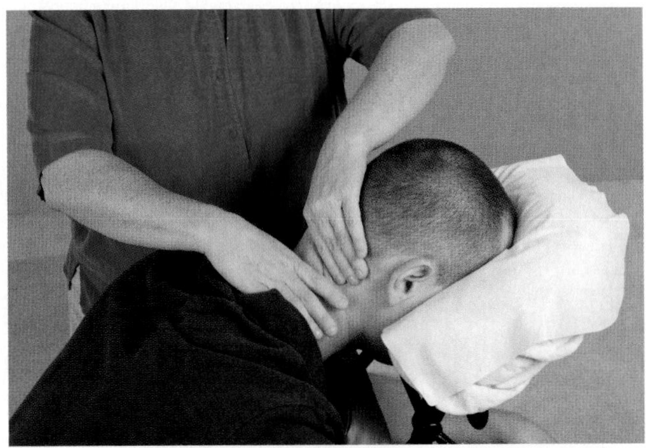

FIGURE 4-29 Kneading the posterior neck muscles.

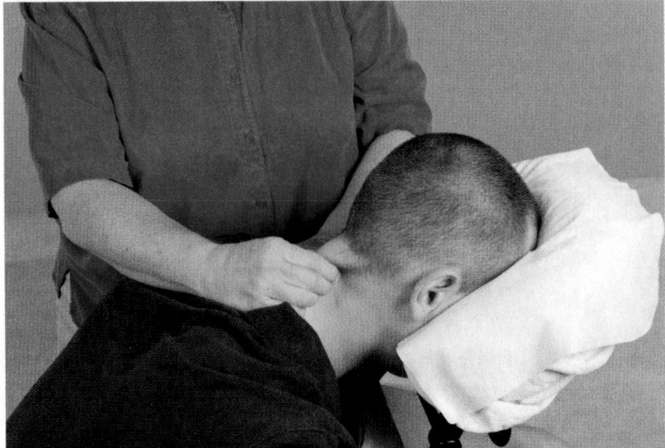

FIGURE 4-30 Gently lifting the lateral portion of the neck muscles away from the nuchal ligament in a pincer grip.

> **Tip** Be mindful that your touch is deeply engaged with the tissue along the occipital ridge so that you do not pull your client's hair, which can feel uncomfortable to the client.

4. Move to the client's right side and repeat Steps 2 and 3.
5. Perform general kneading on the posterior neck.
6. Move to a straight stance in front of your client. Cup both of your hands over the client's scalp, and curve your fingertips to engage the muscles attaching along the occipital ridge (Figure 4-32).
7. Apply slight upward traction while you gently apply circular friction with your fingertips along the entire ridge of the client's occiput from the mastoid process to the midline (Figure 4-33).
8. If it is acceptable to the client to receive scalp massage, massage the entire scalp with gentle circular friction. Be sure to apply pressure deep enough to move the scalp and not just the hair. If the client can tolerate it, pull on the hair very gently as a way to close for this region (Figure 4-34).

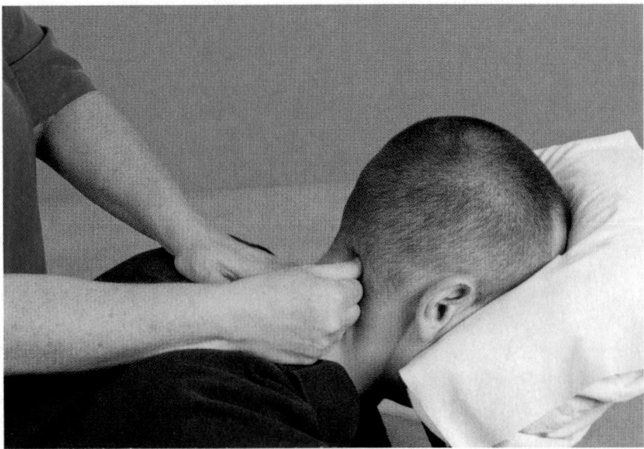

FIGURE 4-31 Using the thumb pad to apply deep specific friction superiorly and inferiorly along the attachment sites on the occipital ridge of the skull.

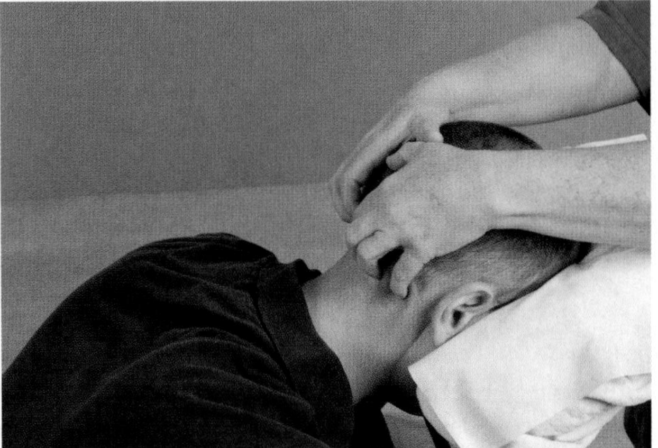

FIGURE 4-32 Cupping both hands over the client's scalp and curving the fingertips to engage the muscles attaching along the occipital ridge.

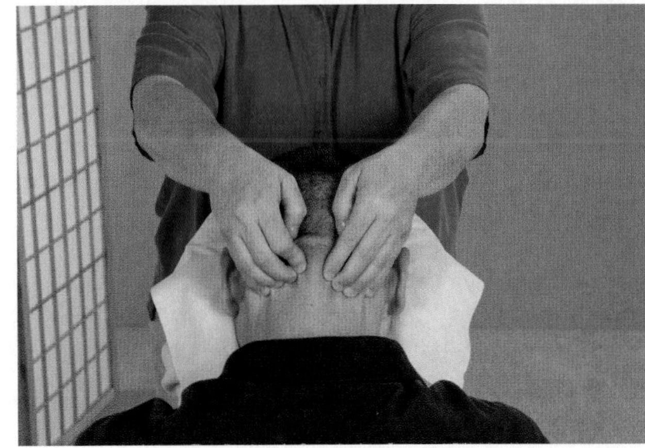

FIGURE 4-33 Applying slight upward traction while gently applying circular friction along the client's occiput.

> **Tip** Scalp massage increases circulation to the head and may help reduce tension headaches.

9. Move to a lunge stance behind your client. Knead the upper trapezius muscles bilaterally to give the client a feeling of connection between the head and neck to the torso.

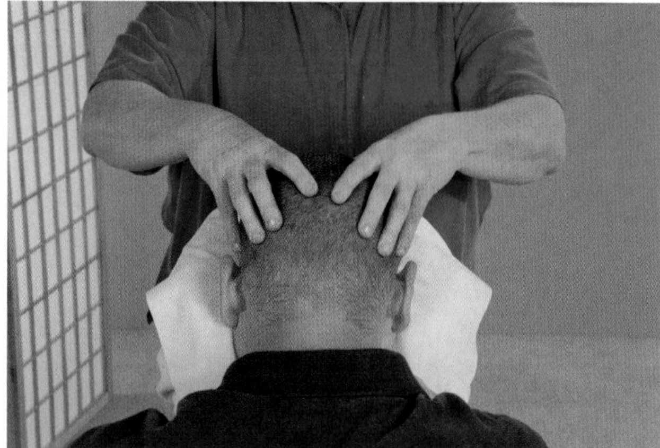

FIGURE 4-34 Scalp massage.

10. Perform percussion followed by brush strokes on the client's back to close the work on this area.

Tsubos

There are several tsubos that practitioners may find helpful to press to alleviate pain and discomfort in the client's head and neck. These are all shown in Figure 4-35.

LI-4: "Union Valley," *Hegu*

This point is located on the highest point of the web of flesh between the thumb and metacarpal II, when the thumb is adducted. It is often effective at stopping headaches. Because it creates a strong downward movement of qi, which may bring on labor prematurely, *this point is not to be used on a pregnant client.* If, however, the baby is overdue, it may be beneficial to press this point, with the mother's consent.

UB-10: "Celestial Pillar," *Tianzhu*

This point is located within the posterior hairline, along the suboccipital groove, approximately ¾ inch lateral to the midline of the posterior neck. It relieves lower back pain, stiff neck, and headache.

SI-3: "Back Ravine," *Houxi*

On a loose fist, this point is proximal to the head of the fifth metacarpal, on the medial side of the hand. It supports the back and spine, and it relieves headache, stiff neck and shoulder, and tight muscles of the elbow, arm, and fingers.

TH-5: "Outer Gate," *Weiguan*

This point is located 1½ inches proximal to the wrist crease in between the radius and the ulna. This point is helpful for headache and pain anywhere in the upper body.

TECHNIQUES FOR THE ARMS AND HANDS

Because the arms and hands are used in virtually every daily activity, it is easy to understand why chair massage clients

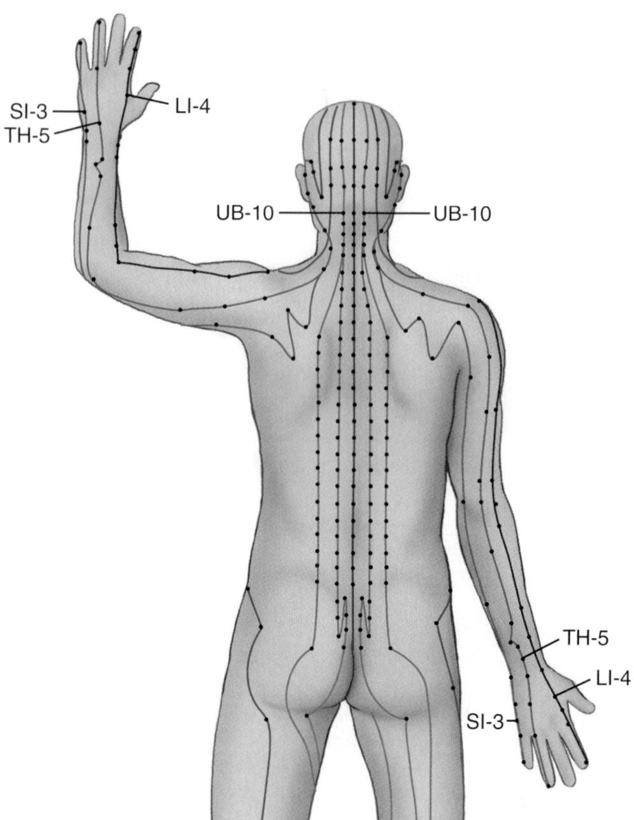

FIGURE 4-35 Tsubos to press to alleviate pain and discomfort in the head and neck. (Modified from Anderson SK: *The practice of shiatsu.* St. Louis, 2008, Mosby.)

are likely to have muscular pain and tension in the muscles of arm and hand movement. Whether clients work 8 hours a day at a computer using a mouse, have jobs requiring physical activity such as carpentry, or are stay-at-home parents who carry toddlers around, they are likely to need specific work on the arms and hands.

The muscles addressed in techniques for the arms and hand are the deltoid, triceps brachii, biceps brachii, brachialis, brachioradialis, pronator teres, pronator quadratus, supinator, wrist flexor group (anterior forearm), and the forearm extensor group (posterior forearm). See Appendix B for the specific attachments and actions of these muscles.

Arm and Hand Conditions

In addition to general muscle tension and fatigue, there are some specific arm and hand conditions that chair massage clients are likely to present with.

Tendinitis and Tenosynovitis

Definition: **Tendinitis** is the inflammation of a tendon; **tenosynovitis** is the inflammation of a tendon sheath.
Symptoms: Pain, swelling (in the acute stage). Pain and tenderness can extend into the surrounding muscles.
Causes: Trauma, repetitive use, and inflammatory diseases such as rheumatoid arthritis. **Lateral epicondylitis (tennis elbow)** is inflammation at the lateral epicondyle of the

humerus, and it is due to repetitive wrist extension or pronation/supination of the forearm. **Medial epicondylitis (golfer's or pitcher's elbow)** is inflammation at the medial epicondyle of the humerus and is due to repetitive wrist flexion.

Treatments: Analgesics, nonsteroidal anti-inflammatory drugs (NSAIDs) such as aspirin or ibuprofen, rest, braces, and gradual return to exercise.

Chair massage considerations: Practitioners should ask clients if they are taking any analgesics or anti-inflammatory medications, even over-the-counter ones. Clients who are taking an analgesic have altered pain perception and may not be able to give accurate feedback about pressure of the techniques being applied during the treatment. Therefore, practitioners should ask clients when they took their most recent dose, and if it is on the same day as the chair massage treatment, practitioners should use lighter pressure to avoid the risk of damaging tissues. Practitioners should ask clients who are taking an anti-inflammatory medication how long they have been taking it, and when they took their most recent dose. Anti-inflammatory medications can alter pain perception, and long-term use can also compromise the integrity of the tissues. If the client has been taking an anti-inflammatory medication for a short time and the most recent dose is taken the same day as the chair massage treatment, or if the client has been taking an anti-inflammatory medication for a long time (three or more months), practitioners should apply lighter pressure to avoid the risk of damaging tissues.

If the tendinitis or tenosynovitis is the result of injury, local massage is contraindicated for 72 hours because of the inflammation; massage would only make it worse. If the tendinitis or tenosynovitis is chronic and in an inflammatory stage, massage is contraindicated. If it is in a non-inflammatory stage, the area can be addressed with deep specific friction on the involved tendons, and a 20-minute follow-up treatment with ice can be recommended to the client.

Clients with adhesive capsulitis (frozen shoulder), discussed under the section "Upper Region of the Posterior Body," can also benefit from massage techniques applied to the biceps brachii, triceps brachii, and deltoid muscles.

Carpal Tunnel Syndrome

Definition: **Carpal tunnel syndrome** is a painful repetitive strain injury of the wrist and hand.

Symptoms: Pain, numbness, tingling, and weakened muscles in the hand and first three digits.

Causes: The carpal tunnel is formed where the transverse carpal ligament connects across carpal bones in the anterior wrist. The tendons of the wrist flexors and the median nerve pass through this tunnel into the hand. Tendinous sheaths may become swollen and irritated through overuse or chronically flexed wrists. The swelling can compress the median nerve. Chronic inflammation can also cause the tendon sheath to thicken, compounding the problem. Common movements that cause carpal tunnel syndrome include typing on a keyboard and passing items over a scanner at a cash register station.

Treatments: Analgesics, anti-inflammatory medications, wearing immobilizing braces on the wrists, massage therapy, surgery to open the transverse carpal ligament.

Chair massage considerations: Practitioners should ask clients if they are taking any analgesics or anti-inflammatory medications, even over-the-counter ones. Clients who are taking an analgesic have altered pain perception and may not be able to give accurate feedback about pressure of the techniques being applied during the treatment. For this reason, practitioners should ask clients when they took their most recent dose, and if it is on the same day as the chair massage treatment, practitioners should use lighter pressure to avoid the risk of damaging tissues. Practitioners should ask clients who are taking an anti-inflammatory medication how long they have been taking it, and when they took their most recent dose. Anti-inflammatory medications can alter pain perception, and long-term use can also compromise the integrity of the tissues. If the client has been taking an anti-inflammatory medication for a short time and the most recent dose is taken the same day as the chair massage treatment or if the client has been taking an anti-inflammatory medication for a long time (three or more months), practitioners should apply lighter pressure to avoid the risk of damaging tissues.

If there is acute inflammation, massage over the wrist is contraindicated. Otherwise, deep specific friction can loosen scar tissue. Passive movements of the elbow, wrist, and finger joints maintain joint range of motion. Massaging the neck, shoulders, and arms can also be helpful to reduce muscle spasms, lengthen shortened muscles, and soften and stretch surrounding connective tissue. If the client has had surgery, the area is contraindicated for massage until healing is complete (i.e., the stitches have been removed and inflammation is gone), approximately 8 to 12 weeks after the surgery. Deep specific friction in the area can help reduce adhesions from surgery.

Treatment Protocol

1. Stand in a straight stance, sit on a stool, or kneel on one knee to the front and right of your client. Place the client's left wrist between the palms of your hands and move your hands briskly back and forth to create a vigorous shaking of the client's entire arm. This technique is referred to as **noodling** because the intent of the movement is to make the arm as limp as a cooked noodle (Figure 4-36).
2. Starting at the top of the client's arm at the deltoid, use both of your hands to perform compressions along the entire length of the arm (Figure 4-37). Be sure the compressions are brisk and rhythmic, particularly over the deltoid, biceps brachii, and triceps brachii muscles.
3. Grasp the client's deltoid with both of your hands so that your thumbs are at the middle fibers of the deltoid

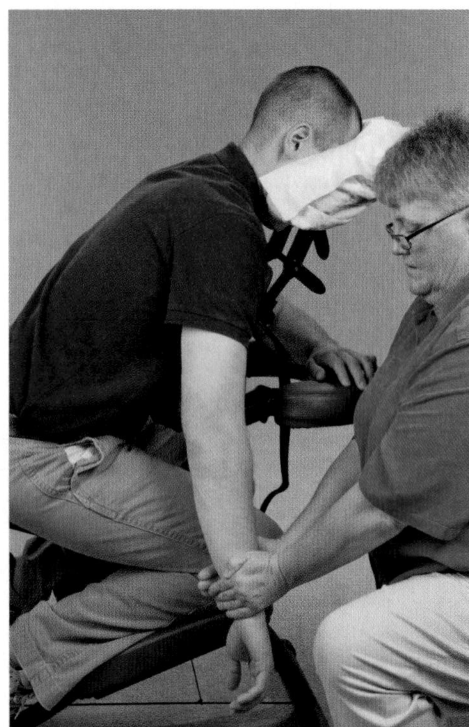

FIGURE 4-36 Noodling the arm.

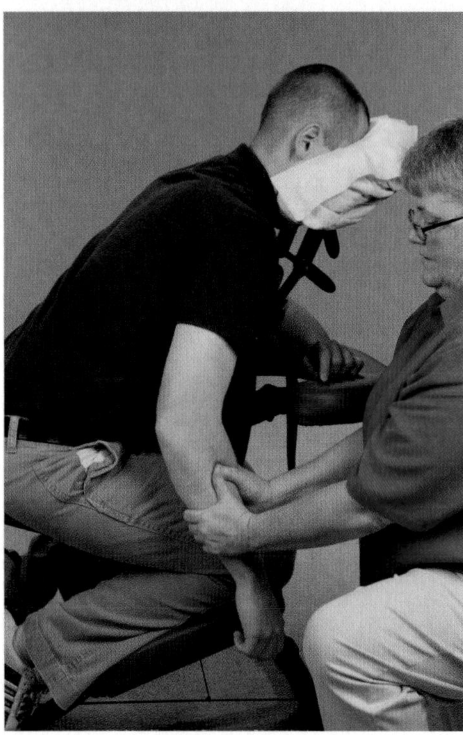

FIGURE 4-37 Using both hands to perform compressions along the entire length of the arm.

and your finger pads are in the triceps brachii. Apply pressure by moving your finger pads laterally from the middle of the arm in a compressive manner (Figure 4-38). Continue applying pressure distally until you reach the elbow. At the elbow, retrace your movements proximally to the deltoid.

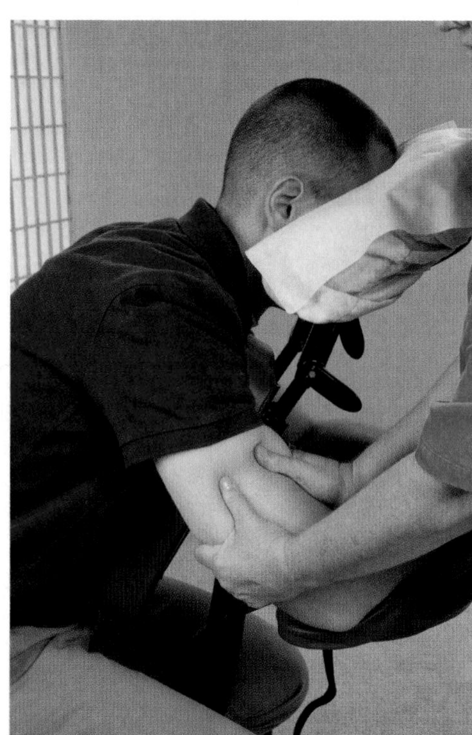

FIGURE 4-38 Applying pressure by moving the finger pads laterally from the middle of the arm in a compressive manner.

Tip Imagine you are spreading out the individual muscle fibers of the upper arm.

4. Palpate the deltoid tuberosity. Use both of your thumb pads to perform circular friction at the tuberosity (Figure 4-39).
5. Perform rhythmic compressions on the entire upper arm.
6. Grasp the client's forearm distal to the elbow with both of your hands, one just distal to the other. Tightly grasp the forearm in a wringing motion to apply deep friction on the client's forearm extensors and flexors. (Figure 4-40). Continue the motion distally to the client's wrist.

Tip This technique is most effective when the hands go in opposite directions as in wringing a towel.

7. Grasp the client's arm at the wrist and noodle the entire arm.
8. Take the client's right hand with your right hand as if you were shaking hands. Grasp the client's arm just below the elbow with your left hand. Perform deep circular friction with your left thumb along the radius from the elbow distally to the wrist. Retrace your movements proximally to the elbow (Figure 4-41). If it is warranted, perform deep specific friction on the medial or lateral epicondyle for medial epicondylitis or lateral epicondylitis, respectively.
9. Perform deep circular friction with your left thumb along the interosseous membrane while adding

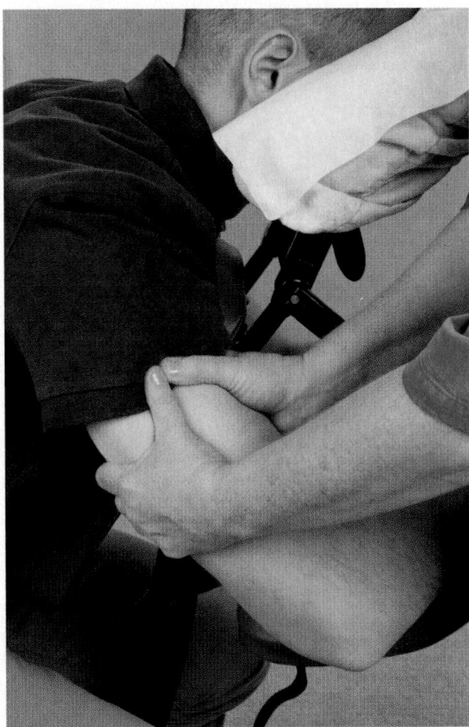

FIGURE 4-39 Circular friction at the deltoid tuberosity.

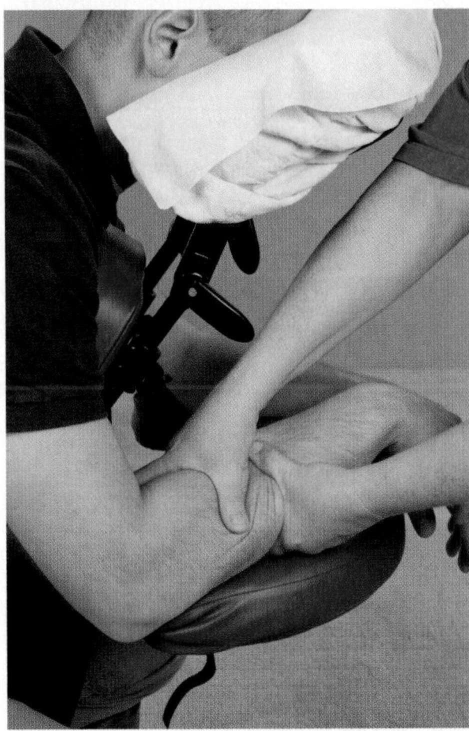

FIGURE 4-40 Grasping the forearm in a wringing motion to apply deep friction.

supinating and pronating with your right hand as you work distally from the elbow to the wrist. Retrace your movements proximally to the elbow.

10. Perform deep circular friction with your thumb along the ulna from the elbow distally to the wrist. Retrace your movements proximally to the elbow.

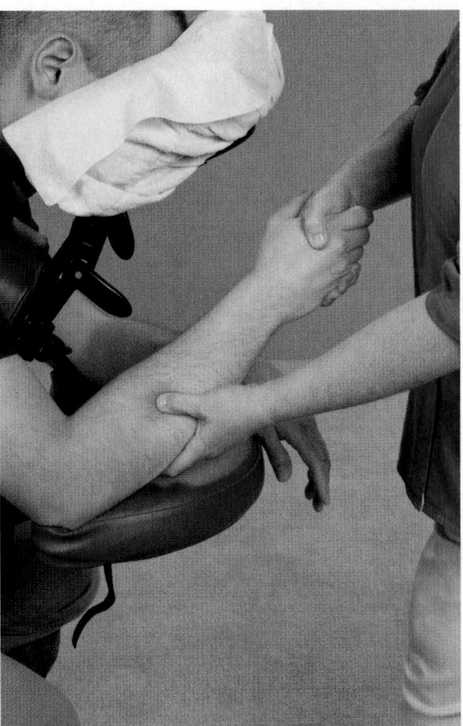

FIGURE 4-41 Deep circular friction along the radius from the elbow distally to the wrist.

11. Grasp the client's forearm with both of your hands, and perform rhythmic compressions from the elbow to the wrist. Perform noodling to shake out the client's entire arm.
12. Move to a straight stance or lunge in front of your client. Take the client's right hand with your right hand and flex the client's elbow. Palpate the brachioradialis with your left hand, then grasp it with a pincer grip and gently knead as much of the muscle as you can (Figure 4-42).
13. With the client's elbow flexed, pin the attachment site of the brachioradialis (just proximal to the elbow) (Figure 4-43 A) while you extend the client's elbow to provide a stretch (Figure 4-43 B). Repeat this stretch two more times.
14. Shake out the client's entire arm. Turn the client's hand palm down and hold it with both your hands. Apply pressure downward and outward to spread the metacarpals apart (Figure 4-44). Repeat two more times.
15. Turn your client's hand palm up. Use your thumb pads to massage the entire palm of your client's hand (Figure 4-45).
16. Interlace your fingers with the client's fingers. Once you have completed the interlacing, both of your thumbs should be on your client's palm (Figure 4-46 A). To stretch the hand, press downward with both of your hands while simultaneously using your thumb pads

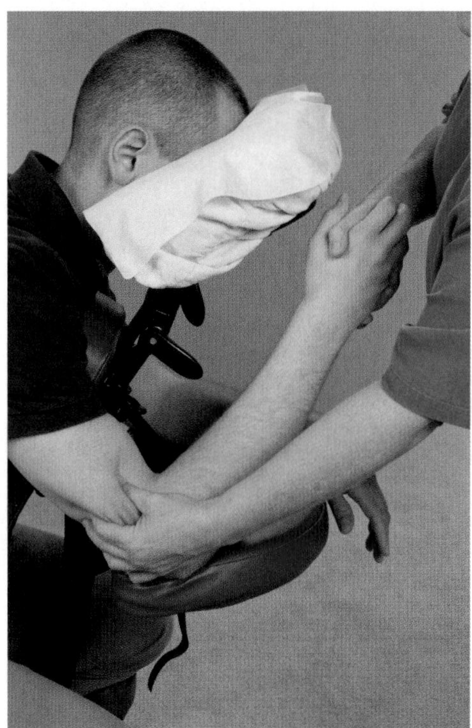

FIGURE 4-42 Grasping the brachioradialis with a pincer grip and gently kneading.

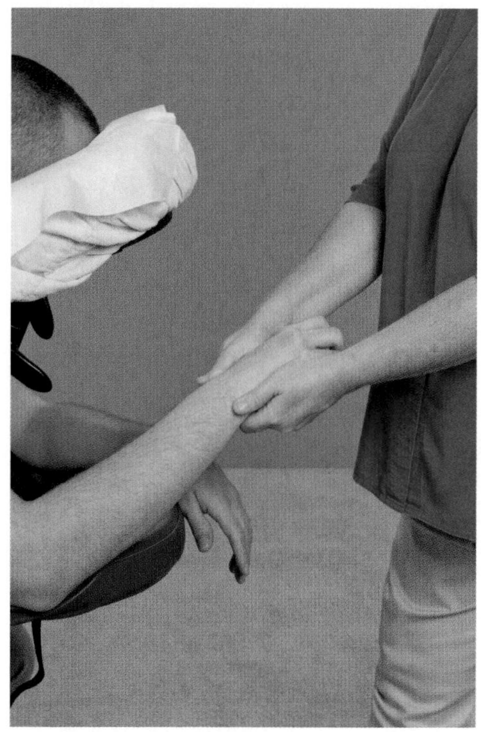

FIGURE 4-44 Spreading the metacarpals.

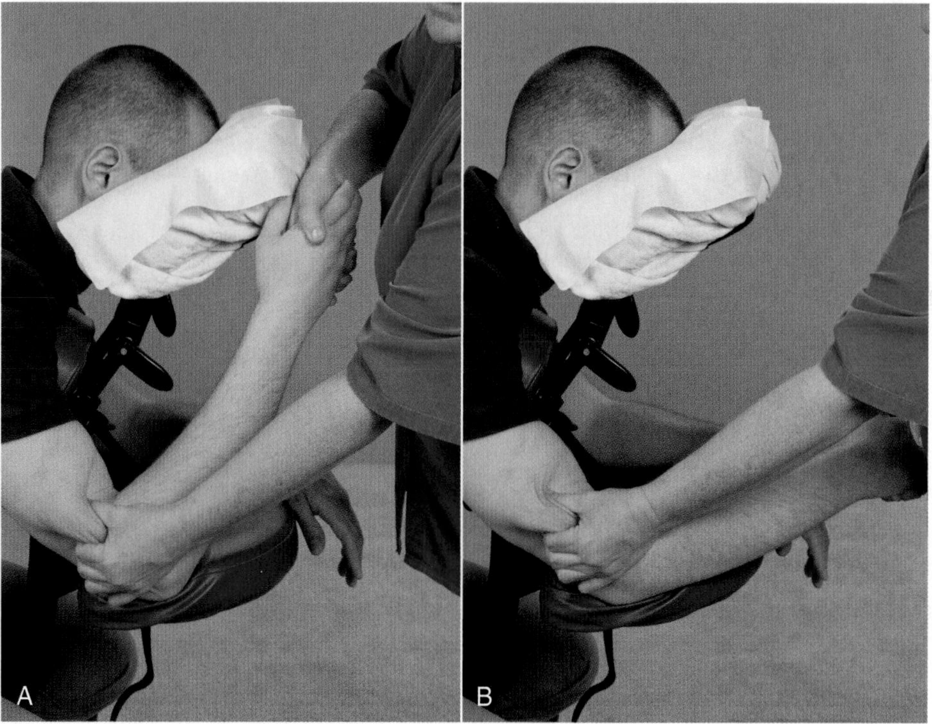

FIGURE 4-43 **A,** Pinning the attachment site of the brachioradialis **B,** Extending the client's elbow to provide a stretch.

to massage the palmar surface of the hand (Figure 4-46 B).

17. Take the client's hand, palm side up, between both your hands. Press downward, spread the client's phalanges, then release the pressure.

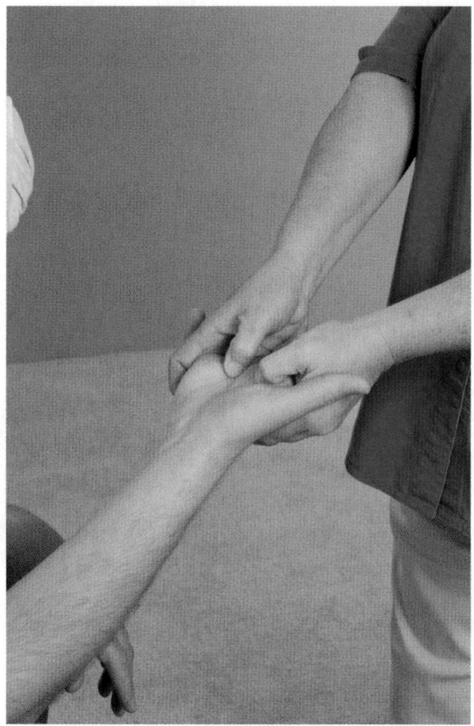

FIGURE 4-45 Massaging the palm with thumb pads.

18. Work each digit of your client's hand by gently grasping each one between your thumb and index finger and briskly gliding from the base of the finger to the tip (Figure 4-47).
19. Noodle the client's arm and place it back on the armrest.
20. Repeat Steps 1 through 19 on the client's right arm.

Tsubos

There are several tsubos that practitioners may find helpful to press to alleviate pain and discomfort in the client's arm and hand. These are all shown in Figure 4-48.

LI-10: "Arm Three Li," *Shousanli*

This point is located in the most lateral depression in the elbow crease on the yang side of the arm. It is a major point for any muscular problems of the forearm and hand.

SI-3: "Back Ravine," *Houxi*

On a loose fist, this point is proximal to the head of the fifth metacarpal on the medial side of the hand. It supports the back and spine, and it relieves headache, stiff neck and shoulder, and tight muscles of the elbow, arm, and fingers.

SI-9: "Shoulder Integrity," *Jianzhen*

This point is located approximately 1 inch superior to the posterior axillary crease. It relieves pain in the scapular area, arm, and hand.

SI-10: "Scapula Hollow," *Naoshu*

This point is located in the depression just inferior and posterior to the acromion process of the scapula, directly

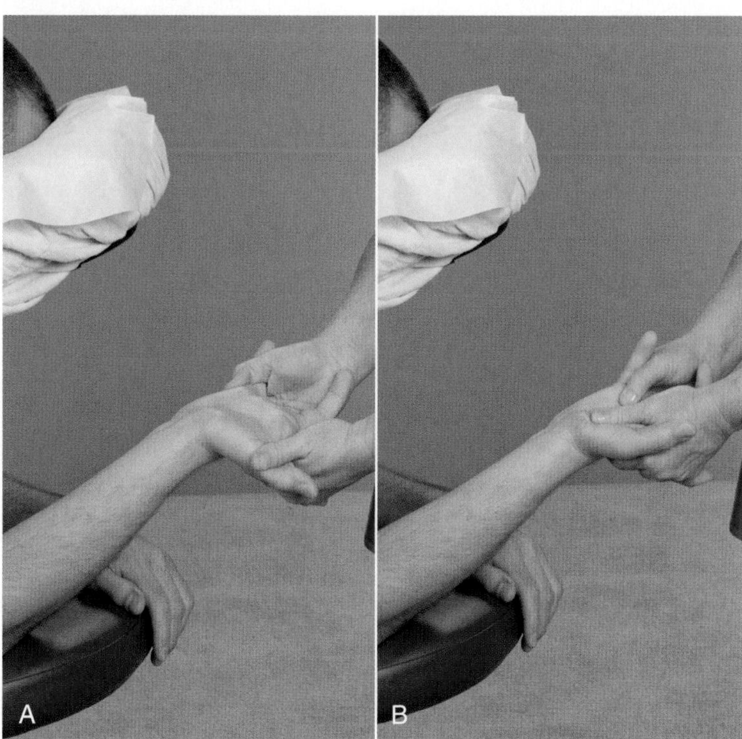

FIGURE 4-46 **A,** Interlacing with the client's fingers. **B,** Pressing downward while using thumb pads to massage the palmar surface of the hand.

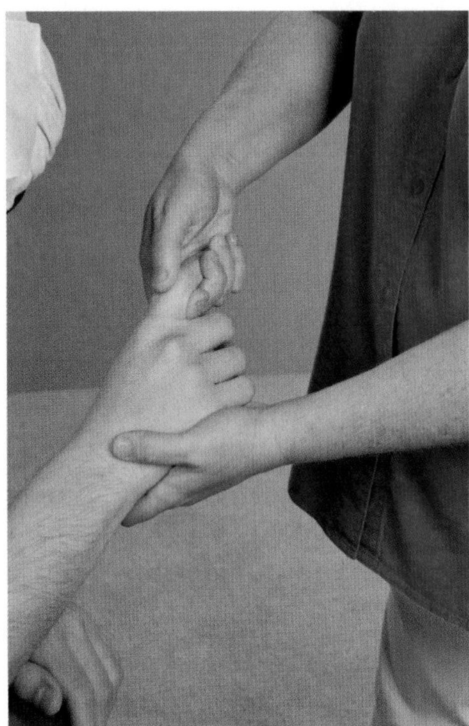

FIGURE 4-47 Gently grasping each digit and gliding from the base of the finger to the tip.

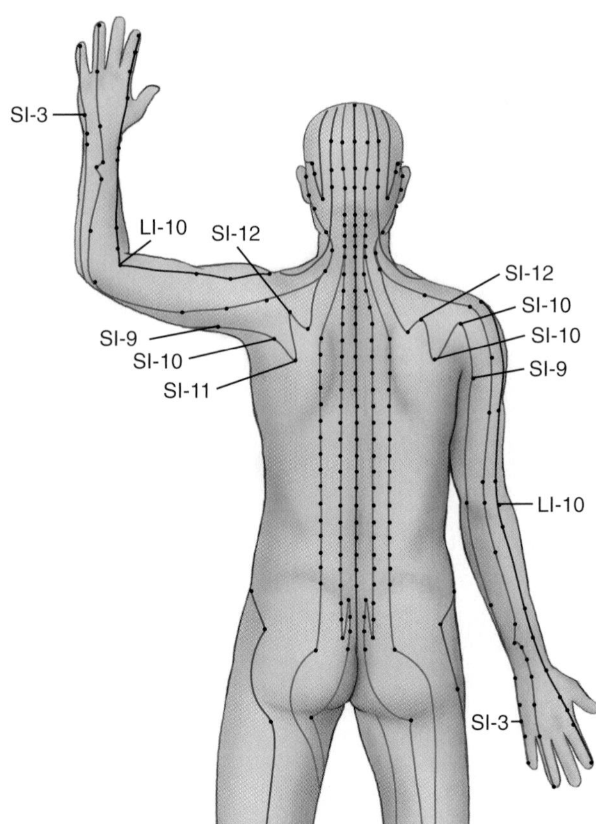

FIGURE 4-48 Tsubos to press to alleviate pain and discomfort in the arm and hand. (Modified from Anderson SK: *The practice of shiatsu.* St. Louis, 2008, Mosby.)

superior to SI-9. It relieves pain and supports the qi in the shoulder and arm.

SI-11: "Celestial Gathering," *Tianzong*

This point is located in the center of the scapula. It is a key point to the back. It diffuses qi stagnation in the chest and ribcage.

SI-12: "Grasping the Wind," *Bingfeng*

This point is located in the suprascapular fossa directly superior to SI-11. It relieves pain and numbness in the shoulder, arm, and hand.

CLOSING THE TREATMENT SESSION

A chair massage session does not end until the client is walking away from the practitioner. This means that the practitioner remains present and in communication with the client even after the hands-on portion is done so the client is not confused about what to do when the practitioner stops working. Practitioners have been known to walk away from the client to wash their hands while the client is still in the chair with his or her face in the face cradle. Imagine how clients might feel when they eventually sit up and notice that the practitioner is no longer around. Confused? Unsure? Abandoned? It is definitely unprofessional on the part of the practitioner.

Helping the Client Out of the Chair

The practitioner should be clear when letting the client know that the treatment session is over by saying something like, "We're done now. It's time for you to lift your head out of the face cradle and sit up straight." As the client does so, the practitioner should hold onto the face cradle covering so that it does not stick to the client's face, then ask the client to slide the legs out from the kneeling pads so that the feet are on the floor. As the client sits for a moment, the practitioner should check to see if the client is experiencing any dizziness or nausea. If so, the client should remain seated until able to stand. The client should be asked if he or she has any questions, and, after answering them, the practitioner should say, "When you are ready, I will help you out of the chair."

The practitioner should explain that the chair will be stabilized so that the client need not worry whether the chair will tip over or cause the client to stumble. The practitioner should also remind the client that the easiest way to exit the chair is by backing off it.

If water is available, the practitioner should then offer the client a drink explain the importance of increasing water intake for the next 24 hours. Sometimes clients who are dehydrated will experience soreness after receiving massage, and drinking water helps alleviate that. Also, clients who have nausea or dizziness from the treatment may be subject to vasovagal syncope (discussed in Chapter 3). Drinking water will help increase blood volume and blood pressure.

Posttreatment Interview

It can be helpful to conduct a posttreatment interview with the client. This interview can consist of one or two questions or be an in-depth interview lasting several minutes. It all depends on the setting in which the chair massage is taking place. For example, at a sports event in which many clients are lined up waiting to receive treatments, the posttreatment interview needs to be short and to the point. At a regularly scheduled corporate office account in which the practitioner has several minutes between each client, the posttreatment interview can last longer.

Generally, the practitioner is looking for feedback on what the client experienced during the treatment. The following are some questions the practitioner can ask:

- How do you feel?
- What methods were most effective for you today?
- Has your pain/discomfort changed? If so, how?
- What might I improve on during the next session? (This question is important if it is likely the practitioner will see this client again.)

SUMMARY

Specific techniques for the neck, shoulders, arms and hands, and the low back, including the gluteals, are designed to address the most common conditions and complaints chair massage clients have in each of these regions. The definition, symptoms, causes, treatments, and chair massage considerations are presented for each condition or complaint.

The muscles addressed in the upper region of the posterior body are the trapezius, the rotator cuff muscles, teres major, and rhomboids. Besides general muscle tension and tightness in the shoulders and upper back, adhesive capsulitis is a shoulder disorder that practitioners may encounter in chair massage clients. The muscles addressed in the mid and low back are the latissimus dorsi, the erector spinae group, quadratus lumborum, gluteus maximus, and gluteus medius. Besides general muscle tension and tightness in the mid and low back, conditions that practitioners may encounter in chair massage clients include muscle strain, sprain, and disk herniation. The muscles addressed in techniques for the neck and head are the upper trapezius, sternocleidomastoid (SCM), splenius capitis and cervicis, semispinalis capitis, scalenes, the suboccipital group, and levator scapula. Besides general muscle tension and tightness in the neck and head, conditions that practitioners may encounter in chair massage clients include tension headache, thoracic outlet syndrome, and torticollis. The muscles addressed in techniques for the arms and hand are the deltoid, triceps brachii, biceps brachii, brachialis, brachioradialis, pronator teres, pronator quadratus, supinator, wrist flexor group (anterior forearm), and the forearm extensor group (posterior forearm). Besides general muscle tension, tightness, and fatigue in the arm and hand, conditions that practitioners may encounter in chair massage clients include tendinitis, tenosynovitis, lateral epicondylitis, medial epicondylitis, and carpal tunnel syndrome.

The practitioner should be clear when letting the client know that the treatment session is over. The practitioner should check to see if the client is experiencing any dizziness or nausea (making sure the client remains seated until able to stand), ask if the client has any questions, and, after answering them, help the client out of the chair, offer the client a drink of water (if possible), and conduct a posttreatment interview.

STUDY QUESTIONS

Answers to Study Questions are located on page 227.

Multiple Choice

1. Which of the following is an example of a repetitive stress injury?
   a. Joint sprain
   b. Adhesive capsulitis
   c. Carpal tunnel syndrome
   d. Tension headache

2. What is the term for the joint trauma that stretches or tears the ligaments of a joint but does not dislocate the bones?
   a. Sprain
   b. Strain
   c. Herniated disk
   d. Tendinitis

3. Which of the following can result from lifting using the small muscles of the back while twisting the torso?
   a. Muscle strain
   b. Low back sprain
   c. Disk herniation
   d. All of the above

4. What is another name for tennis elbow?
   a. Medial epicondylitis
   b. Lateral epicondylitis
   c. Carpal tunnel syndrome
   d. Thoracic outlet syndrome

5. Which of the following tsubos is helpful for relieving headache?
   a. GB-30
   b. TH-5
   c. SI-10
   d. LI-10

Fill in the Blank

1. A(n) ______________ is a point that is an opening or gateway into a channel and is a direct link between the channel and the outside world.

2. The muscle that can be accessed by standing to the client's side and placing straight fingers deep to the erector spinae group in the lumbar region is ______________ ______________.

3. Placing the client's left wrist between the palms of your hands and moving your hands briskly back and forth to create a vigorous shaking of the client's entire arm is referred to as ______________ the arm.

4. The muscles that can be involved in thoracic outlet syndrome are the ______________ and ______________.

5. Two tsubos that should not be used on a pregnant client are ______________ and ______________.

Short Answer

1. Give the definition, symptoms and causes of, and treatments and massage considerations for adhesive capsulitis.

____

____

____

____

____

STUDY QUESTIONS

2. Give the definition, symptoms and causes of, and treatments and massage considerations for carpal tunnel syndrome.

3. Give the definition, symptoms and causes of, and treatments and massage considerations for disk herniation.

4. Give the definition, symptoms and causes of, and treatments and massage considerations for tendinitis and tenosynovitis.

5. Give the definition, symptoms and causes of, and treatments and massage considerations for lateral epicondylitis and medial epicondylitis.

6. Give the definition, symptoms and causes of, and treatments and massage considerations for muscle strain.

7. Give the definition, symptoms and causes of, and treatments and massage considerations for sprain.

8. Give the definition, symptoms and causes of, and treatments and massage considerations for tension headache.

9. Give the definition, symptoms and causes of, and treatments and massage considerations for thoracic outlet syndrome.

STUDY QUESTIONS

10. Describe the factors involved in closing the treatment session.

ACTIVITIES

1. Practice the techniques for the upper region of the posterior body, mid and low back, head and neck, and arm and hand on at least 10 people such as friends and family. Work on people with various body sizes and shapes.
2. Practice locating the tsubos listed in the chapter for each area of the body. Record whether or not pressing the tsubos has the effects described.
3. Practice assisting clients out of the massage chair and conducting posttreatment interviews.

Additional Techniques and Adaptations

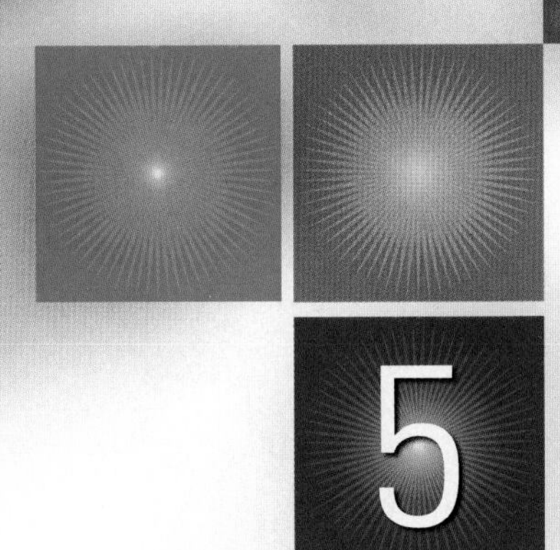

OBJECTIVES

Upon completion of this chapter, the reader will have the information necessary to do the following:

1. Perform stretches for the neck, upper trapezius, pectoralis muscles, shoulders, and arms.
2. Perform specific techniques, other than stretches, for the neck muscles, pectoralis muscles, serratus anterior, iliotibial (IT) band or tract, and the calf muscles.
3. Explain how to move a client to the massage table or futon from the massage chair to receive additional techniques.
4. Perform shiatsu and Thai massage techniques on the client on the futon as an addition to the chair massage treatment.
5. Perform chair massage techniques adapted for clients who use wheelchairs.
6. Perform chair massage techniques adapted for clients in bed.
7. Perform chair massage techniques for clients sitting in straight-backed chairs.

KEY TERMS

Active pin-and-stretch	Myofascial pin-and-stretch
Bulldozing	Passive pin-and-stretch

ADDITIONAL TECHNIQUES

An important distinguishing characteristic of good bodywork practitioners is innovation. Regularly learning new techniques gives practitioners more tools for addressing whatever conditions with which clients present, regular clients benefit from fresh approaches, and learning and practicing new techniques keeps practitioners interested, challenged, and sparks their creativity.

Additional techniques beyond basic chair massage routines can range from stretches for certain areas of the body to detailed work to alleviate conditions the client is experiencing. There are also methods for making a fluid transition from the massage chair to the massage table or futon to continue the therapeutic work being performed. Some Asian bodywork techniques done with the client on a futon can also help to address specific conditions, namely, tightness in the low back, hips, and legs. These methods are all presented in this chapter.

Clients who use wheelchairs, or who are in bed for long periods of time such as for stays in a hospital, hospice, or the home for various medical reasons, can benefit from techniques adapted from chair massage. Ways to perform these types of treatments are also explained in this chapter.

STRETCHES

There are many stretches that practitioners can incorporate into their chair massage treatments. In particular, stretches for the neck, pectoralis muscles, arm muscles, and upper trapezius can be especially useful. These stretches should never be forced; the client is in charge of how far the stretch should be taken. As with all bodywork techniques, if the client is uncomfortable with any of the positions or stretches, the practitioner should either modify them or not do them at all.

Stretches for the Neck

The following are effective stretches for tight neck muscles. Contraindications for neck stretches include any of the following conditions in the client's cervical region:

- Arthritis
- Ankylosing spondylitis
- Herniated disk
- Fused vertebrae (for any reason)
- Osteoporosis
- Nerve impingement in the cervical region
- Any other disorders affecting the cervical vertebrae
- Client hypersensitivity

Lateral Neck Stretch

1. Move your client's arms from the armrest so they are hanging down by the client's sides. Stand behind your client in a straight stance. Have the client bring the right arm up over the side and top of the head so that the right hand touches the left ear (Figure 5-1 A).

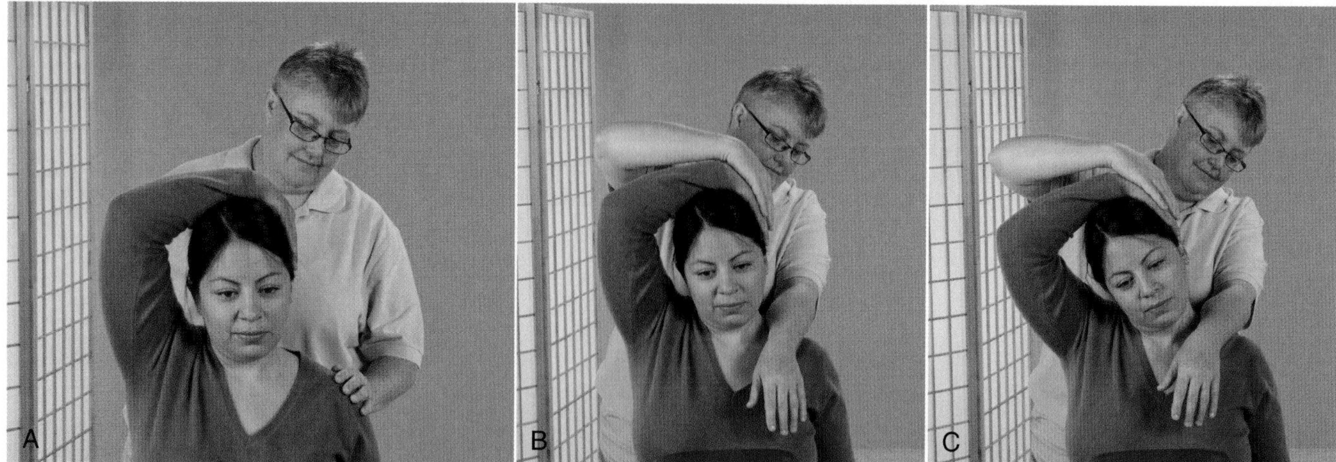

FIGURE 5-1 A, The client reaching the right hand over the head and touching the left ear. **B,** Placing the left forearm on top of the client's left medial upper trapezius, and placing the right hand on top of the client's head to help stabilize the head. **C,** Pulling the client's head over with the right hand as far as is comfortable for the client.

2. Place your left forearm on top of your client's left medial upper trapezius. Place your right hand on top of your client's right hand to help stabilize the head (Figure 5-1 B).
3. Ask your client to take a deep breath. On the exhale, have the client pull the head over with the right hand as far as is comfortable while you drop your weight into your knees and press down with your left forearm. This helps increase the lateral stretch of the neck (Figure 5-1 C). *Do not apply pressure to the client's head with your right hand because you may end up stretching the client's lateral neck more than is comfortable or safe for the client.* The client determines how much he or she wants the neck stretched. If you are concerned that you will apply pressure to the client's head, you can place your right hand on your left forearm instead. Ask your client to tell you when it feels like the stretch has lasted long enough. Have the client release the head and bring it back to center while you release your forearm pressure.
4. Repeat Steps 1 through 3 on the client's right side of the neck.

> **TIP** Be sure that the client's inactive arm is not resting on the armrest or the leg. This will decrease the length, and the effectiveness, of the stretch.

Posterior Neck Stretch

1. Stand behind your client in a straight stance. Have your client sit upright and bring both arms up behind the head, clasping the hands at, and the thumbs below, the occipital ridge. The client should feel like the hands are cradling the head (Figure 5-2 A).
2. Place your arms under each of the client's upper arms with your hands on top of your client's wrists (Figure 5-2 B).
3. Have your client inhale deeply. On the exhale, have the client drop the chin to the chest while you gently press down on the wrists. This assists the posterior neck stretch (Figure 5-2 C). Have the client tell you when there is enough stretch in the posterior neck. Stop applying any more pressure, and hold the stretch for 7 to 10 seconds, then release.
4. When the stretch is completed, have the client bring the head back up and drop the arms.

> **TIP** Bilateral kneading on the upper trapezius at the end of this stretch can be performed as a closing measure.

Techniques for Upper Trapezius

These techniques are effective for loosening tight upper trapezius muscles.

Upper Trapezius Stretch

The contraindications for this stretch include the following:

- Arthritis in the shoulder joint
- Shoulder joint replacement
- Osteoporosis
- Nerve impingement in the cervical or thoracic regions
- Any other disorders affecting the shoulder joint
- Client hypersensitivity in the muscles involved

1. Stand to the left of your client in a straight stance, facing the client. Place your left hand on your client's upper trapezius, palm down. Place your right hand under your

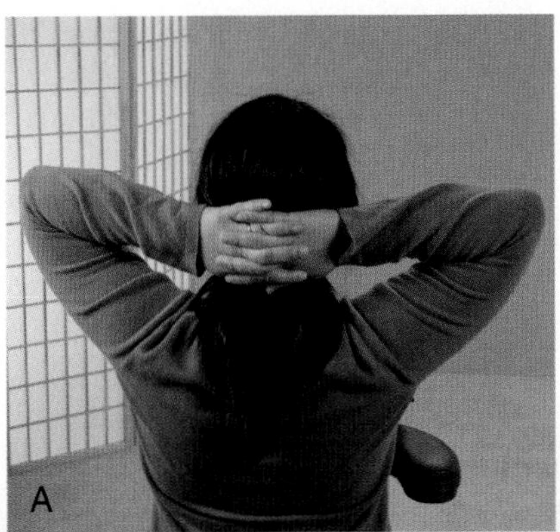

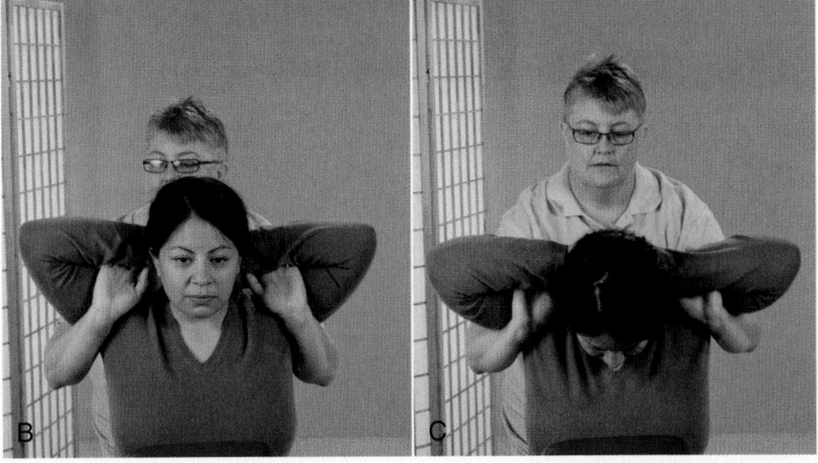

FIGURE 5-2 **A,** The client clasping the hands at the occipital ridge, with the thumbs below the occipital ridge. **B,** The practitioner placing the arms under each of the client's upper arms and the hands on top of the client's wrists. **C,** The client dropping the chin to the chest with the practitioner gently pressing down on the client's wrists.

client's left arm at the inferior angle of the scapula (Figure 5-3 A).

2. Have the client inhale deeply. On the exhale, depress the upper trapezius with your left hand while medially rotating the scapula with your right hand (Figure 5-3 B). Have the client tell you when a stretch is felt. Hold for 7 to 10 seconds, then release.
3. Repeat Steps 1 and 2 on the client's right arm.

Myofascial Pin-and-Stretch of the Lateral Neck Muscles and Upper Trapezius

Myofascial pin-and-stretch is a technique whereby the practitioner stabilizes (pins) the attachment site of a muscle or muscles. Movement of the area then occurs, causing elongation of the muscles involved, thus stretching the associated fascia. If the client creates the movement, it is an **active pin-and-stretch** because the client is using muscular contraction. If the practitioner creates the movement, it is a **passive pin-and-stretch** because the client's muscles stay relaxed while the practitioner moves the body part.

The following myofascial pin-and-stretch techniques of the lateral neck and upper trapezius muscles are active, and they stretch and elongate the fascia overlying these muscles. Because shortened fascia can cause pain and restricted range of motion, pinning and stretching the fascia can be an effective technique. However, some clients may experience some discomfort with the myofascial stretch. This discomfort can be experienced as tightness and possibly a burning sensation as the fascia elongates. Clients should be fully informed about the sensations that can be experienced with this technique and be given the option to decline. With consent, the practitioner should emphasize that in this technique the client is in control of the stretch and that the degree of stretch is determined by how far the client turns the head. Also, the client has the right to tell the practitioner to stop the technique at any time.

Contraindications for this technique include any of the following conditions in the client's cervical region:

- Arthritis
- Ankylosing spondylitis
- Herniated disk
- Fused vertebrae (for any reason)
- Osteoporosis
- Nerve impingement in the cervical or thoracic regions
- Any other disorders affecting the cervical vertebrae
- Client hypersensitivity in the muscles involved

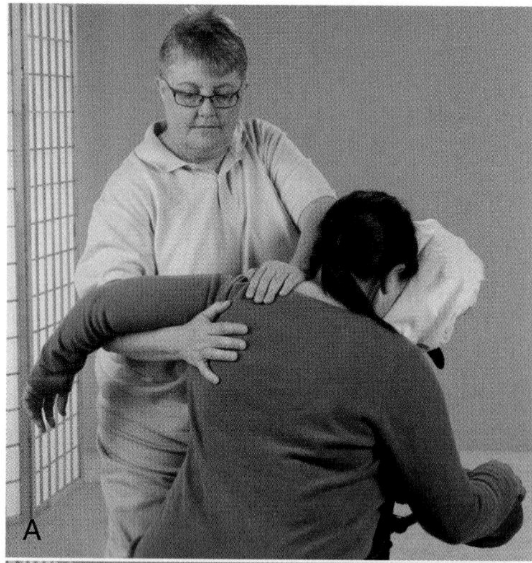

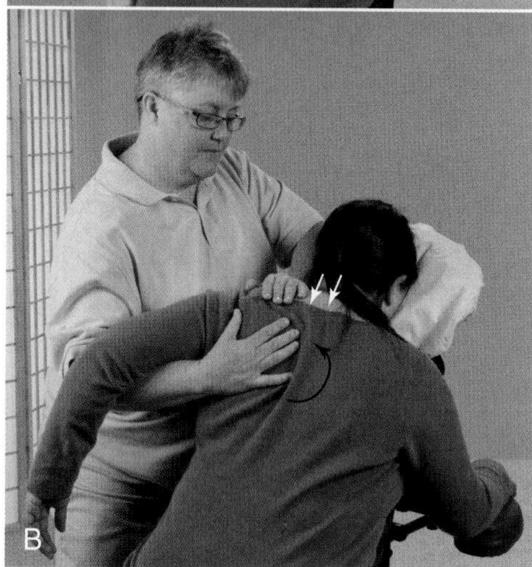

FIGURE 5-3 A, Placing the left hand on the client's upper trapezius and the right hand under the client's left arm at the inferior angle of the scapula. **B,** Depressing the upper trapezius with the left hand while medially rotating the scapula with the right hand.

1. Stand behind your client in a straight stance. Have the client sit upright, and turn the head as far to the right as is comfortable (Figure 5-4 A). This motion creates some slack in the right upper trapezius.
2. With your right hand, tightly grasp, without pinching, as much of the right upper trapezius as you would if you were kneading. Pull the muscle upward. You are essentially pinning the upper trapezius to enhance the stretch. Place your left hand on your client's left upper trapezius to stabilize (Figure 5-4 B).

> **TIP** If the client has a large body, it may be necessary to use both of your hands to pin the right upper trapezius.

3. Have your client inhale deeply. On the exhale, have the client *slowly* turn the head to the left as far as is comfortable (Figure 5-4 C). While this is happening, maintain your grasp on the right upper trapezius for the pin-and-stretch of the lateral neck muscles and upper trapezius. Hold for 7 to 10 seconds.
4. Ask your client to tell you when it feels like the stretch has lasted long enough. Have the client turn the head face forward, and release your gasp on the right upper trapezius.
5. Repeat Steps 1 through 4 on your client's left side.

Stretches for the Pectoralis Muscles

Pectoralis Muscle Stretch

The positioning for and performance of this stretch may not be comfortable for clients who have a larger body size. Practitioners should check in with the client about comfort levels and not perform this technique if the client is not at ease with it. Other contraindications include the following:

- Arthritis in the shoulder, elbow, wrist, or hand joints
- Shoulder joint replacement
- Osteoporosis
- Nerve impingement in the cervical or thoracic regions
- Any other disorders affecting the shoulder, elbow, wrist, or hand joints
- Client hypersensitivity in the muscles involved

1. Stand behind your client in a straight stance. Have your client sit upright. Reach over the front of your client's arms, and then weave your arms back under them (between your client's arms and torso) (Figure 5-5 A). Then clasp your hands between the client's scapulae, effectively pinning your client's arms and opening the chest (Figures 5-5 B and C).
2. Have your client take a deep breath. On the exhale, simultaneously extend your arms while lifting upward to create a stretch in the client's pectoralis muscles (Figure 5-5 D). Hold for 7 to 10 seconds, then release.

Pectoralis Stretch with Client's Hands Clasped behind Head

Contraindications for this stretch include the following:

- Arthritis in the shoulder, elbow, wrist, or hand joints
- Shoulder joint replacement
- Osteoporosis
- Nerve impingement in the cervical or thoracic regions
- Any other disorders affecting the shoulder, elbow, wrist, or hand joints
- Client hypersensitivity in the muscles involved

1. Stand behind your client in a straight stance. Have the client sit up with the hands clasped behind the head (Figure 5-6 A).
2. Grasp your client's elbows, and gently lean back to stretch the pectoralis muscles (Figure 5-6 B). Hold for 7 to 10 seconds, then release.

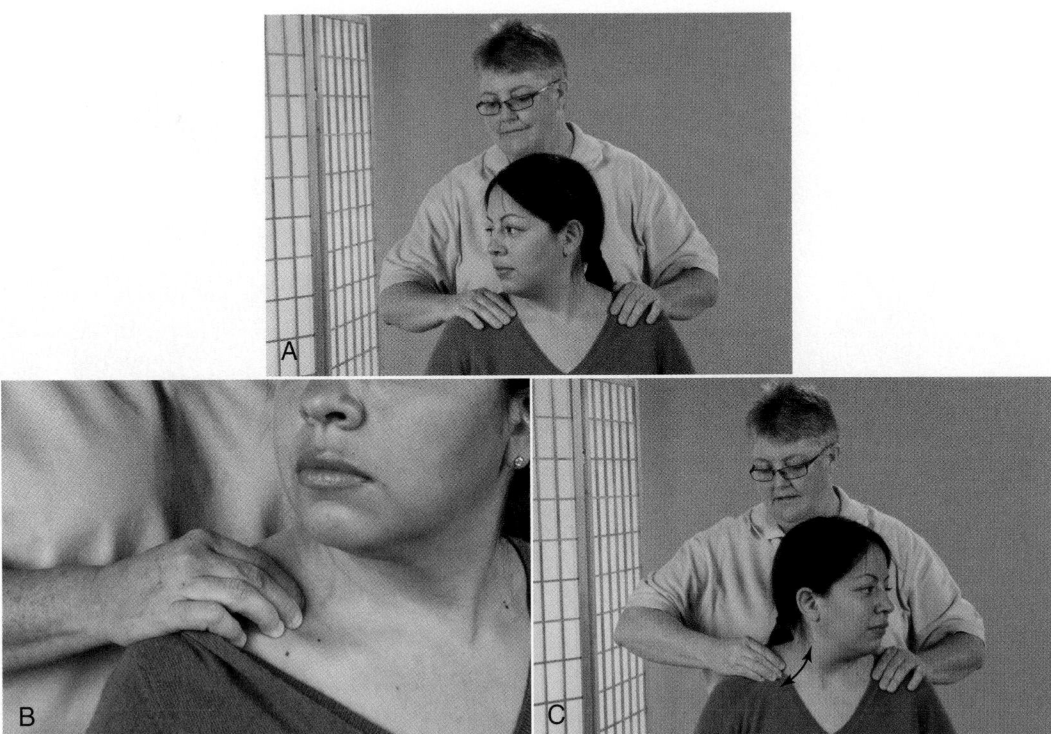

FIGURE 5-4 **A,** The client turning the head as far to the right as is comfortable. **B,** Grasping, without pinching, the client's right upper trapezius and pulling the muscle upward, and placing the left hand on the client's left upper trapezius to stabilize. **C,** The client slowly turning the head to the left while exhaling.

3. This stretch can be modified by placing your foot on the back of the seat of the chair so that your flexed knee provides a support for your client to lean into, thus deepening the stretch (Figure 5-6 C).

If there is not enough room on the seat to easily support your foot, *do not use this modification of the technique.* It is unprofessional to ask your client to scoot forward or to slide your foot around on the seat while finding somewhere to place it.

Shoulder and Arm Stretches

These stretches are effective for loosening tight muscles of the shoulders and arms. Contraindications for these stretches include the following:

- Arthritis in the shoulder, elbow, wrist, or hand joints
- Shoulder joint replacement
- Osteoporosis
- Nerve impingement in the cervical or thoracic regions
- Any other disorders affecting the shoulder, elbow, wrist, or hand joints
- Client hypersensitivity in the muscles involved

Arm Stretch at the Shoulder Joint

1. Stand on the right side of your client, facing forward, in a lunge position with your right leg forward and your left leg back. With your left hand, grasp your client's right arm at the biceps brachii so that your hand is on the inside of your client's arm (Figure 5-7 A). Lift your client's arm and grasp it mid-forearm or at the wrist with your right hand. Whether to grasp it mid-forearm or at the wrist is based on which position gives you the most control during the stretch.
2. Ask the client to take a deep breath. On the exhale, continue lifting the arm upward as you lunge forward as far as is comfortable for the client (ask the client to tell you when this is), thus stretching the arm forward (Figure 5-7 B). Latissimus dorsi will be stretched also. Hold for 7 to 10 seconds, then release.
3. Repeat Steps 1 and 2 on the client's right arm.

Arm Stretch While Standing in Front of Client

1. Stand in front and to the right of your client in a lunge position with your left leg forward and your right leg back. Interlock your flexed right elbow with the client's flexed right elbow, and have the client's hand point downward. Grasp the client's right wrist with your left hand to stabilize the arm (Figure 5-8 A).
2. Lift the client's arm upward and anteriorly while you lean backward as far as is comfortable for the client (ask the client to tell you when this is) (Figure 5-8 B). The client should feel the shoulder girdle open with this stretch. Hold 7 to 10 seconds, then release.
3. Repeat Steps 1 and 2 on the client's right arm.

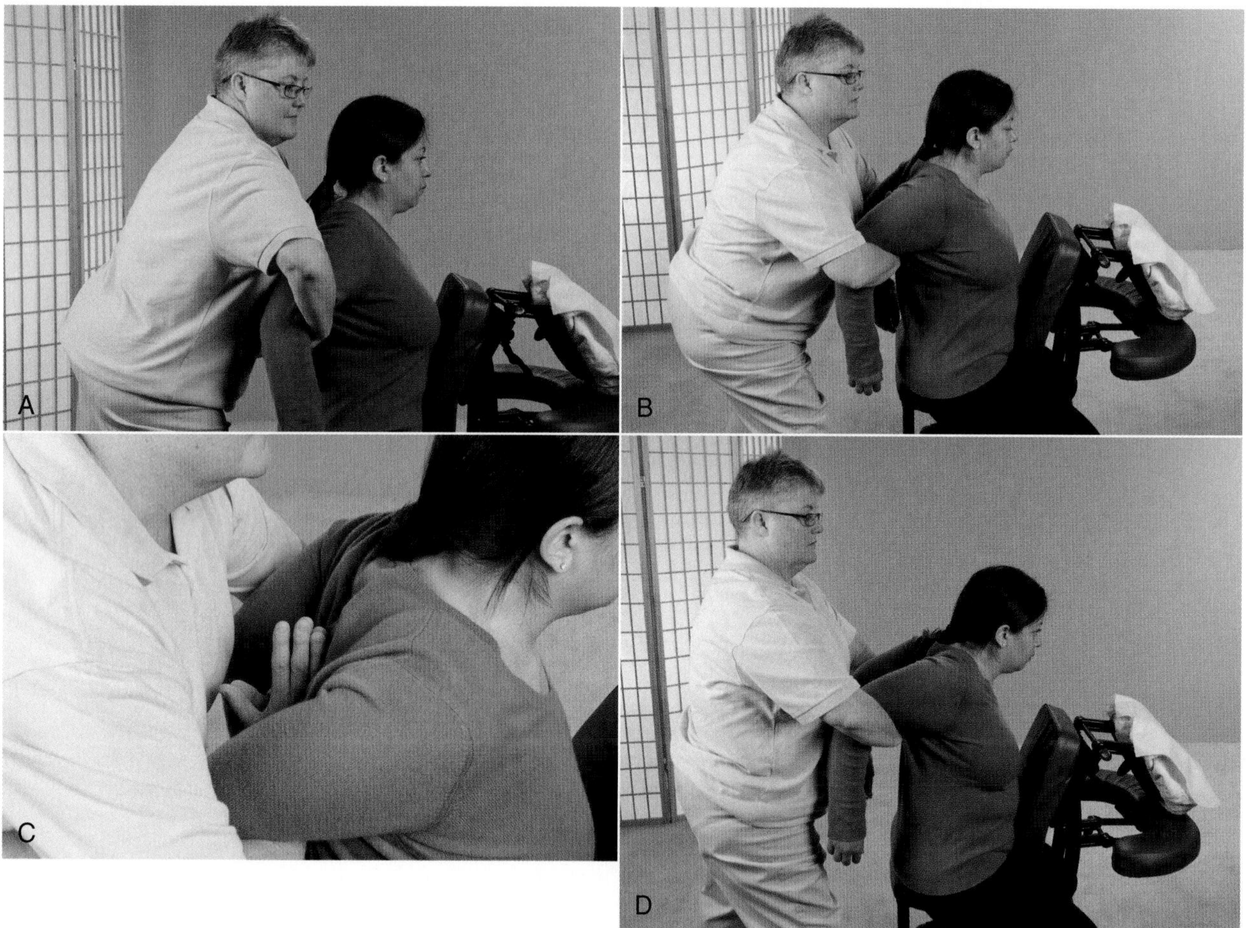

FIGURE 5-5 **A,** The practitioner reaching the arms over the front of the client's arms, then weaving back under them. **B** and **C,** The practitioner clasping the hands between the client's scapulae. **D,** As the client exhales, the practitioner extending the arms while lifting upward to create a stretch in the client's pectoralis muscles.

Triceps Brachii Stretch

1. Stand behind and to the right side of your client. Raise the client's right arm with the elbow flexed until the point of the elbow is up alongside the head and the client's hand is just inferior to the posterior neck. (The client should look as if giving oneself a pat on the back.) (Figure 5-9 A.)
2. Place your right hand on the client's elbow and your left hand on the client's right upper trapezius to stabilize (Figure 5-9 B).
3. Ask your client to inhale deeply. On the exhale, press the client's elbow posteriorly as far as is comfortable for the client (ask the client to tell you when this is). (Figure 5-9 C). Hold for 7 to 10 seconds, then release.

   This stretch can be modified by pressing the elbow laterally to engage different muscles fibers of the triceps brachii, as well as the rhomboids (Figure 5-9 D). Hold for 7 to 10 seconds, then release.
4. Repeat Steps 1 through 4 on the client's left arm.

Triceps Brachii Stretch with Sustained Pressure in Upper Trapezius

This stretch is similar to the triceps brachii stretch just described. In this instance, pressure from the elbow is added so that the practitioner can apply two techniques at the same time: sustained pressure in the client's upper trapezius while stretching the client's triceps brachii.

1. Before bringing the client's arm upward, place your flexed right elbow in the client's left upper trapezius at the attachment site of the levator scapula or anywhere in the area between the clavicle and the scapula.
2. Bring the client's arm upward so that both your hands are grasping the elbow (Figure 5-10 A). Ask your client to take a deep breath. On the exhale, depress your right elbow into the upper trapezius while moving the client's elbow posteriorly to create the stretch (Figure 5-10 B). Hold 7 to 10 seconds, then release.
3. Repeat Steps 1 and 2 on the client's right arm.

TECHNIQUES FOR OTHER AREAS OF THE BODY

Other areas of the client's body that can benefit from specific techniques performed during chair massage, besides stretches, include the serratus anterior, anterior and lateral neck muscles, pectoralis muscles, iliotibial (IT) band or tract, and the calf muscles.

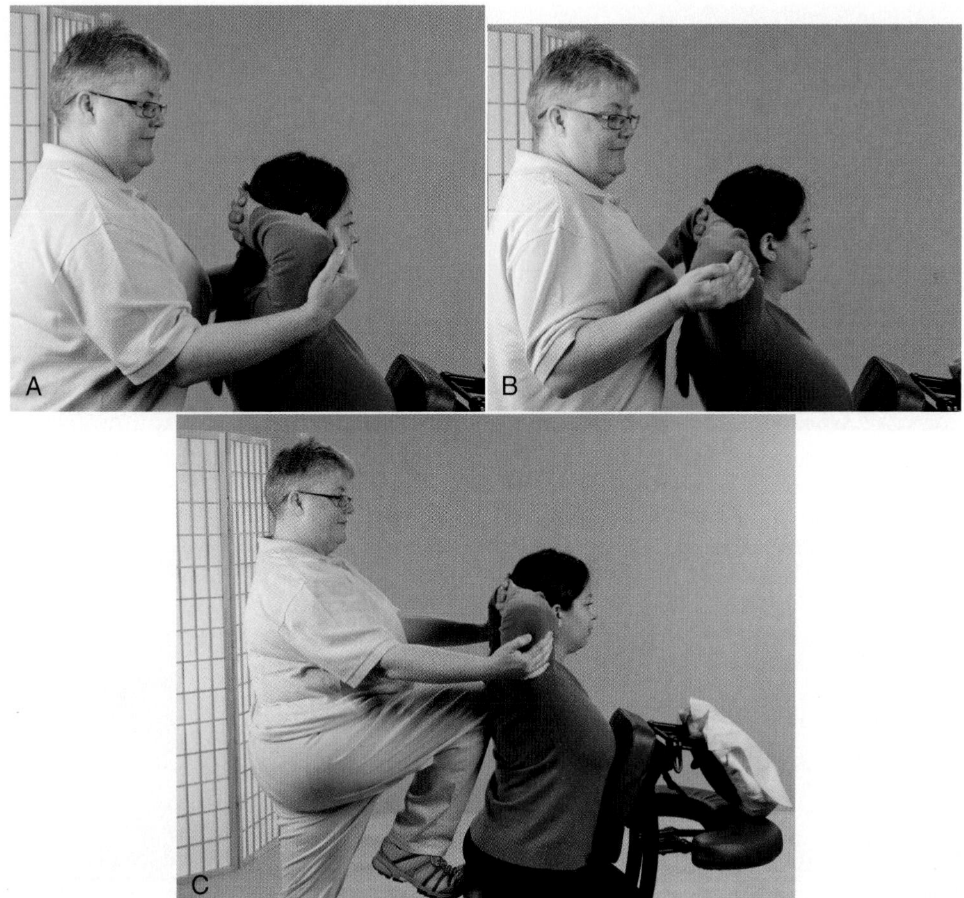

FIGURE 5-6 **A,** The client clasping the hands behind the head. **B,** Grasping the client's elbows and gently leaning back to stretch the pectoralis muscles. **C,** The practitioner placing the foot on the back edge of the chair seat so that the flexed knee provides a support for the client to lean into, thus deepening the stretch.

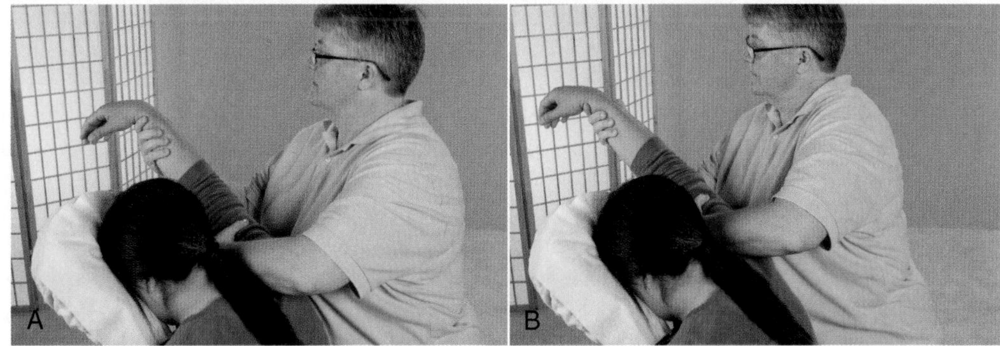

FIGURE 5-7 **A,** Grasping the right arm at the biceps brachii so that the hand is on the inside of the client's arm, and lifting the client's arm and grasping it at the wrist with the right hand. **B,** On the exhale, continuing to lift the arm upward while lunging forward, thus stretching the arm forward.

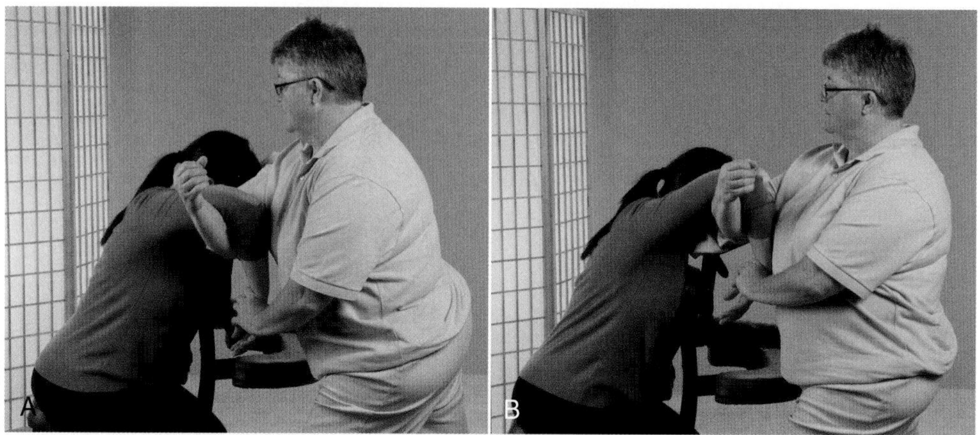

FIGURE 5-8 **A,** Interlocking the flexed elbow with the client's flexed elbow, and the hand pointing downward, and grasping the wrist with the hand to stabilize the arm. **B,** Lifting the client's arm upward and anteriorly while leaning backward.

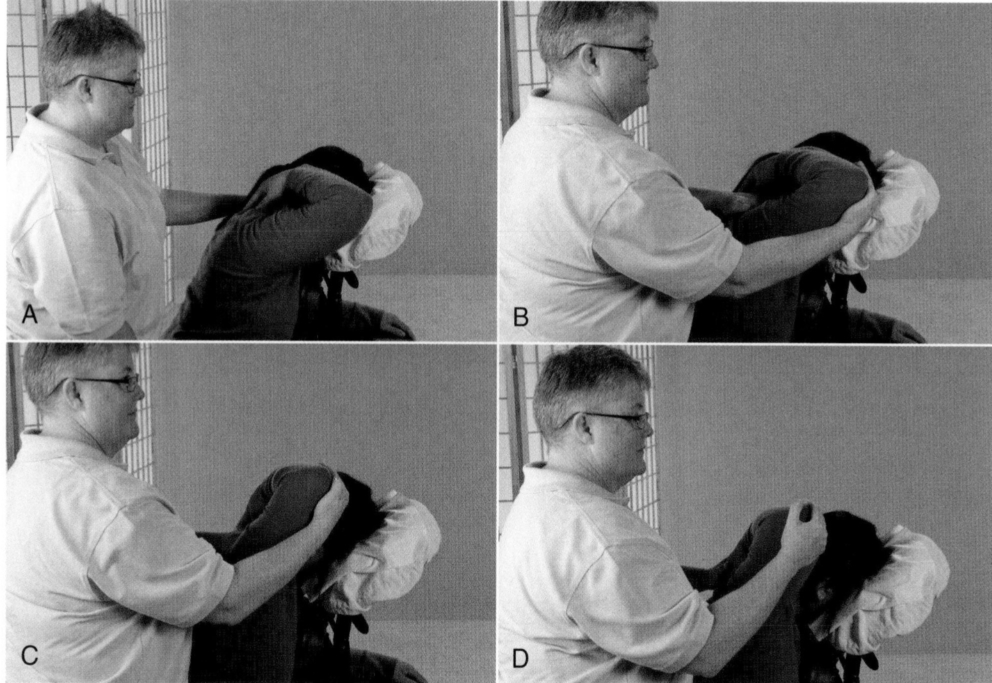

FIGURE 5-9 **A,** The point of the client's elbow is alongside the client's head, and the client's hand is just inferior to the client's posterior neck. **B,** The practitioner placing one hand on the client's elbow and the other hand on the upper trapezius to stabilize. **C,** Pressing the client's elbow posteriorly. **D,** Pressing the client's elbow laterally to engage different muscle fibers of the triceps brachii, as well as the rhomboids.

Serratus Anterior

When the client is positioned on the massage chair with the arms on the armrest, the serratus anterior can be accessed quite easily. Clients who have some limited scapular mobility can benefit from having the serratus anterior worked specifically. Contraindications for these techniques include the following:

- Osteoporosis (deep pressure is contraindicated; lighter pressure may be applied)
- Nerve impingement in the cervical or thoracic regions
- Client hypersensitivity in the muscles involved

Effective techniques to address tightness in the serratus anterior include **bulldozing**—that is, gliding deeply with the fingertips of straightened fingers along the muscle fibers to, and possibly under, the lateral border of the scapula (Figure 5-11 A); compressions (Figure 5-11 B); and deep friction (Figure 5-11 C).

Positioning the Client Backward on the Massage Chair

To perform more specific work on the anterior and lateral neck muscles and the pectoralis muscles, the client should

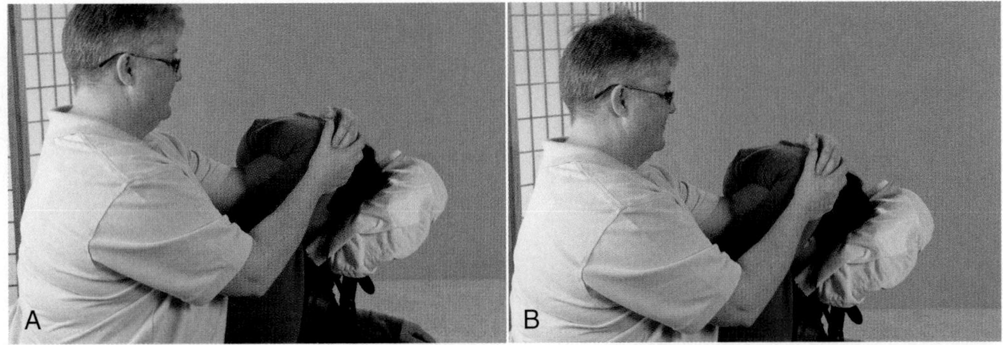

FIGURE 5-10 **A,** Bringing the client's arm upward so that both hands are grasping the elbow. **B,** Depressing the right elbow into the upper trapezius while moving the elbow posteriorly to create the stretch.

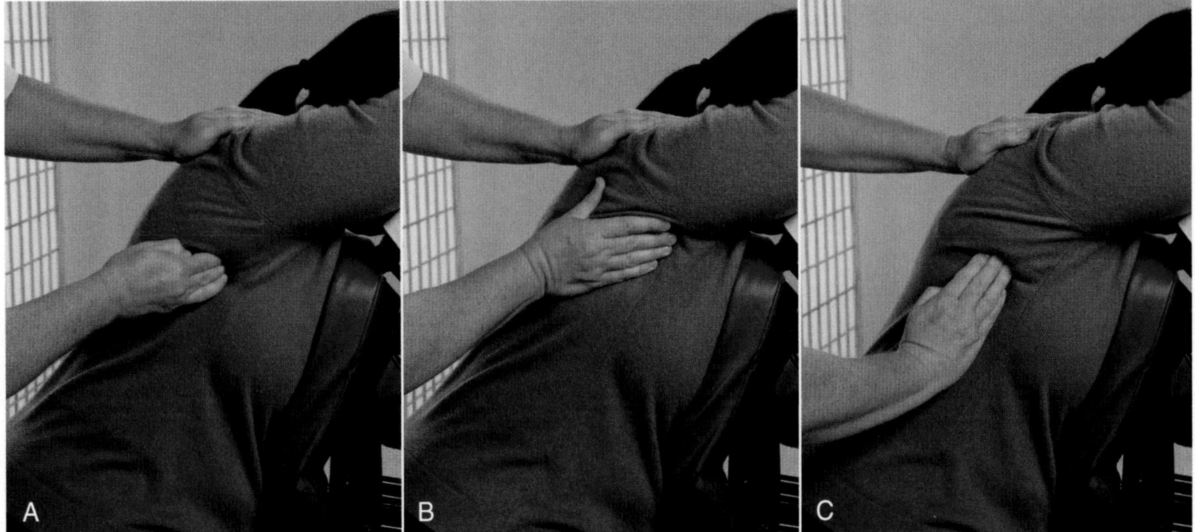

FIGURE 5-11 **A,** Bulldozing along the muscle fibers of the serratus anterior to lateral border of the scapula. **B,** Compressions on the serratus anterior. **C,** Deep friction on the serratus anterior.

be sitting backward on the chair. Depending on the therapeutic needs of the client, the chair massage treatment can either start or finish with the client seated this way. If the treatment starts this way, before the client sits down, the practitioner should loosen the cam locks and place the face cradle and face cradle tubes in the downward position so they are out of the way. If necessary, adjust the seat so that the client can place the feet flat on the floor. The practitioner should then hold on to the side of the chair to stabilize it (so that the client need not worry whether the chair will tip over or cause the client to stumble) while the client sits down and becomes comfortable (Figure 5-12).

If the treatment is to end with the client seated backward on the chair, the practitioner should ask the client to lift the head out of the face cradle and sit up straight. As the client does so, the practitioner should hold onto the face cradle covering so that it does not stick to the client's face. The practitioner then asks the client to slide the legs out from the kneeling pads so that the feet are on the floor. As the client sits for a moment, the practitioner should check in to see if the client is experiencing any dizziness or nausea.

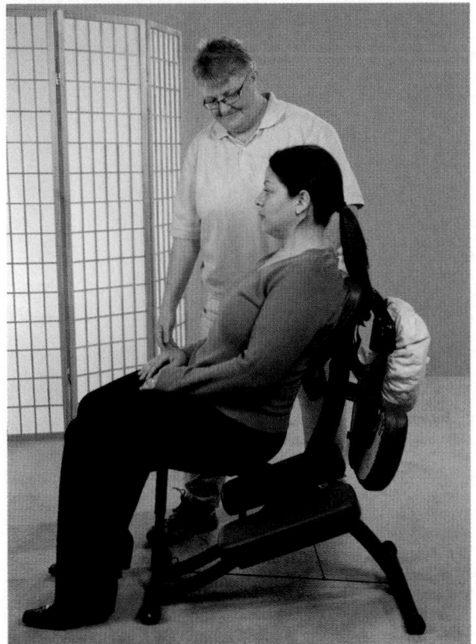

FIGURE 5-12 Client sitting backward on the chair.

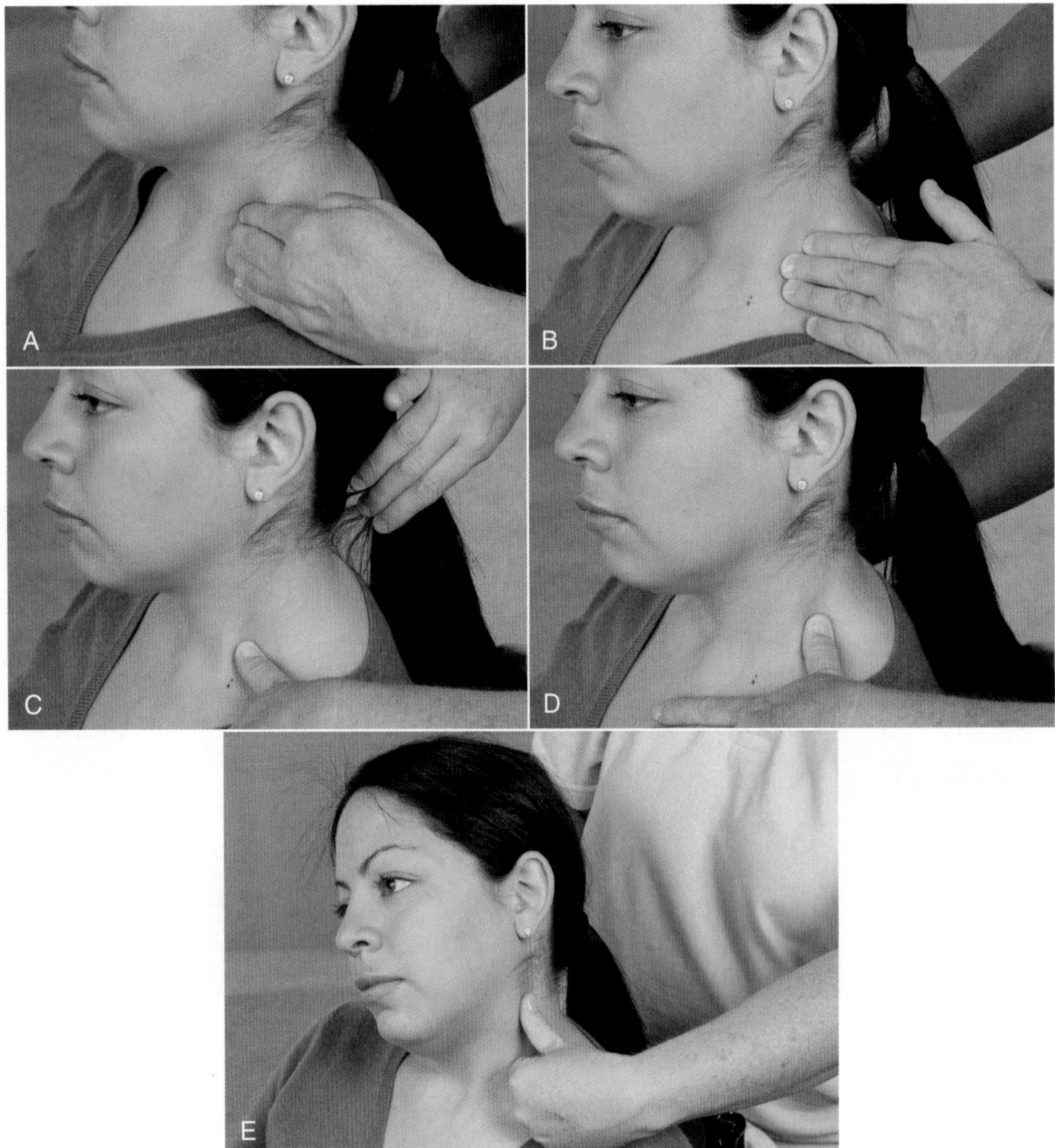

FIGURE 5-13 **A,** Deep circular friction with finger pads on SCM. **B,** Deep circular friction with finger pads on the scalenes. **C,** Deep thumb glides on SCM. **D,** Deep thumb glides on the scalenes. **E,** Deep thumb glides on the scalenes with lateral neck stretch.

If so, the practitioner should make sure the client remains seated until able to stand. When the client is ready, the practitioner should help the client out of the chair by stabilizing the chair so that the client need not worry whether the chair will tip over or cause the client to stumble as the client exits the chair by backing off it. The practitioner should then loosen the cam locks and place the face cradle and face cradle tubes in the downward position so they are out of the way. The practitioner should hold on to the side of the chair to stabilize it while the client sits down and becomes comfortable.

Anterior and Lateral Neck Muscles

Clients generally benefit from working the anterior and lateral neck muscles, especially the sternocleidomastoid (SCM) and scalene muscles, more specifically. Contraindications for these techniques include any of the following conditions in the client's cervical region:

- Arthritis
- Ankylosing spondylitis
- Herniated disk
- Fused vertebrae (for any reason)
- Osteoporosis (deep pressure is contraindicated; lighter pressure may be applied)
- Nerve impingement in the cervical region
- Any other disorders affecting the cervical vertebrae
- Client hypersensitivity in the muscles involved

Techniques to loosen sternocleidomastoid (SCM) and the scalene muscles include deep circular friction using the thumb or finger pads (Figures 5-13 A and B) and deep glides along the muscle fibers using the thumb (Figures 5-13 C and D). When applying a deep glide on the scalenes, the

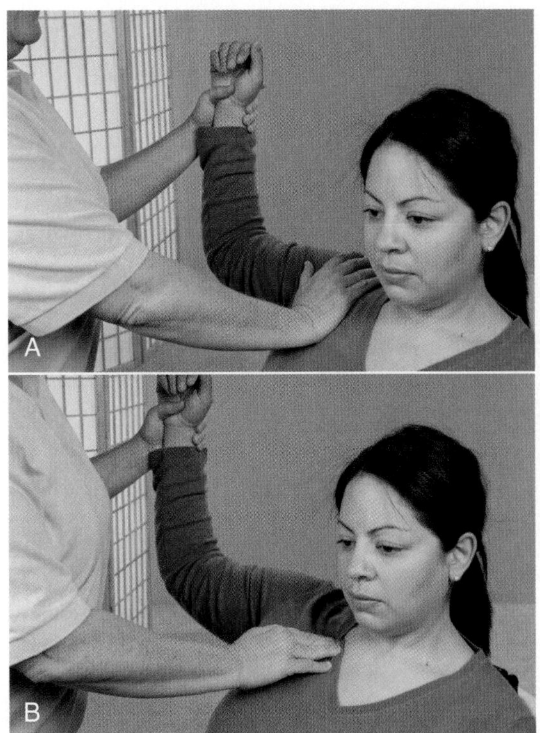

FIGURE 5-14 **A,** Compressions on the pectoralis major. **B,** Deep friction just under the clavicle.

effectiveness of the technique can be enhanced by stretching the lateral neck by placing your other hand on the upper trapezius and gently pressing down (Figure 5-13 E).

Pectoralis Muscles

Contraindications for using the following techniques on the pectoralis muscle (major) include the following:

- Osteoporosis (deep pressure is contraindicated; lighter pressure may be applied)
- Nerve impingement in the cervical or thoracic regions
- Client hypersensitivity in the muscles involved

Techniques to loosen the pectoralis major muscle include compressions (Figure 5-14 A), soft fist kneading, thumb pressure, and deep friction (Figure 5-14 B) along the muscle, especially just under the clavicle.

Iliotibial (IT) Band

Clients who experience hip and leg muscle tightness may benefit from having their IT bands worked. With the client positioned in the massage chair, the IT band is easily accessible to perform techniques that can loosen it, alleviating tightness in the gluteal, hamstrings, and quadriceps femoris muscles. Contraindications for techniques for the IT band include the following:

- Osteoporosis (deep pressure is contraindicated; lighter pressure may be applied)
- Client hypersensitivity in the IT band

Work along the length of the IT band using compressions (Figure 5-15 A), thumb pressure (Figure 5-15 B), soft fist kneading (Figure 5-15 C), or vibration. The forearm can be rolled along the IT band (Figure 5-15 D), and more specific pressure can be applied using the elbow (Figure 5-15 E). Because the IT band is a sensitive area for most clients, practitioners should check in with the client about the pressure applied and modify it as necessary.

The Calf Muscles

When the client is positioned on the massage chair, tight calf muscles can be addressed, including gastrocnemius, soleus, tibialis posterior, and fibularis (peroneus) longus and brevis. Contraindications for working deeply include the following:

- Osteoporosis (deep pressure is contraindicated; lighter pressure may be applied)
- Deep venous thrombosis (DVT)
- Vascular disorders (deep pressure is contraindicated; lighter pressure may be applied)
- Client hypersensitivity in the muscles involved

Techniques to loosen the calf muscles include palming, compressions (Figure 5-16 A), kneading (Figure 5-16 B), soft fist kneading (Figure 5-16 C), thumb and finger pressure, especially between the heads of gastrocnemius and between the individual muscles (Figure 5-16 D), and circular and deep specific friction (Figure 5-16 E).

PERFORMING ADDITIONAL TECHNIQUES ON THE MASSAGE TABLE AND FUTON

There are a variety of reasons for including a chair massage in a full-body massage table (or futon) treatment session. Sometimes, a particular area of the body can be more effectively addressed with the client in a sitting position, such as the neck, shoulders, or quadratus lumborum. Positioning the client on the massage chair allows the practitioner better angles of access to work more deeply into the muscle tissue than a prone client on a massage table would allow.

Another reason to use both a massage chair and a table is to serve a client who, for whatever reason, does not want to lie facedown on the massage table but does want a full-body treatment. In this case, treatment can be done on the chair to address the client's posterior body, and then the anterior can be addressed with the client on the table.

An alternative to a massage table is a futon on the floor. Asian bodywork techniques from shiatsu and Thai massage, including stretches and range-of-motion techniques, can help to loosen tightness in the client's low back, hips, quadriceps femoris, hamstring and calf muscles, and the feet and ankles in a very effective manner.

It is important that the practitioner communicate clearly to the client why the treatment is either starting out or finishing with the client on the massage chair. It is also important that the practitioner explain to the client how the transition from the massage chair to the massage table or futon (or vice versa) will take place. If the treatment plan includes having the client move from chair to table (or

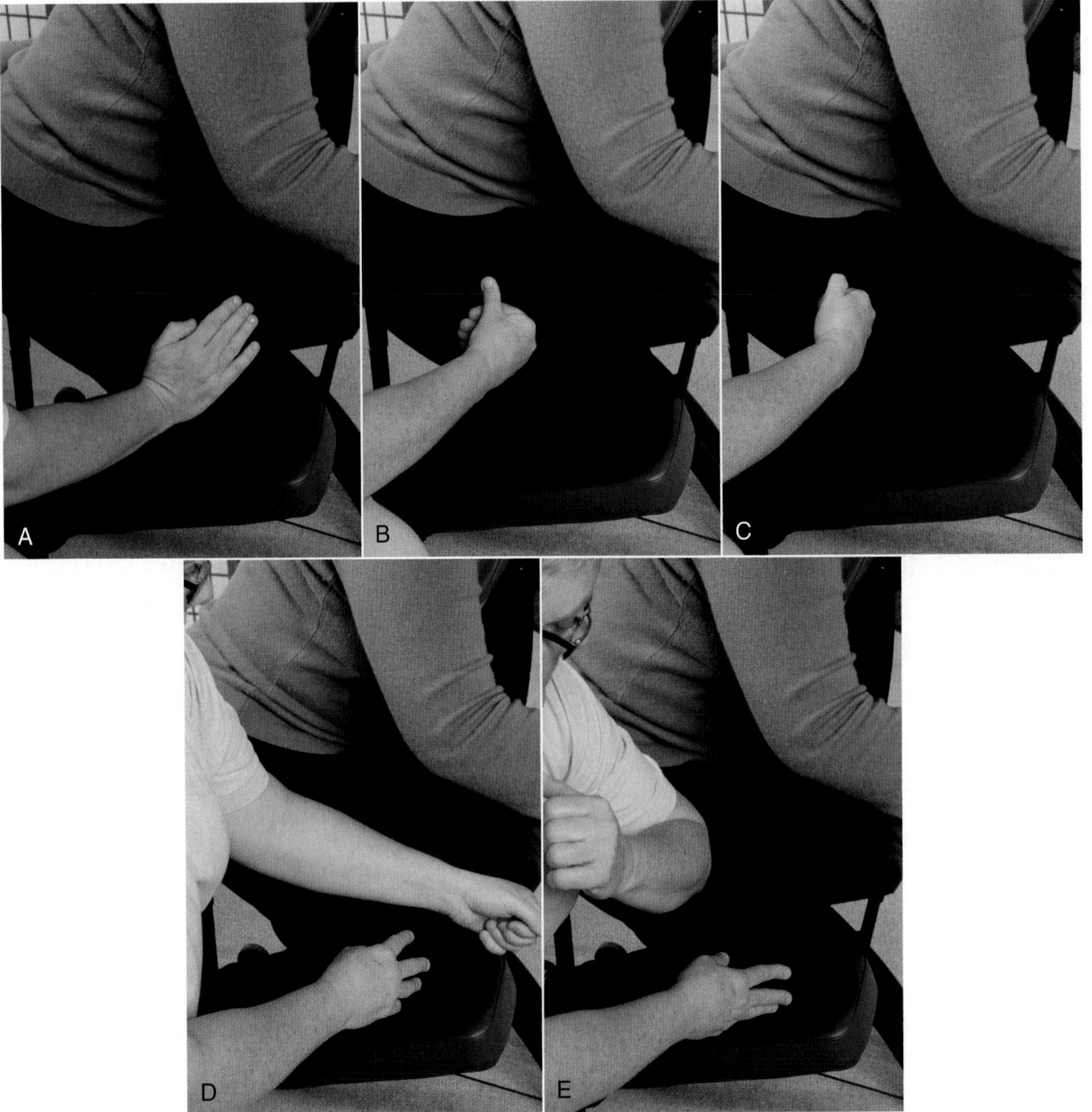

FIGURE 5-15 **A,** Compressions along the IT band. **B,** Thumb pressure along the IT band. **C,** Soft fist kneading along the IT band. **D,** Rolling the forearm along the IT band. **E,** Elbow pressure along the IT band.

futon) at some point in the session, the practitioner should make sure this is clear during the pretreatment interview so that the client knows what to expect. This is especially important if the client will be disrobing for the table massage. Be clear about how the client's privacy will be maintained for undressing and getting under the sheet on the table. Informed consent can include that the treatment would have two phases, one phase on the massage chair and another on the massage table or futon. Informed consent should also include that the time of the treatment may be extended or not, dependent on the agreement between the client and practitioner.

Transition from the Massage Chair to the Massage Table

Before the client's treatment session begins, everything necessary to perform the treatment on the massage table should be in place (i.e., the massage table is set up, linens are on the massage table, lubricant and hand cleaner are within easy reach for the treatment, and so forth). Setting everything up ahead of time ensures a smooth transition, and the client receiving an efficient treatment within the allotted treatment time.

Once the chair massage techniques are complete, inform the client and ask the client to sit up. The practitioner

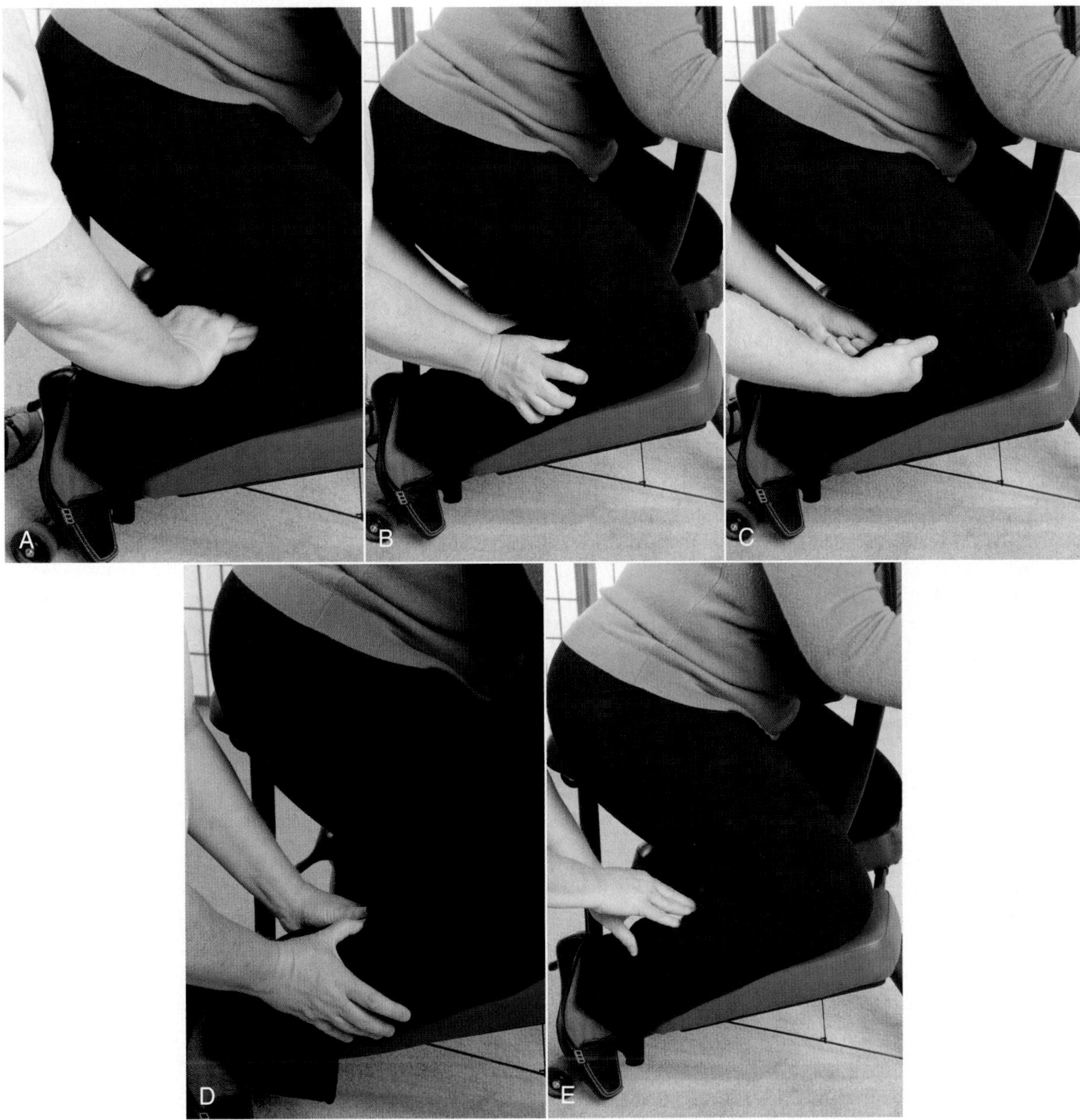

FIGURE 5-16 **A,** Compressions on the calf muscles. **B,** Kneading the calf muscles. **C,** Soft fist kneading on the calf muscles. **D,** Thumb pressure between the heads of gastrocnemius. **E,** Circular friction on the calf muscles.

should remind the client that the practitioner will be leaving the treatment room while the clients disrobes to a comfortable level and gets on the massage table underneath the top sheet. If necessary, the practitioner should help the client get off the massage chair before leaving the room. The practitioner should also let the client know that the practitioner will knock before coming back in.

Transition from the Massage Chair to the Futon

As noted previously in the discussion about moving from chair to table, before the client's treatment session begins, have everything necessary for the futon portion of the treatment in place (i.e., the futon is laid out with fresh linen, hand cleaner is positioned within easy reach, and so forth).

Shiatsu and Thai massage techniques require that both the practitioner and the client wear comfortable, loose-fitting shirts and pants. The best types of pants to wear are those with an elastic or drawstring waist. Because the nature of the stretches and joint range-of-motion (ROM) techniques performed, jeans and pants with zippers should not be worn because they inhibit movement and the zippers can pinch the skin. Skirts and shorts are not advisable either because they can be too revealing during the stretches and joint range-of-motion techniques. In the event the client has brought a change of clothes for the futon work, have the client change once the pretreatment interview is completed and before the session begins, to ensure an easy transition from chair to futon without having to take time then to change.

Once the chair massage techniques are complete, the practitioner should inform the client, ask the client to sit up, help the client get off the massage chair, and then the client can simply move to the futon and lie down.

Shiatsu and Thai Massage Techniques

All of the following stretches, unless otherwise noted, begin with the client supine on the futon:

1. *Straight-leg stretch for the low back and hamstrings.* Grasp around your client's ankles and pick up the legs. While keeping your client's legs straight, stand up. Place one of your feet on the futon behind the client's gluteals and your other foot on the futon at the level of the client's hip, with the foot parallel to the client's body. Holding the client's legs together, gently push them forward as the client exhales, leaning forward as you do so, as far as is comfortable for the client (ask the client to tell you when this is) (Figure 5-17). Hold for a few seconds, then release. Repeat two more times.
2. *Hip range-of-motion technique.* Half-kneel by your client's legs. Supporting under the heel and knee, bring your client's leg into a flexed hip and knee position. Move your hand from under the knee to on top of the knee. Use the hand on top of the knee to guide as you move the leg clockwise several times in a wide range of motion (within your client's tolerance). Then move the leg counterclockwise several times in a wide range of motion (within your client's tolerance). Make sure you move your body as well; this should not be done in a static position (Figure 5-18). Repeat on your client's other leg.
3. *Knee-to-chest stretch.* Get into a half-kneeling position (your inside knee is on the futon; your outside foot is flat on the futon at the level of the client's hip) facing your client's head. Tuck your client's leg in between your leg and torso. Place your inside hand on your client's opposite thigh and your outside hand on top of the knee. Watch for your client to inhale. On the exhale, gently lunge forward to stretch the hip as far as is comfortable for the client (ask the client to tell you when this is). Hold for few seconds, then release (Figure 5-19). Lay your client's leg out straight. Repeat on your client's other leg.
4. *Range-of-motion technique to loosen the low back.* Stand in a wide straight stance at your client's feet. Flex your client's knees and place your hands on top of the knees. While keeping your client's legs together, move the legs clockwise several times in a wide range of motion (within your client's tolerance), then move the legs counterclockwise several times in a wide range of motion (within your client's tolerance). Make sure you move your body as well; this should not be done in a static position (Figure 5-20).
5. *Across-the-body stretch to loosen the low back.* Standing in a wide straight stance at your client's fee, push both of your client's knees to one side of the body, bracing the feet inside your calf. Perform an across-the-body stretch by placing one hand on your client's shoulder and your other hand on the lateral side of your client's knee that is on top. Gently press down as far as is comfortable for client (ask the client to tell you when this is). Hold for a few seconds, then release. Bring your client's knees to center and repeat with the knees on the other side of the client's body. Lay your client's legs out straight (Figure 5-21).
6. *Ankle-loosening techniques.* With one hand, cup the heel of one of the client's feet and grasp along the sole with your other hand. Plantarflex then dorsiflex your client's ankle several times to stretch it and to stretch the anterior and posterior lower leg muscles. Move the foot clockwise several times in a wide range of motion (within your client's tolerance), then move the foot counterclockwise several times in a wide range of motion (within your client's tolerance) (Figure 5-22). Repeat on your client's other foot.
7. *Bilateral leg stretch for the hips and low back.* Kneel at your client's feet. Grasp both feet at the heels, then gently pull backward. *Do not lift the legs off the futon.* Lifting the legs can compromise your client's back (Figure 5-23). Hold for several seconds, then release.

   Use these techniques with the client prone:
8. *Three-way quadriceps stretch.* This stretch is performed while supporting the client's ankle with one hand and stabilizing the sacrum with your other hand. Make sure you move your body as well; these movements should not be done in a static position.
   a. Flex your client's knee and point the foot toward the center of the gluteals (Figure 5-24 A). Lean gently but firmly, then slide your hand toward the toes to stretch the ankle in plantar flexion (within

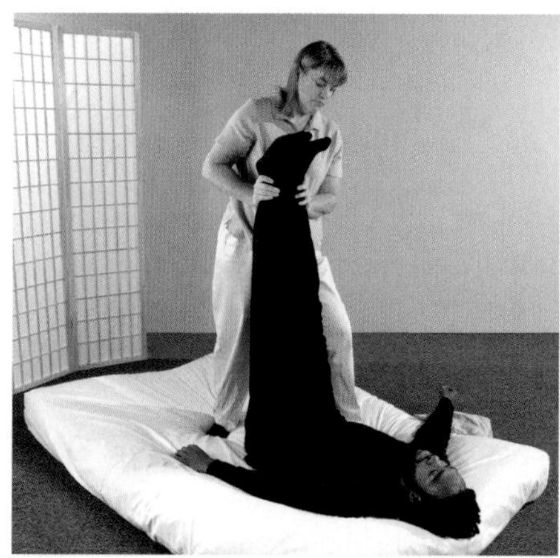

FIGURE 5-17 Straight leg stretch for the low back and hamstrings. (From Anderson SK: *The practice of shiatsu.* St. Louis, 2008, Mosby.)

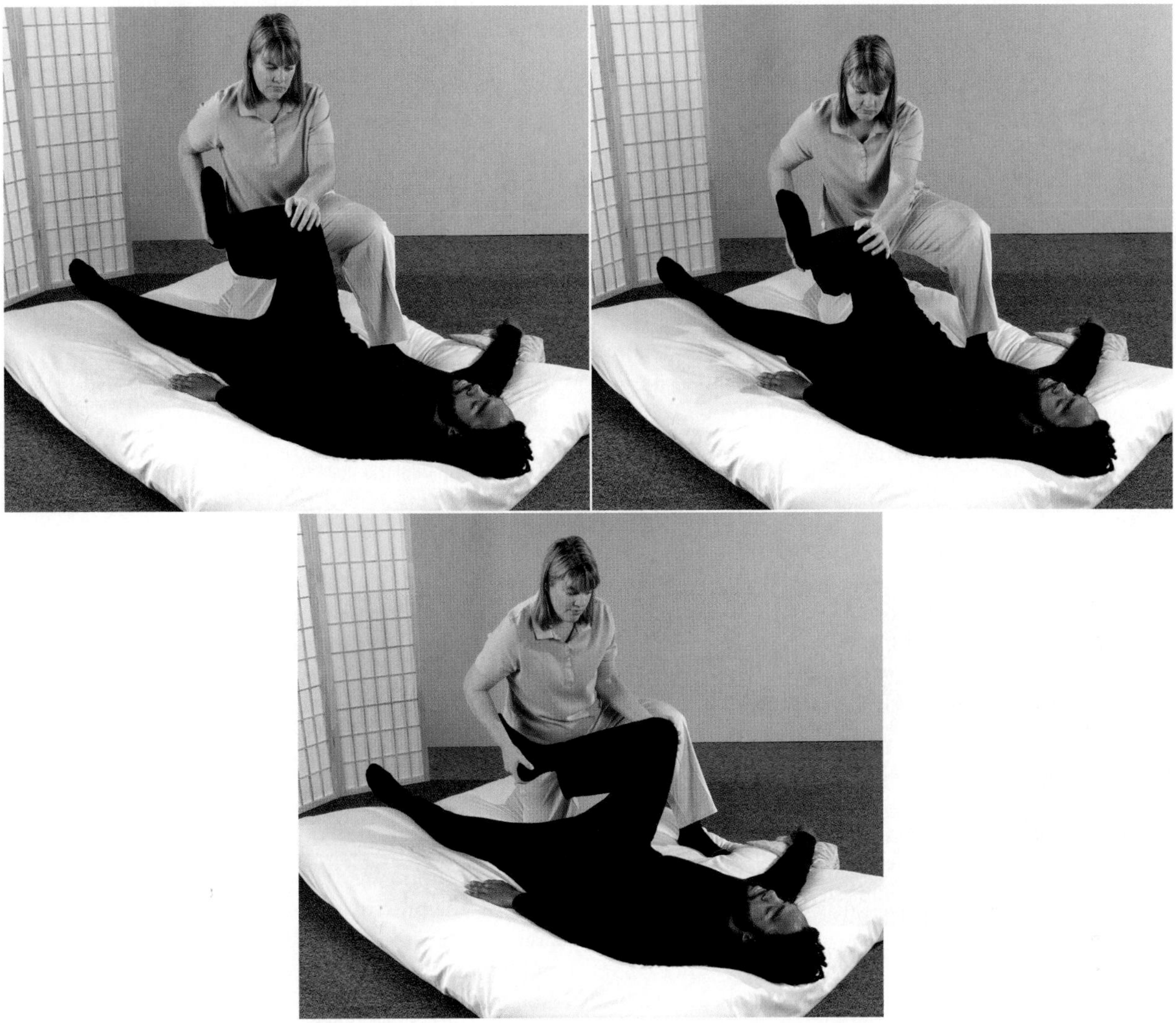

FIGURE 5-18 Hip range-of-motion technique. (From Anderson SK: *The practice of shiatsu.* St. Louis, 2008, Mosby.)

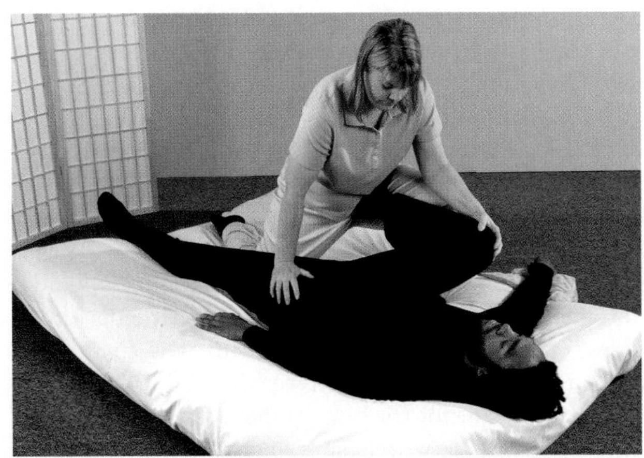

FIGURE 5-19 Knee-to-chest stretch. (From Anderson SK: *The practice of shiatsu.* St. Louis, 2008, Mosby.)

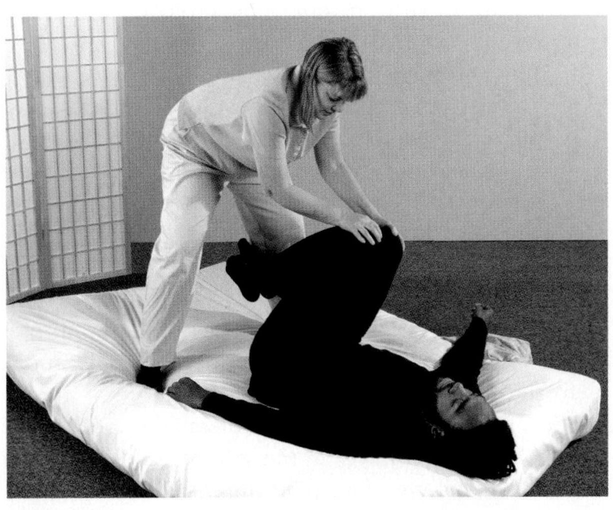

FIGURE 5-20 Range-of-motion technique to loosen the low back. (From Anderson SK: *The practice of shiatsu.* St. Louis, 2008, Mosby.)

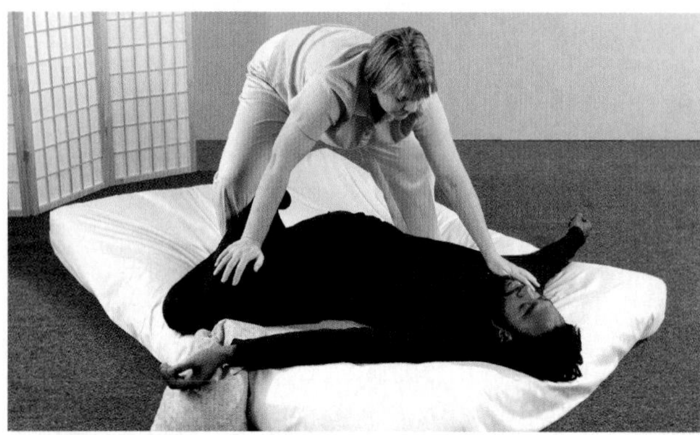

FIGURE 5-21 Across-the-body stretch to loosen the low back. (From Anderson SK: *The practice of shiatsu.* St. Louis, 2008, Mosby.)

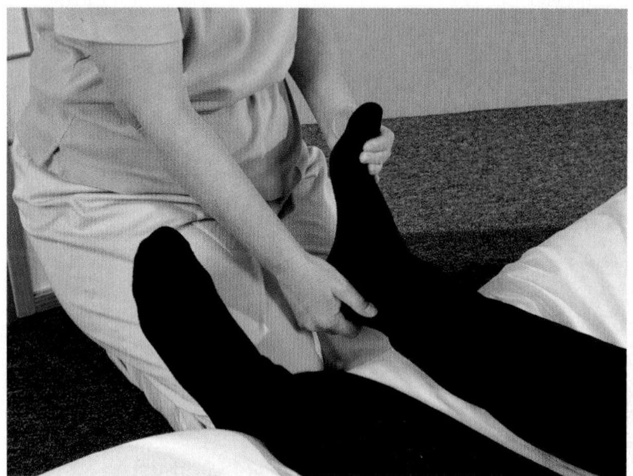

FIGURE 5-22 Ankle loosening techniques. (From Anderson SK: *The practice of shiatsu.* St. Louis, 2008, Mosby.)

your client's tolerance). Hold for several seconds, then release.

b. Flex your client's knee and point the foot across to the opposite gluteals (Figure 5-24 B). Lean gently but firmly (within your client's tolerance). Hold for several seconds, then release.
c. Move your client's leg in a clockwise movement to perform range of motion of the leg toward you, then place it along the lateral side of the gluteals (Figure 5-24 C). Lean gently but firmly (within your client's tolerance). Hold for several seconds, then release. Lay your client's leg out straight.

Repeat Steps 8 a through c on your client's other leg.

9. *Work the soles of the feet.* Either bilaterally or unilaterally, knead the soles of your client's feet. Use thumb pressure, finger pressure, the backs of your hands, and so forth (Figure 5-25).
10. *Kneel on the client's feet.* If it is tolerable to your client, kneel with your knees in the soles of the client's feet. Place each of your hands on the client's calves (Figure 5-26). Remain in this position for approximately a minute or longer.

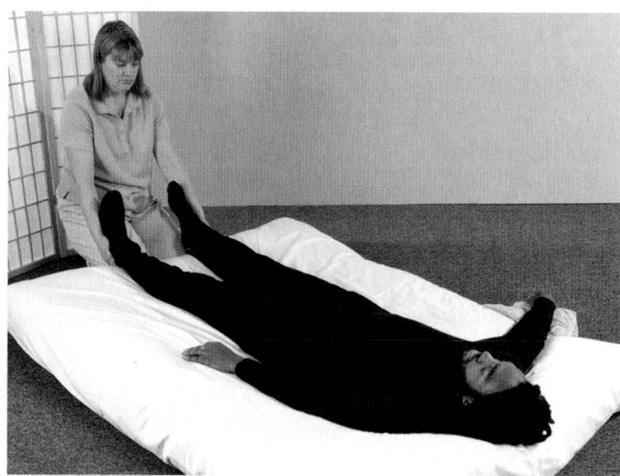

FIGURE 5-23 Bilateral leg stretch for the hips and low back. (From Anderson SK: *The practice of shiatsu.* St. Louis, 2008, Mosby.)

ADAPTATIONS FOR CLIENTS IN WHEELCHAIRS

It is very possible for clients who use wheelchairs to receive an effective posterior neck and back massage. Often the low- and midback muscles are tight because of long-term sitting. If it is possible for the client to lean forward, the practitioner can access the posterior neck and many of the back muscles. The key for an effective treatment is to have proper propping for the client. If the client cannot lean forward, the practitioner can still work on the upper trapezius muscles, the pectoralis muscles, the shoulders, arms and hands, the thighs, and possibly the anterior lower leg. Practitioners also need to be mindful of body mechanics so that they do not hurt the client or injure themselves.

Propping the Client

There are two ways to forward-prop the client. One is with the use of a tabletop massage support. Generally, depending on the manufacturer, the equipment can be fastened to a desk or tabletop, and the client is able to lean forward securely (Figure 5-27). However, as the arms are folded in front to support the client's body, the amount of arm flexibility and strength the client has determines whether this is a good method of propping.

Pillows are another way of propping a person in a wheelchair in order to receive work on the back. Pillows are piled on the client's lap until they are level with the sternum, or a pillow or pillows can be placed on a tabletop. If the client is using a scooter, a pillow can be placed on the handles. The client then leans forward, places the arms on the pillows, and rests the head on the arms. The client's head will be turned to one side for breathing (Figure 5-28).

It is important for the practitioner to make sure that all controls of electric wheelchairs or scooters are turned off so that no switches are accidentally moved during the treatment. All wheelchairs, electric and manual, need to be

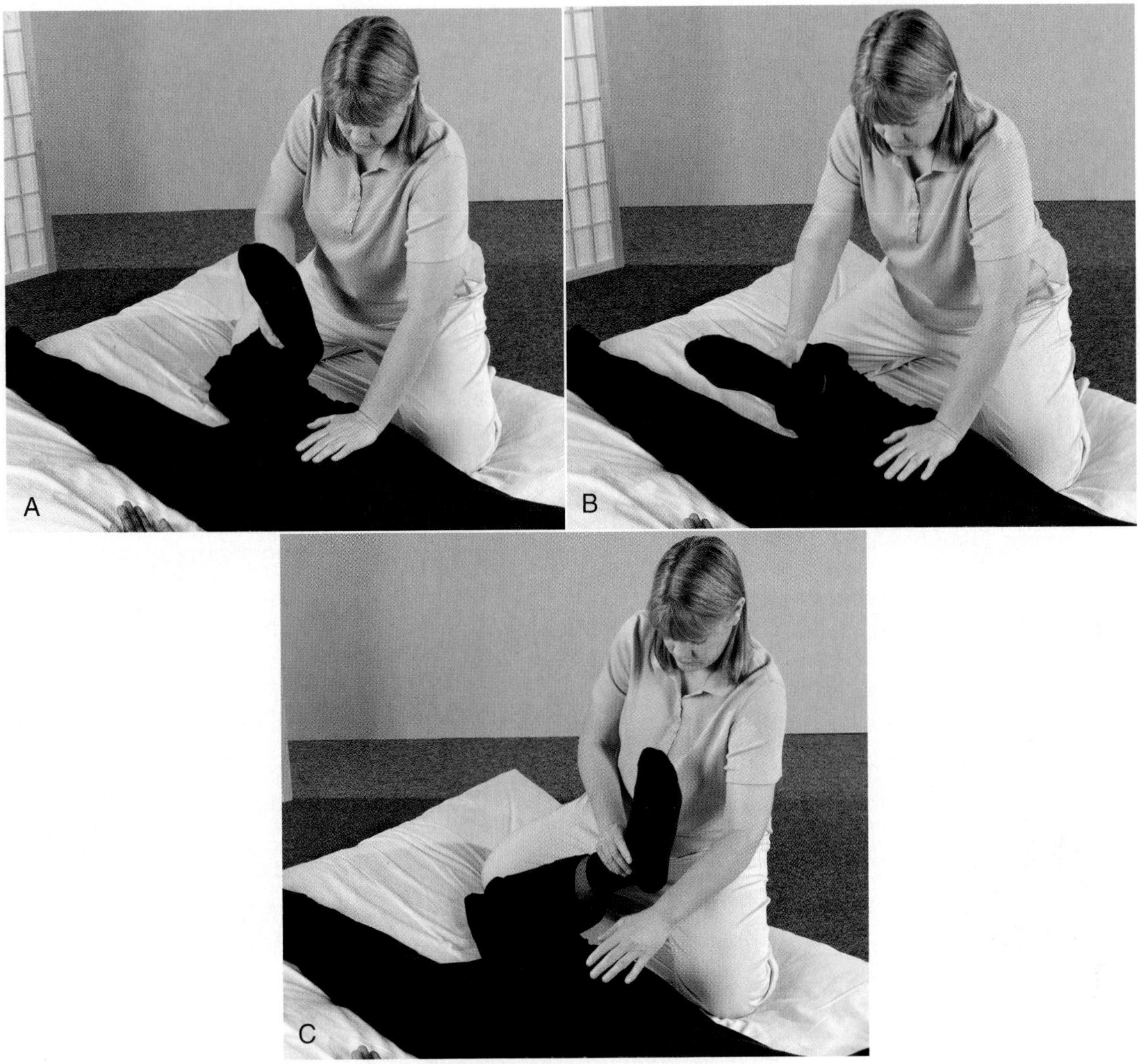

FIGURE 5-24 **A,** Three-way quadriceps stretch, first position. **B,** Three-way quadriceps stretch, second position. **C,** Three-way quadriceps stretch, third position. (From Anderson SK: *The practice of shiatsu.* St. Louis, 2008, Mosby.)

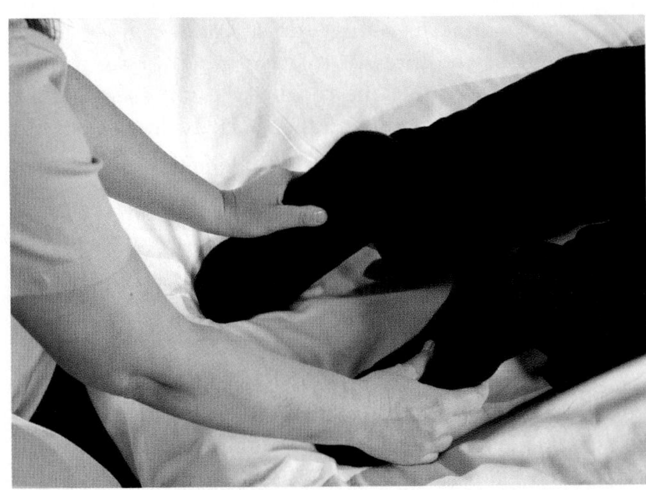

FIGURE 5-25 Work the soles of the feet. (From Anderson SK: *The practice of shiatsu.* St. Louis, 2008, Mosby.)

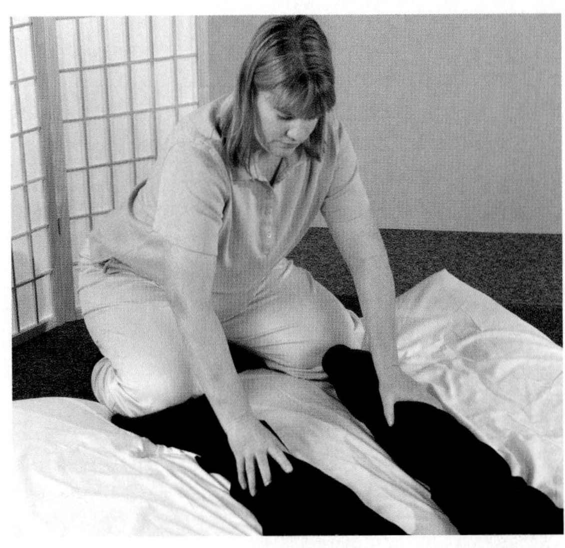

FIGURE 5-26 Kneeling on the client's feet. (From Anderson SK: *The practice of shiatsu.* St. Louis, 2008, Mosby.)

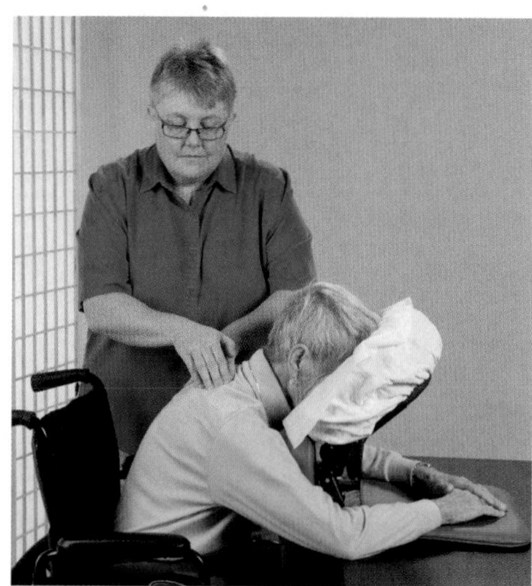

FIGURE 5-27 Tabletop massage support for a client in a wheelchair.

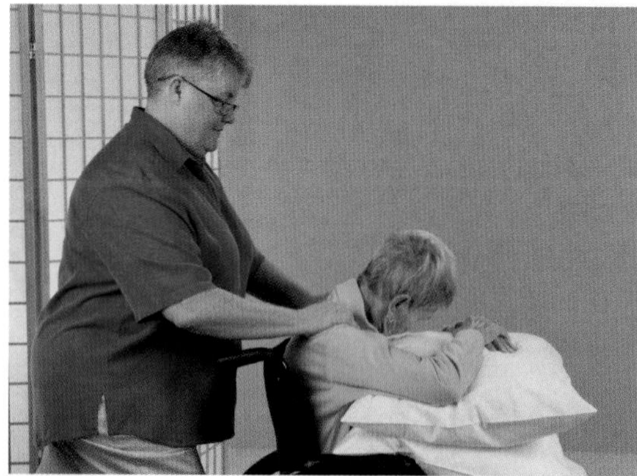

FIGURE 5-28 Propping with pillows for a client in a wheelchair.

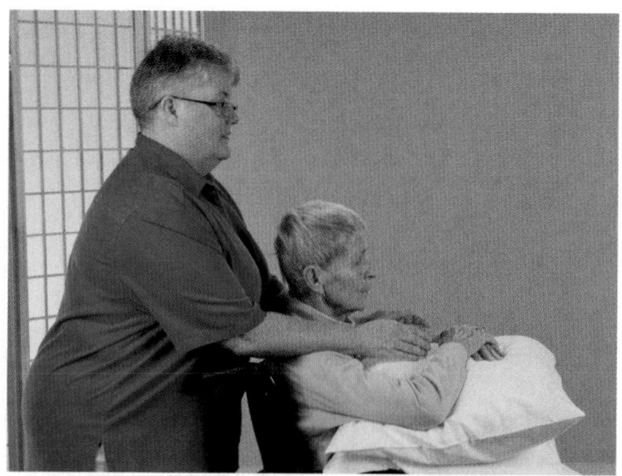

FIGURE 5-29 Applying pressure downward into the upper trapezius bilaterally with the forearms.

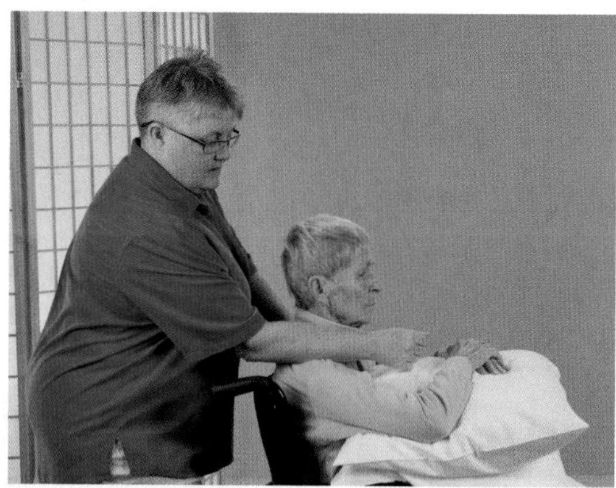

FIGURE 5-30 Rocking the forearm along the client's upper trapezius laterally and then back medially.

locked into position so that they do not move during the treatment.

Treatment Protocol

Many of the techniques presented throughout this text can be adapted for clients in wheelchairs. What follows is a suggested treatment protocol practitioners can use as a basic routine. Practitioners are also encouraged to use their creativity and design their own treatments.

1. Stand behind the client's wheelchair in a straight stance. Place both of your forearms on the client's right and left upper trapezius. Simultaneously apply pressure downward into the muscle tissue by dropping your weight into your knees and flexing them slightly, then release (Figure 5-29). Move your forearms laterally along the upper trapezius and then back medially as you continue to apply pressure, then release. You should be able to create a rhythm with this stroke as you press downward and move outward. Repeat three more times.
2. Stand to the back and right side of your client in a lunge position with your right leg forward and your left leg back. Place your left hand on the client's left shoulder to stabilize the client's arm while you place your right forearm on the client's right upper trapezius, midway between the shoulder joint and the neck. Apply pressure with your forearm in a rocking motion (Figure 5-30). Make sure to lunge forward and back with each motion of the forearm to create rhythm along with pressure. Continue the rocking motion as you move your forearm laterally and then back medially along the upper trapezius. Repeat three more times.

> **TIP** If your back heel is leaving the floor as you lean forward, then you are applying good pressure into the tissue while using proper body mechanics.

3. Either stay in the lunge position or stand behind the client's left shoulder. Knead the upper trapezius with both of your hands, making sure to fully grip as much of the tissue as you can (Figure 5-31). Continue kneading until you feel the muscle tissue soften.

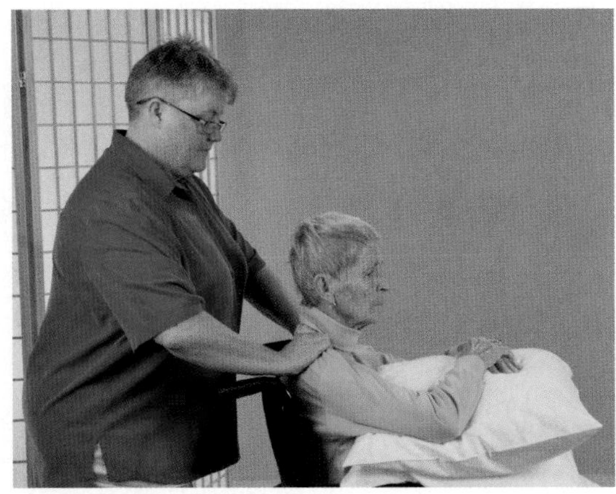

FIGURE 5-31 Kneading the client's upper trapezius with both hands.

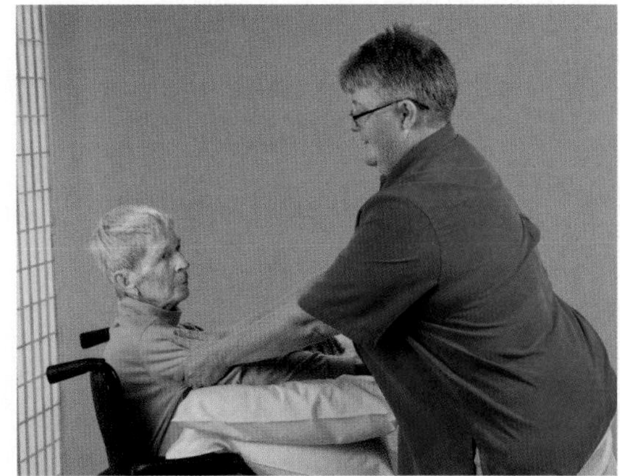

FIGURE 5-33 Applying compressions down the arm.

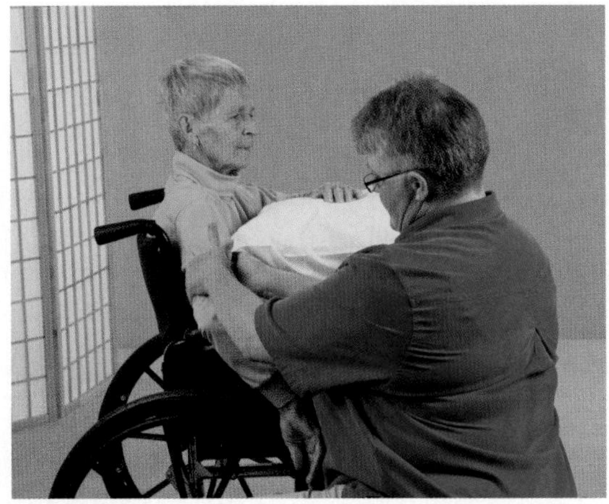

FIGURE 5-32 Grasping the client's arm with both hands at the deltoid, and gently jostling it.

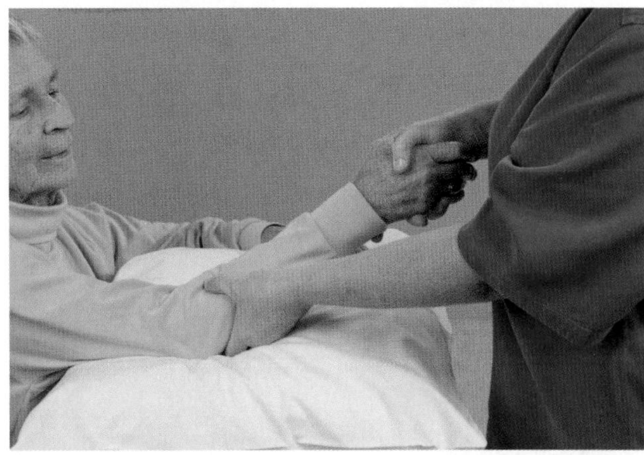

FIGURE 5-34 Applying circular friction along the radius.

4. Move to stand, kneel on one knee or sit on a stool in front of your client on the right side. Grasp the client's left arm with both of your hands at the deltoid, and gently shake it to jostle it as you move down the client's arm to the wrist (Figure 5-32). Be mindful that your grasp is not too tight. The intent is to allow the client's arm to be loose as you are shaking and rolling it. Repeat two more times.
5. With both hands, grasp the client's left arm so that your thumbs are on the deltoid. Use your thumb pads to apply circular friction at the attachment of the deltoid to the deltoid tuberosity. Apply compressions down the entire length of the client's arm to the wrist (Figure 5-33). When you reach the wrist, compress proximally back up to the deltoid. Repeat two more times.
6. Move to a lunge position in front of your client and grasp your client's right hand in a handshake with your right hand. Use your left hand to grasp the client's forearm just distal to the elbow with your thumb on the medial surface of the arm. While applying compressions, apply circular friction with your thumb pad distally along the ulna, then the radius, then the interosseus membrane (Figure 5-34).
7. Use your left thumb to apply pressure along the length of the interosseus membrane while your right hand gently supinates and pronates the client's forearm (Figure 5-35). This motion will allow you to apply deeper pressure into the tissue of the forearm. Make sure you are rocking back and forth to create a sense of movement with these techniques on the forearm.
8. Turn your client's right hand palm down. Grasp it with both of your hands and your thumbs parallel on the back of the hand. Gently apply pressure outward and downward to spread the metacarpals apart (Figure 5-36). Repeat two more times.
9. Turn the client's hand palm up and hold it with both of your hands. Use both of your thumb pads to massage the palm until you feel the entire palm has been addressed (Figure 5-37).
10. Turn the client's hand palm down. Holding the client's wrist with your left hand, use your right hand to gently grasp each finger between your thumb and index finger

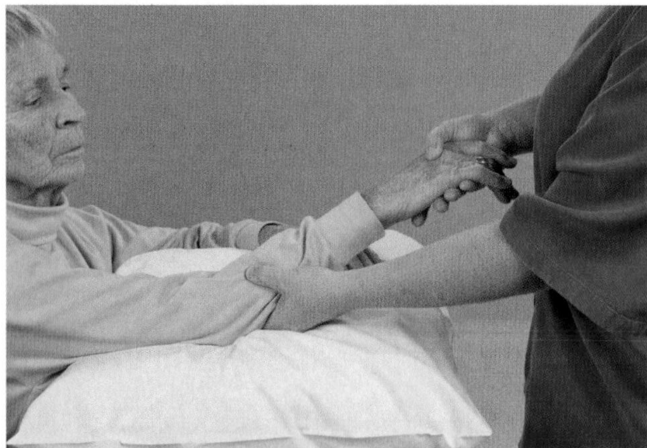

FIGURE 5-35 Applying pressure along the length of the interosseus membrane while supinating and pronating the forearm.

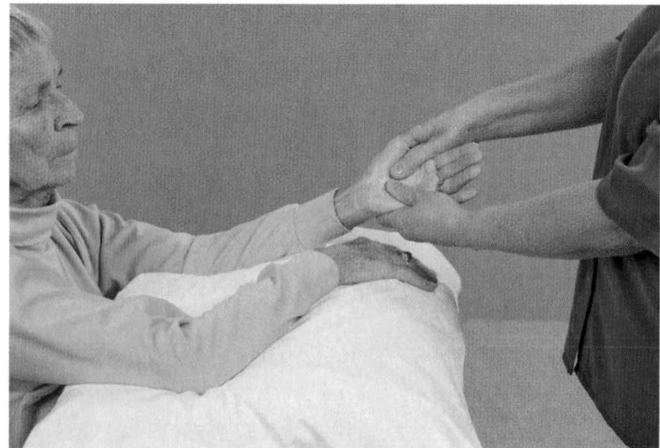

FIGURE 5-37 Massaging the palm with the thumb pads.

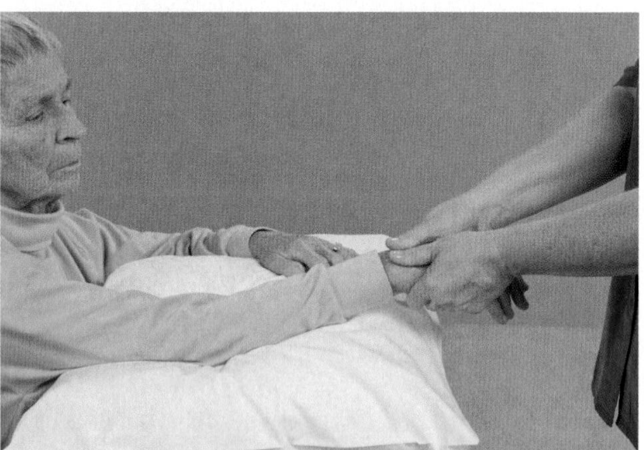

FIGURE 5-36 Spreading apart the metacarpals.

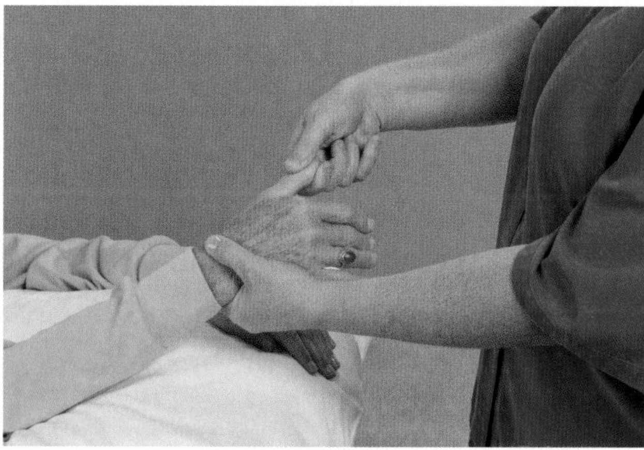

FIGURE 5-38 Gently grasping each finger with a rolling motion, moving from the base of the finger to the tip.

with a rolling motion, moving from the base of the finger to the tip (Figure 5-38). Repeat for each finger.

11. Finish working the hand by doing another metacarpal spreading as in Step 8.
12. Return to the right side of the client. Grasp the client's right arm with your two hands, and gently shake the arm out once more as a finishing technique. Place the client's arm back on the client's lap or on the armrest of the wheelchair.
13. Move to stand behind the client. Knead the client's upper trapezius bilaterally.
14. Repeat Steps 2 through 12 on the client's left side.
15. Move to stand behind the client. Knead the client's upper trapezius to connect the client's two sides and to provide closure to the shoulder and arm massage.
16. Standing behind your client, place your left hand on the client's forehead to stabilize the head. Use your right hand to knead all of the posterior neck muscles (Figure 5-39). Continue kneading until you feel the muscles soften.
17. Holding the client's hair out of the way with your left hand, gently grasp the client's right posterior neck muscles between your right thumb and index finger. Roll the muscle tissue back and forth as you move inferiorly from the base of the client's head down to the level of C-7 (Figure 5-40). Repeat the rolling motion superiorly to the base of the head. Repeat two more times.

    Repeat the technique using your left thumb and index finger on the client's left posterior neck.
18. Finish working the neck by repeating Step 16. This creates a sense of connection between the left and right sides of the neck for the client.

If it is possible for the client to lean forward, then the back muscles can be addressed. Either use the desktop table support or pillows as discussed under "Propping the Client," and have the client lean forward until comfortable.

1. Stand in a lunge to the back and right side of your client. Place your right hand on the client's deltoid to

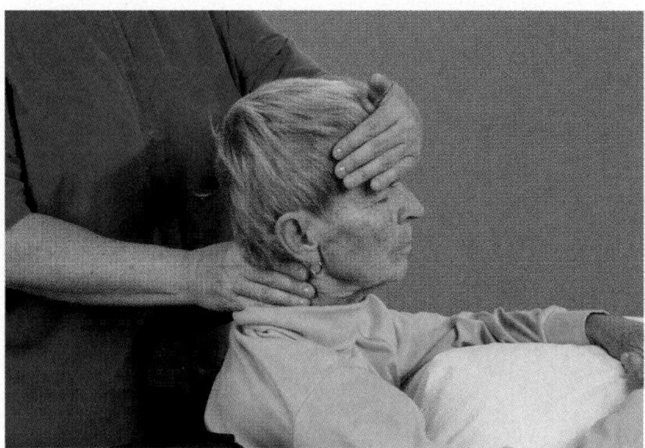

FIGURE 5-39 Kneading all of the posterior neck muscles.

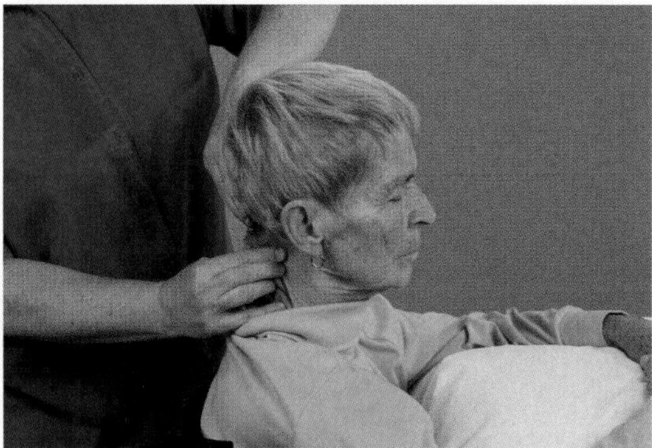

FIGURE 5-40 Rolling the posterior neck muscle tissue back and forth between the thumb and index finger.

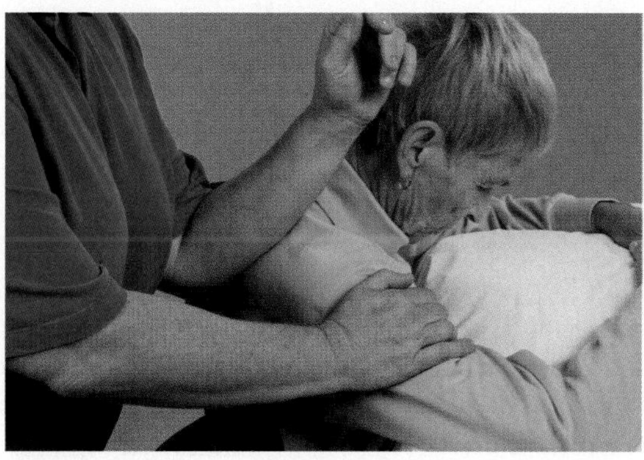

FIGURE 5-41 Applying deep circular friction with the forearm on the middle trapezius and rhomboids.

stabilize while applying deep circular friction with your left forearm on the client's middle trapezius and rhomboids (Figure 5-41).

2. Move to a straight stance, stack your hands on top of each another, and apply more specific circular pressure with your fingertips along the medial border of the client's scapula and infraspinatus and supraspinatus (Figure 5-42). Use your fingertips to address the entire shoulder girdle region, softening tight muscle tissue as you find it. You can also use your thumb pads.

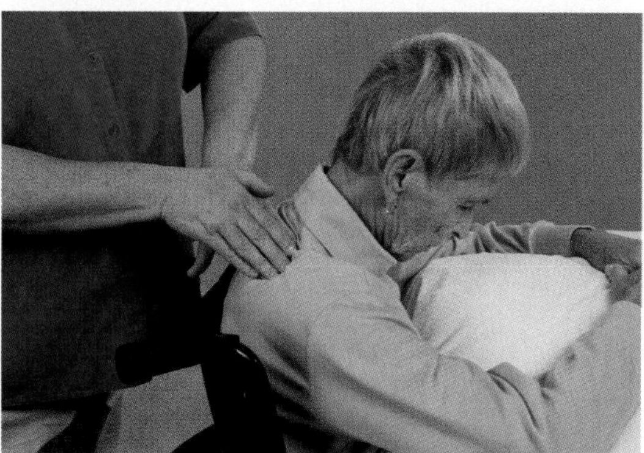

FIGURE 5-42 Stacking the hands on top of each another to apply more specific circular pressure along the medial border of the scapula and infraspinatus and supraspinatus.

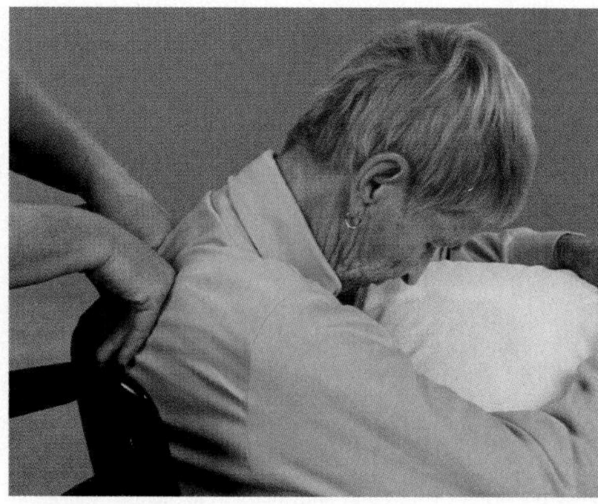

FIGURE 5-43 Using the backs of the hands to lean in and bilaterally engage the tissue of the rhomboids.

3. Repeat Steps 1 and 2 on the client's right side.
4. Move back to a lunge stance. Use the backs of your hands to lean in and bilaterally engage the tissue of the rhomboids. Then move the tissue downward until the area feels stretched (Figure 5-43). Repeat three more times or until you feel the muscle tissue of the low back soften.

   Repeat on the client's left side.

TIP Make sure to flex your knees as you lean downward into the tissue while doing this technique.

5. Perform brush strokes over the client's entire back followed with percussion.
6. Have the client sit up in the chair. To ensure your client's comfort, check to see if a drink of water or anything else is needed.
7. Stand in a straight stance behind your client. Massage the client's face by gliding upward with the palms of your hands (Figure 5-44). Ask if it is comfortable for the client to lightly lean back into you as you perform this technique. Having the client lean into you can

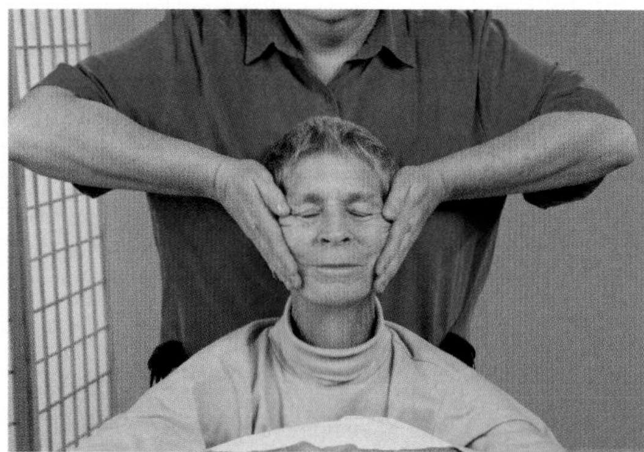
FIGURE 5-44 Massaging the client's face by gliding upward with the palms of the hands.

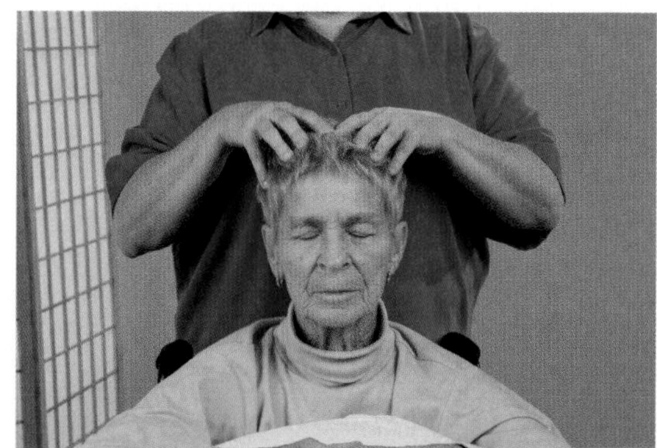
FIGURE 5-46 Massaging the client's entire scalp by performing circular motions and kneading with the fingertips.

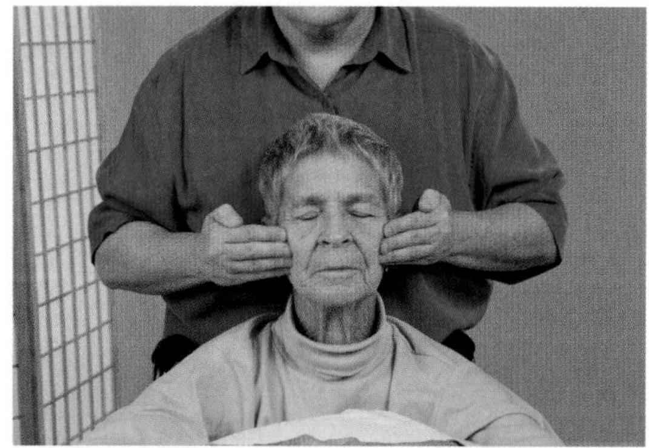
FIGURE 5-45 Performing circular motions on the client's cheeks with the fingertips.

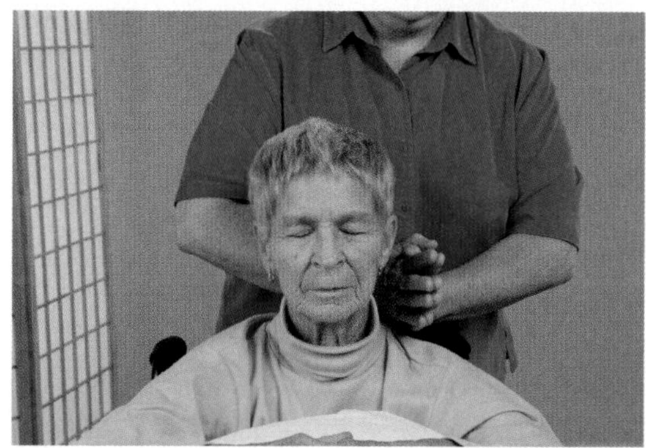
FIGURE 5-47 Applying quacking percussion on the upper trapezius.

sometimes make clients feel more supported, although not all clients like this.

8. Perform circular motions on the client's cheeks with your fingertips (Figure 5-45). Follow this with finger pad presses along the cheekbones, moving medial to lateral. Continue with circular motions on the client's temples.
9. Massage the client's entire scalp by performing circular motions and kneading with your fingertips (Figure 5-46).
10. Apply quacking or other type of percussion on the client's left, and then right, upper trapezius (Figure 5-47). Remember to keep the emphasis on the upstroke.

ADAPTATIONS FOR CLIENTS IN BEDS

It is possible to adapt chair massage techniques for clients who are in bed, whether at home, in an assisted-care facility, in hospice, or in a hospital. These clients would, of course, need to be vital enough to receive massage and not have any conditions that are contraindicated for massage. It is essential that the practitioner receive written clearance from the client's physician to perform the treatment. In some municipalities, a prescription for massage may be necessary. The treatment session needs to be documented properly, which includes the client filling out a pretreatment (intake) form and the practitioner writing session notes for every treatment performed. Feedback forms that the client fills out for each session are also important. Practitioners should take scrupulous care in maintaining the client's records, as the client's physician can request these at any time or, in fact, they may be required to be submitted after each treatment.

Proper propping is important to ensure that the client is comfortable and without risk of injury from any propped position, and so that practitioners can use effective body mechanics to minimize their risks of injury. Additionally, the client may have IVs, ports, catheters, and other medical equipment attached to the body, or places of recent surgery or invasive procedures; the practitioner needs to take great care working around these areas. Some of these items or areas may not be readily visible, so the practitioner should find out from the client and the client's healthcare providers any cautionary and contraindicated areas for massage on the client's body.

If the client is able to sit on the side of the bed with the feet on the floor, it is possible to prop with pillows and a chair. The chair is placed with its back to the client. Pillows are placed across the top of the back of the chair, and the weight of the client leaning forward onto the pillows keeps the chair from moving forward (clearly—do not use a chair with wheels). With permission from the client, the practitioner would kneel on the bed (shoes off) behind the client and address the client's back muscles.

If the client is able to sit up in bed, it is possible to place the pillows in front so that the client can lean forward while the practitioner addresses the back muscles. The practitioner would work on one side of the client's back at a time, as the practitioner will need to stand to the side of the bed to perform the treatment. The practitioner can work on the client's arms and hands while the client is lying down.

Practitioners must be especially conscious of their body mechanics while working on clients in beds, as it is easy to not notice a strained posture while focusing on the client. Practitioners should take care not to compromise their own health by moving their bodies into, and staying in, stressful positions. When working on a client in a hospital bed, it is also helpful for practitioners to become familiar with how to adjust the bed height so that they can then easily adjust the bed to the proper height to work on the client.

Sometimes healthcare settings such as hospitals, hospice centers, and assisted-living centers cause clients to have dry skin. An option practitioners can consider is to bring a massage lotion and massage it into the client's skin during the treatment. Massage oil is not recommended because it tends to leave residue on the skin.

Practitioners should note that performing treatments on clients in a hospital environment requires much sensitivity to the client's level of physical, emotional, and mental stamina. Most hospital stays are stressful, and the client is usually not feeling well. Some people respond to the situational stress with emotional outbursts (tears or anger) or become depressed or sad. As with any other client in any other setting, the practitioner should not take things personally and remain professional at all times.

Hospitals, assisted-living facilities, and hospice centers are environments where one is likely to encounter pathogens. Therefore, it is essential that practitioners take proper steps to maintain good health. They should practice standard precautions at all time and be aware of their own state of health before going into the hospital setting. If they are feeling run-down or sick, they should not perform treatments.

Practitioners should also be aware that working in healthcare settings may impact them emotionally. Not everyone is comfortable working in hospitals, assisted-living facilities, and hospice centers. It can sometimes be difficult to provide massage to those who are sick or dying. Practitioners should do an honest self-evaluation to see if they are comfortable working in these settings. It is better not to perform treatments there at all if the practitioner feels there is a chance the environment and conditions would make it difficult to do the work.

Treatment Protocol

Many of the techniques presented throughout this text can be adapted for clients in beds. What follows is a suggested treatment protocol practitioners can use as a basic routine. These techniques are for the client in a hospital bed who is able to sit upright and who is able to move to the side of the bed and place the feet on the floor. Practitioners are also encouraged to use their creativity and design their own treatments.

1. Begin the session by having the client sit on the edge of the bed and with feet flat on the floor (Figure 5-48).
2. Standing in a lunge in the front and to the left of the client, grasp the client's left arm at the deltoid with both of your hands. Apply compressions down the entire length of the client's arm to the wrist (Figure 5-49). When you reach the wrist, compress proximally back up to the deltoid. Repeat two more times.
3. Hold the client's left hand with your left hand, and perform single-handed kneading with your right hand distally on your client's right upper arm from the shoulder to the elbow (Figure 5-50 A). Move your right

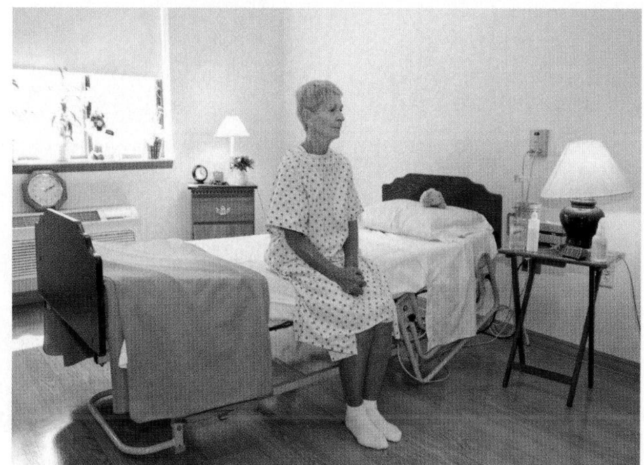

FIGURE 5-48 Client sitting on the edge of the bed with feet placed flat on the floor.

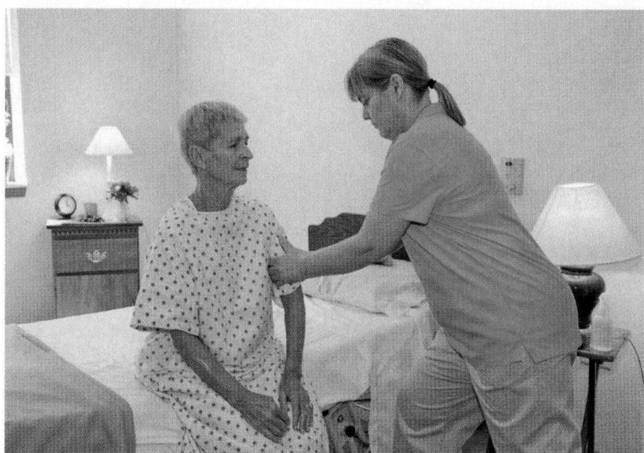

FIGURE 5-49 Applying compressions down the entire length of the arm.

hand back up to the client's shoulder and repeat two more times.

Continue single-handed kneading with your right hand distally on your client's forearm from the elbow to the wrist (Figure 5-50 B). Move your right hand back up to the client's shoulder and repeat two more times.

TIP Be careful to not pinch the client's arm while performing single-handed kneading.

4. Turn your client's left hand palm down. Grasp it with both of your hands and your thumbs parallel on the back of the hand. Gently apply pressure downward and outward to spread the metacarpals (Figure 5-51). Repeat two more times.
5. Turn your client's hand palm up. Interlace the fingers of both your hands with your client's fingers. Spread the palm to stretch it, then use both of your thumb pads to massage the surface of the palm while maintaining the stretch (Figure 5-52).
6. Turn the client's hand palm down. Holding the client's wrist with your left hand, use your right hand to gently grasp each finger between your thumb and index finger with a rolling motion, moving from the base of the finger to the tip. Repeat for each finger.
7. Hold your client's left hand with your left hand. Use your right hand to gently brush the entire length of your client's arm (Figure 5-53). Give the arm a slight shake to signal completion of work, and place it down at the client's side.

TIP Optional
If the client would like it, lubricant can be applied to the client's arm and then the arm can be massaged (Figure 5-54).

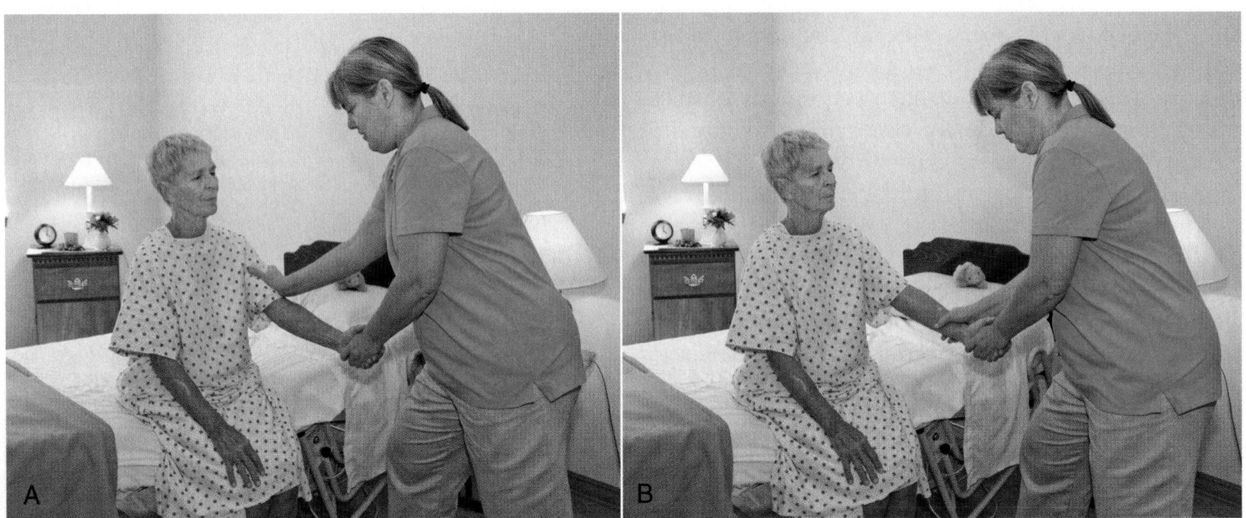

FIGURE 5-50 **A,** Performing single-handed kneading on the upper arm from the shoulder to the elbow. **B,** Continuing single-handed kneading distally on the forearm from the elbow to the wrist.

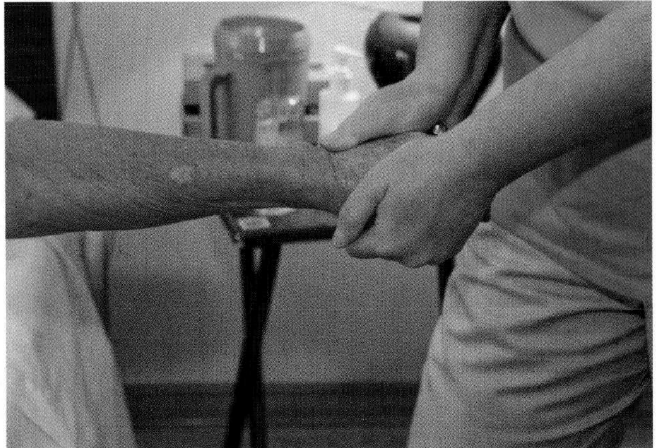

FIGURE 5-51 Gently applying pressure downward and outward to spread the metacarpals.

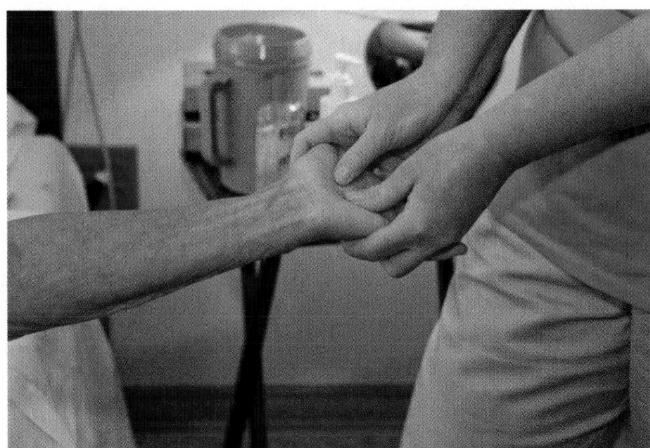

FIGURE 5-52 Interlacing the fingers, spreading the palm to stretch it, and using both thumb pads to massage the surface of the palm.

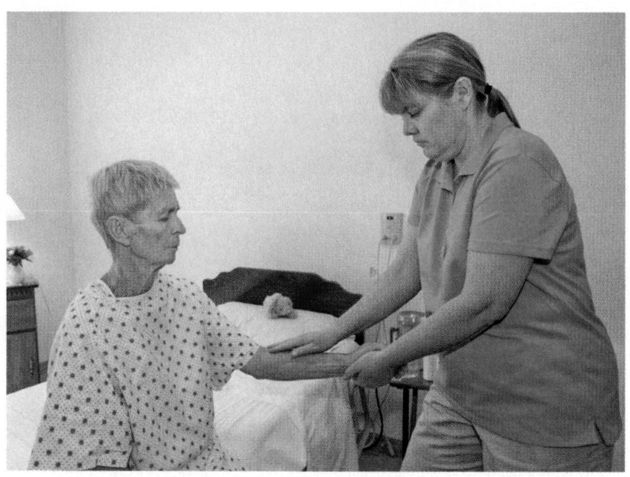

FIGURE 5-53 Gently brushing the entire length of the arm.

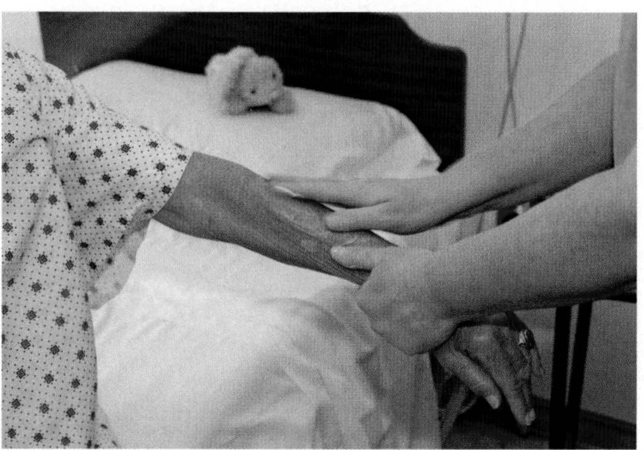

FIGURE 5-54 Applying lubricant and massaging the arm.

8. Repeat Steps 2 through 7 on the client's right side.
9. With your client's permission, kneel behind your client on the hospital bed (be sure to remove your shoes first). Place your forearms on either side of your client's neck on the upper trapezius. Apply pressure downward as you move your forearms laterally and then back medially to cover the entire area (Figure 5-55). Repeat three more times.
10. Lightly knead the client's upper trapezius bilaterally until you feel the tissue soften.
11. Place your left elbow on the client's right upper trapezius in the space between the clavicle and the scapulae. Keeping the client's elbow flexed, use your right hand to grasp the client's right hand and gently raise and shake the arm upward as you apply light pressure downward onto the upper trapezius with your left elbow. Once the hand is raised high enough, grasp the client's wrist with your left hand while continuing to grasp the client's hand with your right hand (Figure 5-56). This technique allows for stretching of the triceps brachii while pressure is applied to the upper trapezius. Check in with the client about the depth of pressure and whether the stretch is comfortable; modify the technique as needed. Return the arm to the client's side, and lightly knead the upper trapezius.
12. Sink back to sit on your heels. With your right hand in a soft fist, perform circular friction on the client's upper right quadrant. Hold the client's left shoulder with your left hand to provide stability as pressure is applied (Figure 5-57).
13. Press and perform circular friction with your thumb pads along the attachment sites of the client's scapula to soften tight muscle tissue (Figure 5-58).

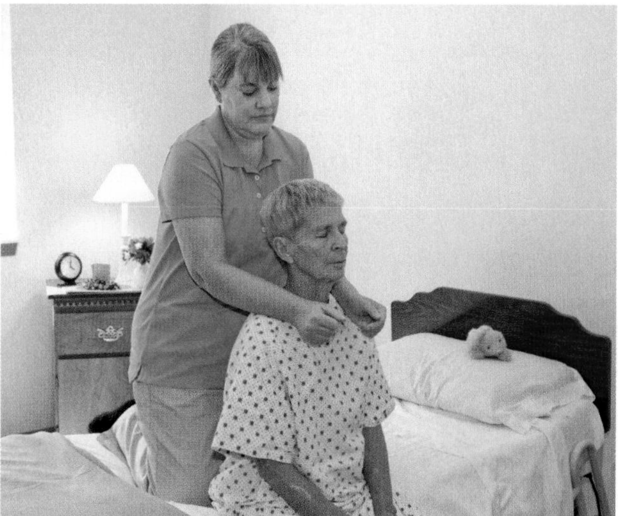

FIGURE 5-55 Applying pressure downward while moving the forearms laterally and then back medially.

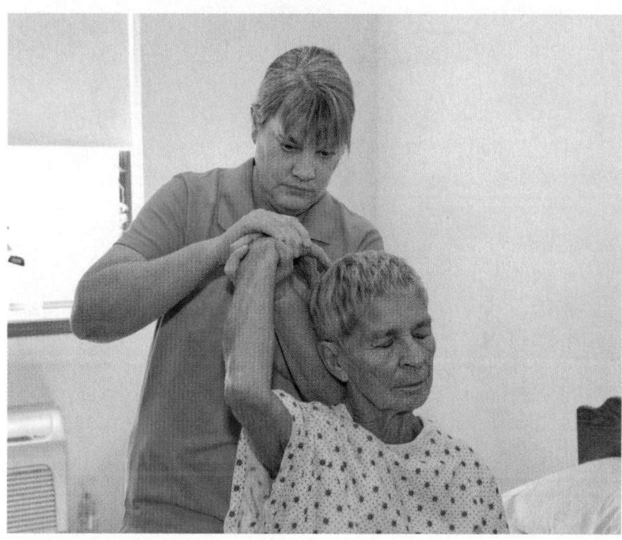

FIGURE 5-56 Applying light pressure downward onto the upper trapezius with the practitioner's elbow while keeping the client's elbow flexed and grasping the client's hand and wrist.

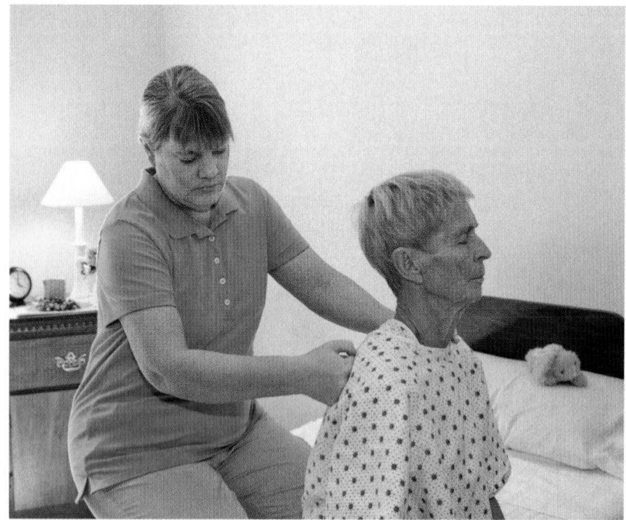

FIGURE 5-57 Performing circular friction on the upper right quadrant.

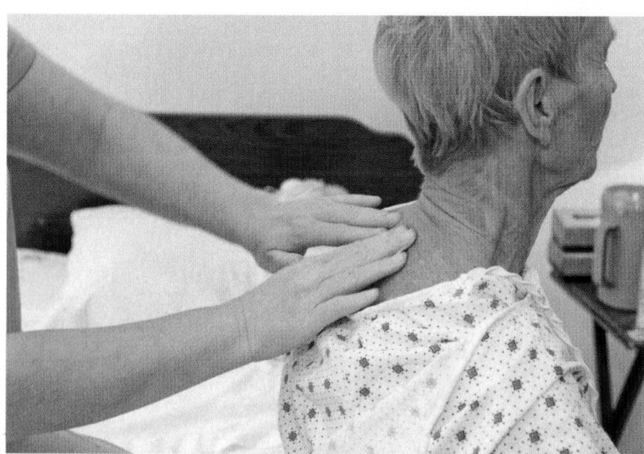

FIGURE 5-59 Applying lubricant and massaging the upper back.

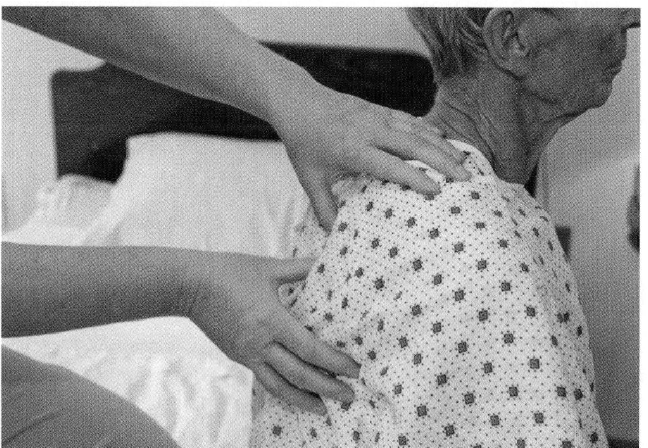

FIGURE 5-58 Pressing and performing circular friction with the thumb pads along the attachment sites of the scapula.

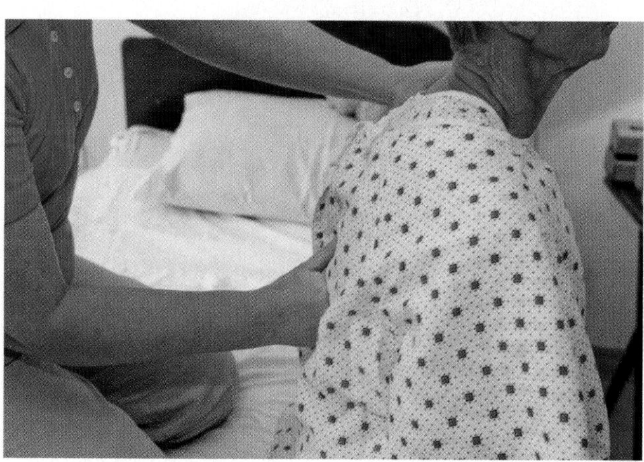

FIGURE 5-60 Performing circular friction movements in a soft fist in the mid and low back.

TIP Optional
If the client would like it, the hospital gown can be loosened and lubricant can be applied to the upper back. Gliding and kneading strokes can then be applied (Figure 5-59).

14. Holding the client's left shoulder with your left hand to stabilize the client's torso, perform circular friction movements with your right hand in a soft fist in your client's mid and low back from the level of approximately T-6 inferiorly to the posterior iliac crest, then superiorly back up to the level of T-6 (Figure 5-60). Repeat two more times.
15. Engage the tissue of the client's low back with the back of your right hand, and compress and stretch inferiorly (Figure 5-61). Hold for a few seconds, then release. Repeat three more times throughout the low back area or until you feel the muscle tissue of the low back soften.
16. Repeat Steps 11 through 15 on your client's right side.
17. Perform percussion to close the work on your client's back (Figure 5-62).
18. Move to the front of your client, and kneel with one knee on the floor. Perform gentle compressions on the client's right medial and lateral lower leg (Figure 5-63).
19. Interlace your fingers and place the heels of your hands on the medial and lateral sides of the calf directly posterior to the tibia and fibula and just distal to the popliteal fossa. Compress and gently pull the calf away from the bones (Figure 5-64), then release. Move slightly distal and repeat. Repeat the movements distally to the Achilles tendon and then back proximally.
20. Hook the fingers of both your hands in the center line between the heads of gastrocnemius just distal to the popliteal fossa. Gently pull simultaneously with both hands toward the bone (Figure 5-65), then release. Move slightly distal and release. Repeat the movements distally to the heel and then back proximally.

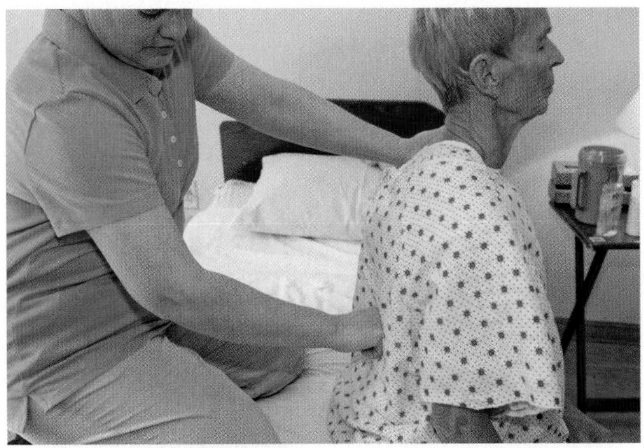

FIGURE 5-61 Engaging the tissue of the low back with the back of the hand, compressing and stretching inferiorly.

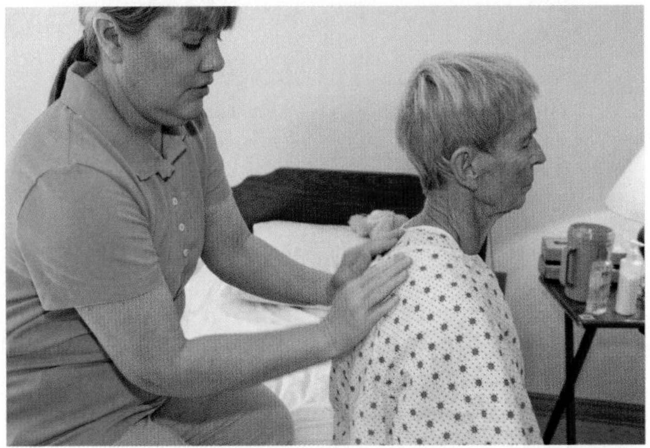

FIGURE 5-62 Cupping percussion on the back.

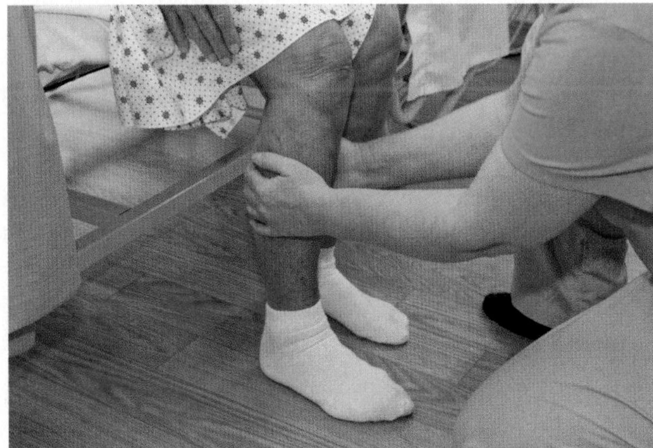

FIGURE 5-63 Performing gentle compressions on the lower leg.

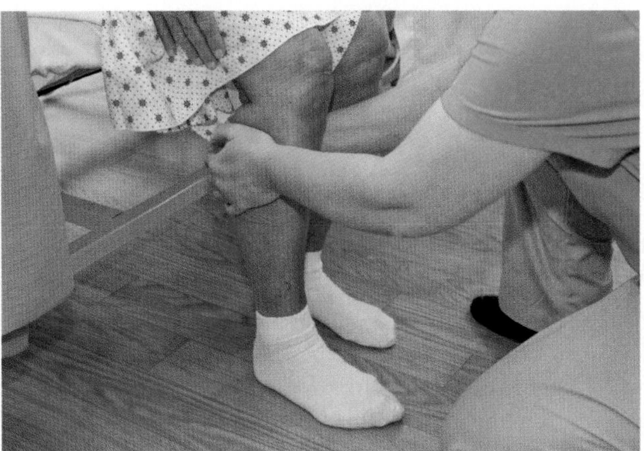

FIGURE 5-64 Compressing and gently pulling the calf away from the bone.

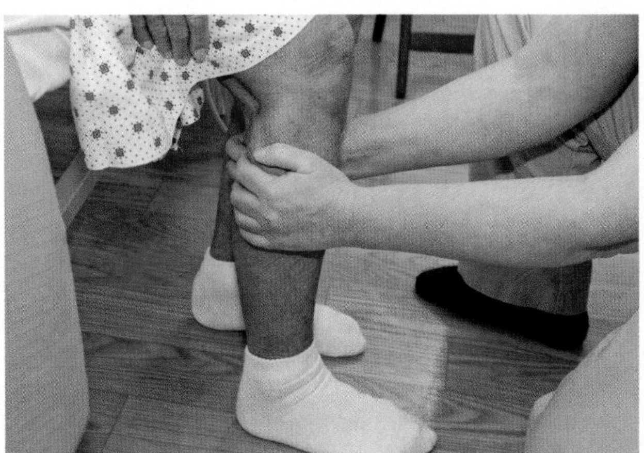

FIGURE 5-65 Hooking the fingers between the gastrocnemius and gently pulling toward the bone.

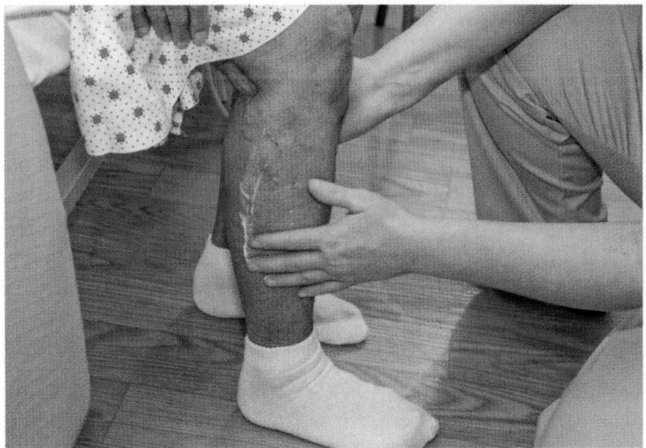

FIGURE 5-66 Applying lubricant and massaging the leg.

> **TIP Optional**
> If the client would like it, lubricant can be applied to the client's leg and then the leg can be massaged (Figure 5-66).

21. Repeat Steps 18 through 20 on the client's other leg.
22. Either kneel behind or sit next to your client, and gently knead your client's posterior neck.
23. Place your right thumb on the edge of your client's occipital ridge. Perform circular friction or deep spe-

cific friction along the occipital ridge, moving laterally and then back medially.

24. Place your hands on your client's scalp, and gently massage using circular or kneading motions with your fingertips.

MASSAGE USING A STRAIGHT-BACKED CHAIR

It is possible to provide chair massage treatments without the use of a manufactured massage chair. With creativity and a kitchen table or office desk, a chair with a back, and a pillow, effective seated massage treatments can be given. Ideally, the chair should have no arms and no wheels. Recall from Chapter 2 that one method is to place pillows on a table, then have the client sit on a stool or chair and lean forward onto the pillows, or if more propping is required, bolsters made from specially shaped foam rubber or other materials can be purchased and used for client comfort. The client raises the arms onto the pillow, rests one arm over the other, and then leans forward, turning the head so that the cheek rests on the arm. The practitioner asks the client to shift posture until comfortable. Because there is no face cradle, the practitioner should ask how the client is doing throughout the treatment to ensure that the client's neck does not get stiff from being turned to one side. The practitioner should let the client know it is all right to turn the head from one side to the other if needed.

In another method of propping the client sits in the chair backward, straddling the seat. A pillow is placed between the client and the back of the chair for comfort as the client leans forward into the support of the chairback. The client keeps the head upright during the treatment.

The body mechanics the practitioner should use when providing massage with this type of improvised setup are the same as used during treatments given to clients sitting on the manufactured massage chair. These include lunges, softly flexed knees, relaxed arms when applying pressure, allowing gravity to work rather then "muscling" the tissue, and keeping the shoulders relaxed.

Treatment Protocol

Many of the techniques presented throughout this text can be adapted for clients in a straight-backed chair. Practitioners are also encouraged to use their creativity and design their own treatments. What follows is a suggested treatment protocol practitioners can use as a basic routine. Practitioners should be mindful of the legs of the chair so as not to trip over them while working.

1. Stand behind the client with in a straight stance. Knead the client's upper trapezius bilaterally (Figure 5-67).
2. Move to a lunge position. Place both of your palms flat with your fingers spread on either side of your client's spine at the level of T-6. Keep your back leg straight as you apply pressure straight into the erector spinae muscle group. Palm-press inferiorly to your client's midback (Figure 5-68 A). At the midback, to prevent hyperextension of your wrists, change your hand position to soft fists with your thumbs on top. Continue applying pressure straight into the back muscles until you reach your client's posterior iliac crest (Figure 5-68 B). Press superiorly back up to the level of T-6. Repeat two more times.

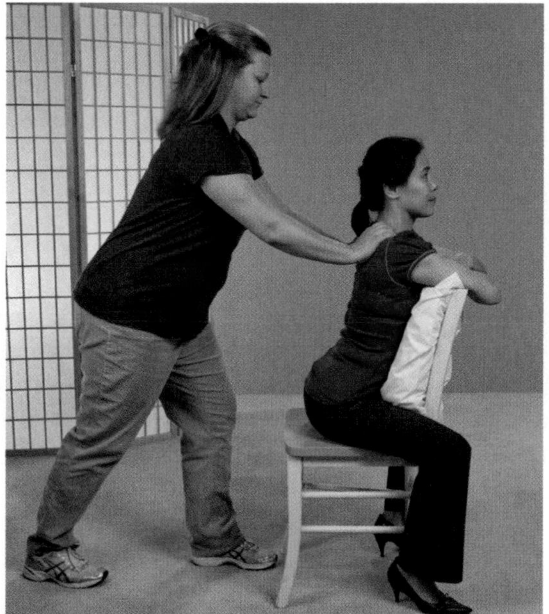

FIGURE 5-67 Kneading the upper trapezius bilaterally.

3. Move to the right of your client, and place your left forearm on your client's right upper trapezius. Sink into your lunge as you apply pressure with your forearm directly downward into the upper trapezius, then release (Figure 5-69). Repeat as you move your forearm laterally along the upper trapezius until you reach the shoulder joint, then move medially back toward the neck. Repeat three more times.
4. Place your left forearm along your client's rhomboids and press firmly. Use the broad surface of your forearm to apply pressure (Figure 5-70 A). Address the entire upper right quadrant of your client's back by changing the angle and position of your forearm and by moving to the side of your client (Figure 5-70 B).
5. Move to your client's left side, and repeat Steps 3 and 4.
6. Stand behind your client, and repeat Step 2. This connects the upper and lower quadrants of the back as you prepare to work on your client's low back.
7. Move to a half-kneeling position. Starting at your client's midback, use soft fists to apply pressure straight into the erector spinae muscles bilaterally until you reach your client's posterior iliac crest (Figure 5-71). Press superiorly back up to the midback. Repeat two more times.

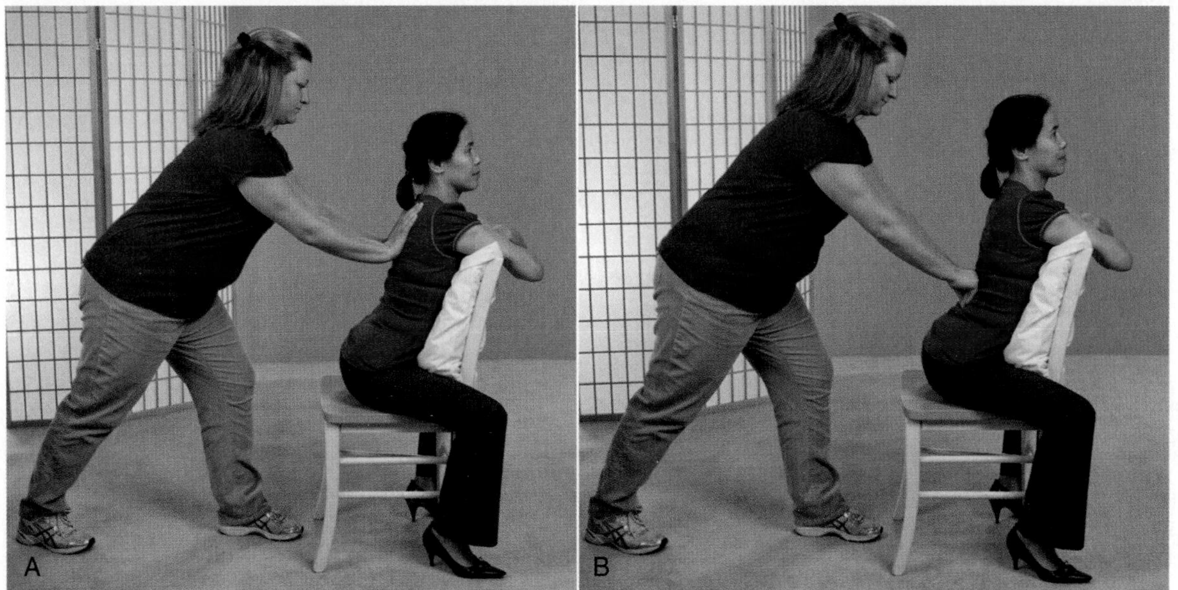

FIGURE 5-68 **A,** Palm-pressing inferiorly to the client's midback. **B,** Applying pressure with soft fists down to the posterior iliac crest.

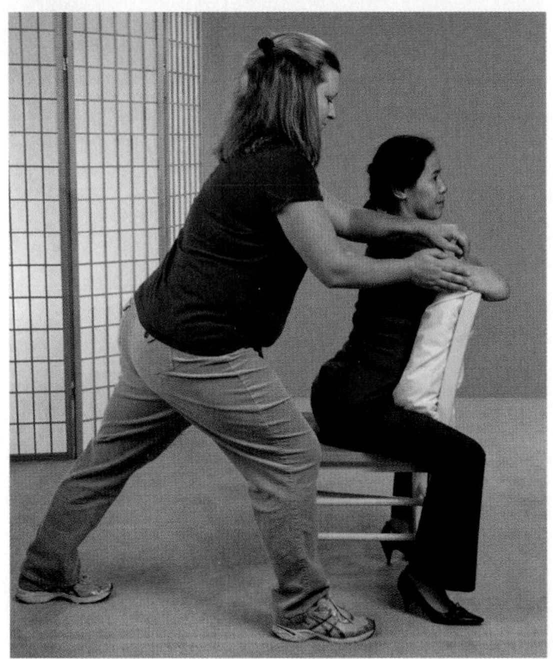

FIGURE 5-69 Applying pressure with the forearm directly downward into the upper trapezius.

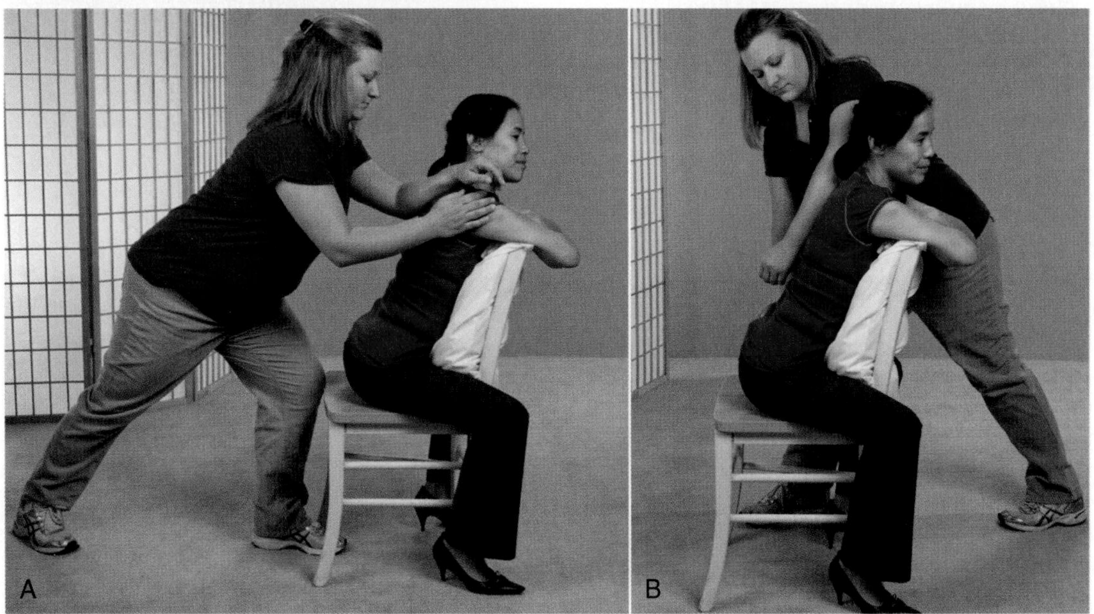

FIGURE 5-70 **A,** Using the forearm to apply pressure on the rhomboids. **B,** Moving to the side of the client and using the forearm to apply pressure on the rhomboids.

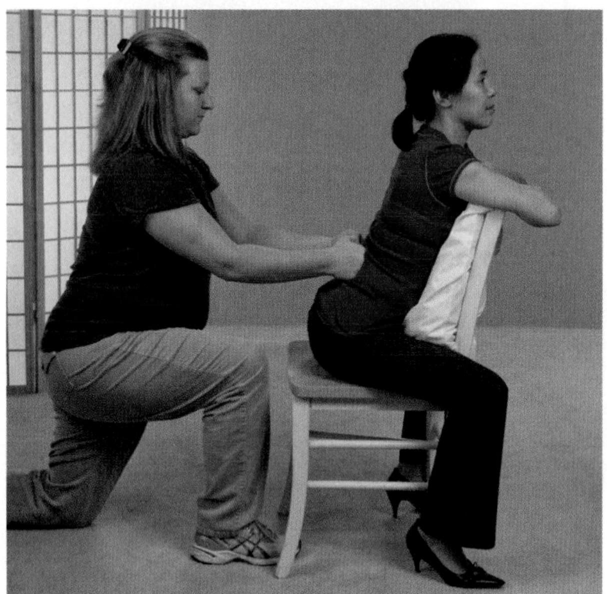

FIGURE 5-71 Using soft fists to apply pressure straight into the erector spinae muscles bilaterally.

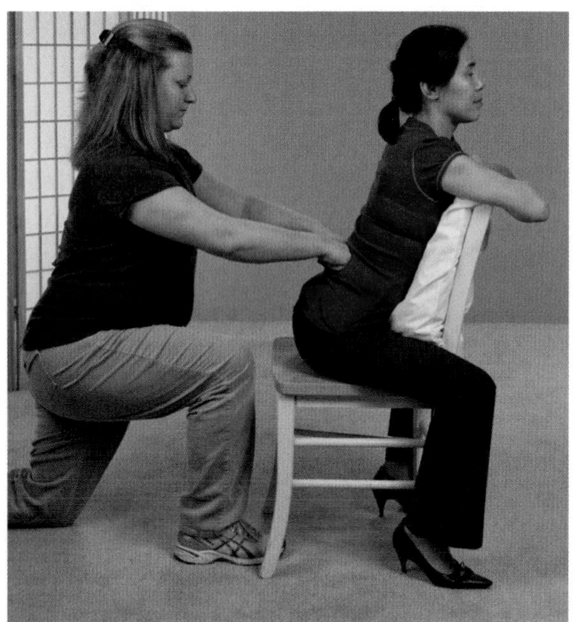

FIGURE 5-72 Using soft fists to apply pressure in a circular motion.

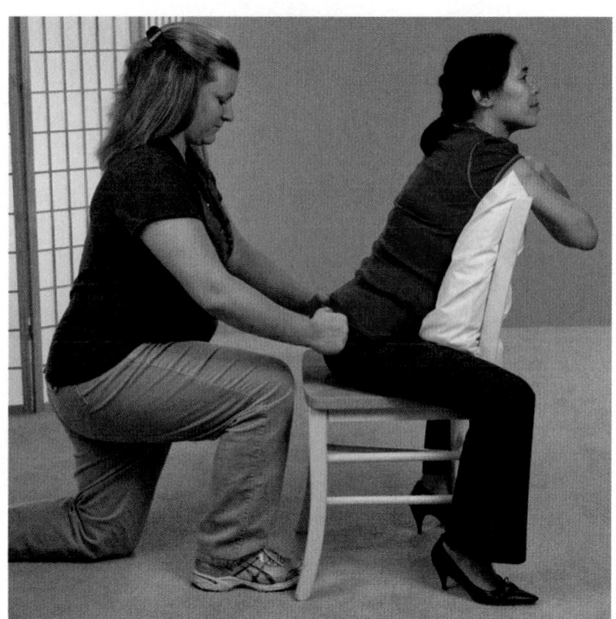

FIGURE 5-73 Continuing circular movements laterally along the iliac crest to the greater trochanter of the hip.

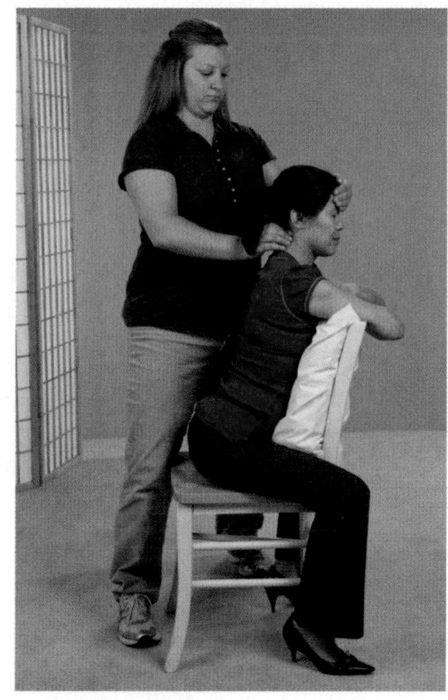

FIGURE 5-74 Placing the hand on the client's forehead and performing general kneading of the posterior neck.

8. Use soft fists to apply pressure in a circular motion (Figure 5-72). This moves the tissue in different directions as you move inferiorly to the posterior iliac crest, then superiorly up to the midback area. Repeat two more times.
9. Use soft fists to apply pressure in a circular motion inferiorly to the posterior crest again, and when you reach the posterior iliac crest, continue the circular movements laterally along the iliac crest to the greater trochanter of the hip (Figure 5-73). You may use both of your soft fists on your client's right side and then move to the left side, or you may choose to work the left and right side simultaneously. The intention is to address all of the low back muscle attachments at the posterior iliac crest.
10. Once you have completed work on your client's low back, stand in a straight stance and perform brush strokes along the clients' entire back to close the work.
11. Stand to the left of your client. Place your left hand on the client's forehead to provide stability while you perform general kneading of the posterior neck (Figure 5-74).

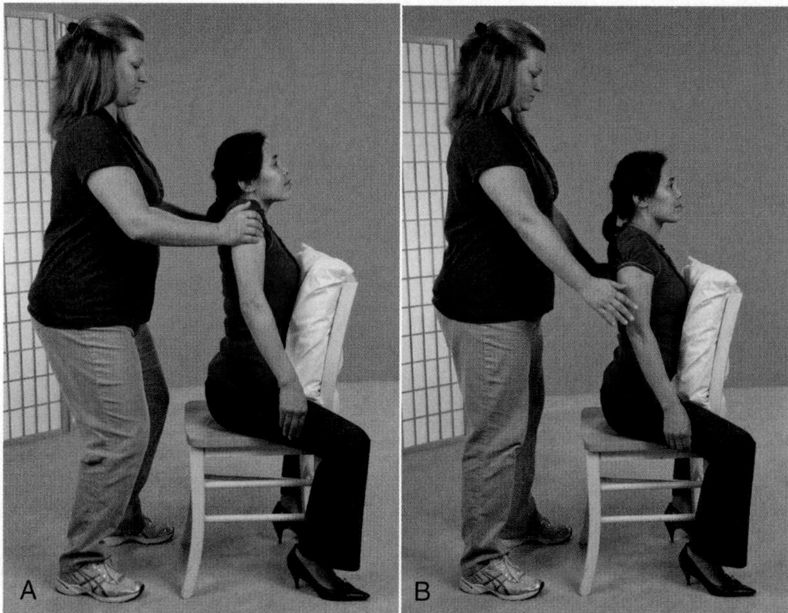

FIGURE 5-75 A, Grasping and lifting both of the shoulders upward simultaneously. **B,** On the exhale, releasing both shoulders simultaneously.

12. Stand in a straight stance behind your client, and grasp both of your client's arms at the deltoids. Have the client inhale while you lift the shoulders upward simultaneously (Figure 5-75 A). On the exhale, release both shoulders simultaneously (Figure 5-75 B). Repeat two more times.
13. Move to the right front of your client and stand in a lunge position. Pick up your client's arm and make sure that the elbow is extended with fingers pointing to the ground. Grasp the upper arm with both of your hands just below the axillary fold. Pull the arm slightly laterally (so that the client's hand does not hit the chair), and gently vibrate the arm by rolling the upper arm between both of your hands (Figure 5-76).
14. Place your thumbs side by side as you use both hands to do compressions from the deltoid to the wrist (Figure 5-77).
15. Take the client's right hand with your right hand as if you were shaking hands. With your left hand, perform one-hand kneading on the client's upper arm (Figure 5-78), then perform deep circular friction with your thumb along the radius from the elbow distally to the wrist (Figure 5-79). Retrace your movements proximally to the elbow. Repeat along the ulna and then along the interosseus membrane.
16. Turn your client's right hand palm down. Grasp it with both of your hands and your thumbs parallel on the back of the hand. Gently apply pressure downward and outward to spread the metacarpals (Figure 5-80). Repeat two more times.
17. Turn your client's hand palm up. Interlace the fingers of both your hands with your client's fingers. Spread the palm to stretch it, then use both of your thumb pads to massage the surface of the palm while maintaining the stretch (Figure 5-81).

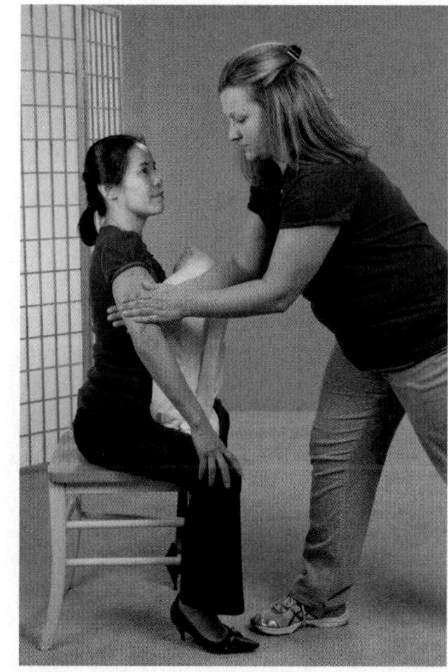

FIGURE 5-76 Rolling the arm between both hands.

18. Turn the client's hand palm down. Holding the client's wrist with your left hand, use your right hand to gently grasp each finger between your thumb and index finger with a rolling motion, moving from the base of the finger to the tip (Figure 5-82). Repeat for each finger.
19. Repeat Steps 13 through 18 on the client's left arm.
20. Move to either a straight stance or lunge behind your client. Place your hands on your client's scalp, and

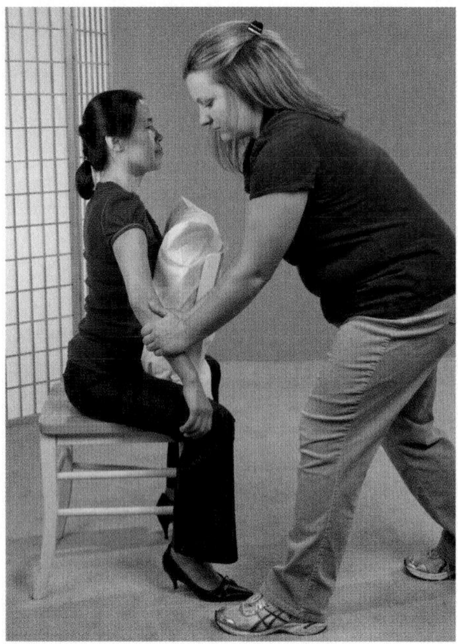

FIGURE 5-77 Compressions from the deltoid to the wrist.

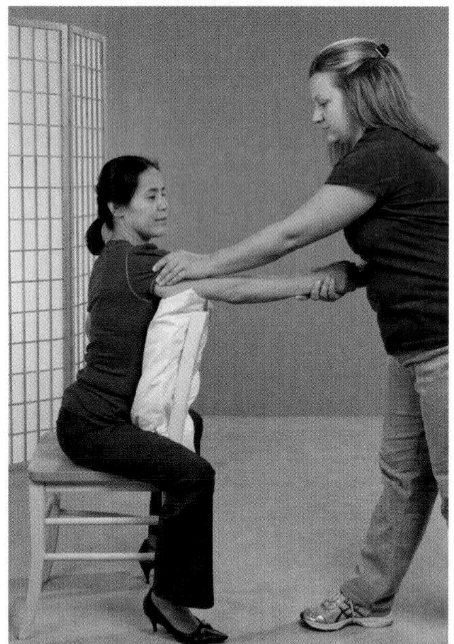

FIGURE 5-78 One-handed kneading on the upper arm.

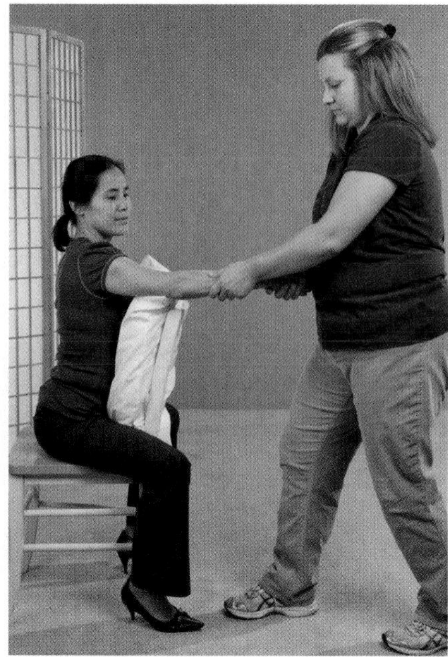

FIGURE 5-79 Circular friction along the radius.

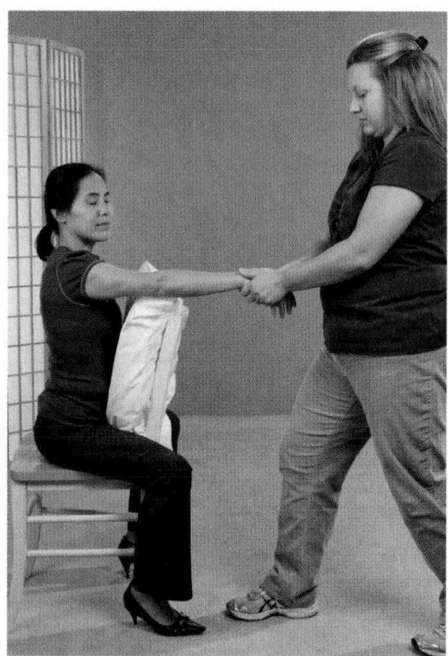

FIGURE 5-80 Gently applying pressure downward and outward to spread the metacarpals.

gently massage using circular or kneading motions with your fingertips (Figure 5-83).

21. Perform percussion on the client's left, and then right, upper trapezius, and along the upper back along the scapulae (Figure 5-84). Be sure to emphasize the upward stroke.
22. Perform brushing strokes on the client's entire back to close the treatment (Figure 5-85).

SUMMARY

Stretches that practitioners can incorporate into their chair massage treatments include those to the neck, pectoralis muscles, arm muscles, and upper trapezius. Other areas of the client's body that can benefit from specific techniques, other than stretches, include the anterior and lateral neck muscles, pectoralis muscles, serratus anterior, iliotibial (IT) band, and the calf muscles. These techniques

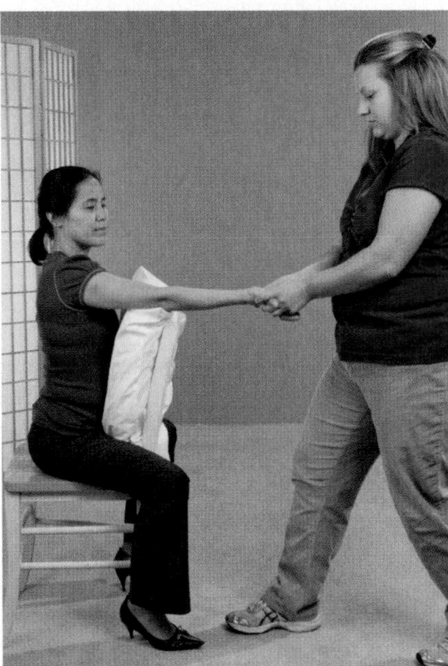

FIGURE 5-81 Interlacing the fingers, spreading the palm to stretch it, and using both thumb pads to massage the surface of the palm.

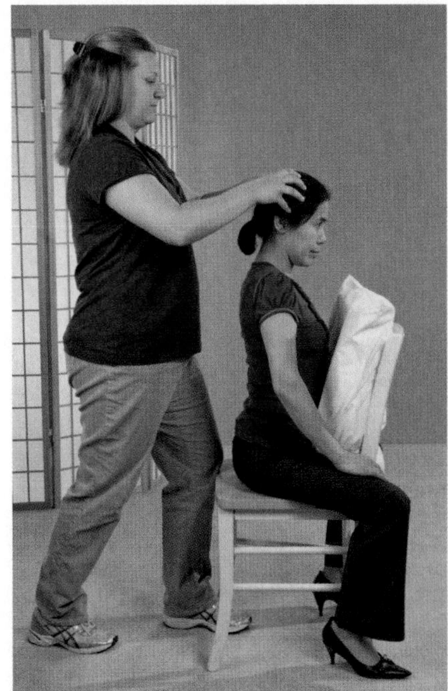

FIGURE 5-83 Massaging the client's scalp.

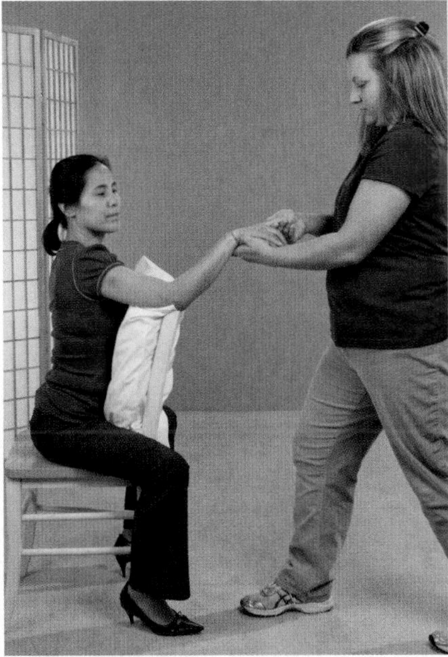

FIGURE 5-82 Gently grasping each finger with a rolling motion, moving from the base of the finger to the tip.

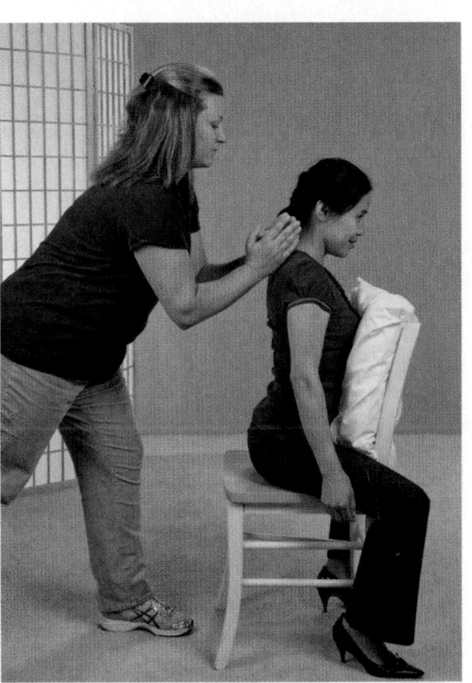

FIGURE 5-84 Performing quacking percussion.

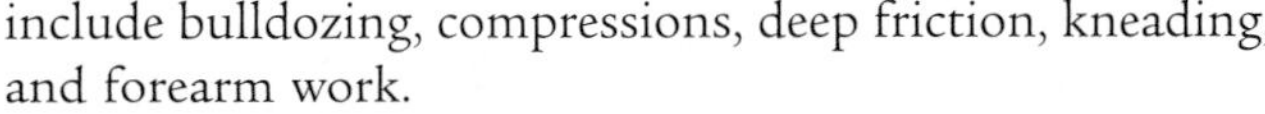

include bulldozing, compressions, deep friction, kneading, and forearm work.

Chair massage work can be supplemental to treatments on a massage table or futon in cases where, for example, an more optimal angle to address the client's neck is needed, the client is uncomfortable lying facedown on a massage table, or additional stretches for the low back and legs are warranted. Practitioners need to communicate clearly to the client why the treatment is either starting out or finishing with the client on the massage chair and to explain how the transition from the massage chair to the massage table or futon (or vice versa) will take place. Shiatsu and Thai massage techniques on the futon help loosen and stretch the low back, legs, and ankles.

Techniques can be adapted for clients who use wheelchairs. A tabletop massage support can be used, or the

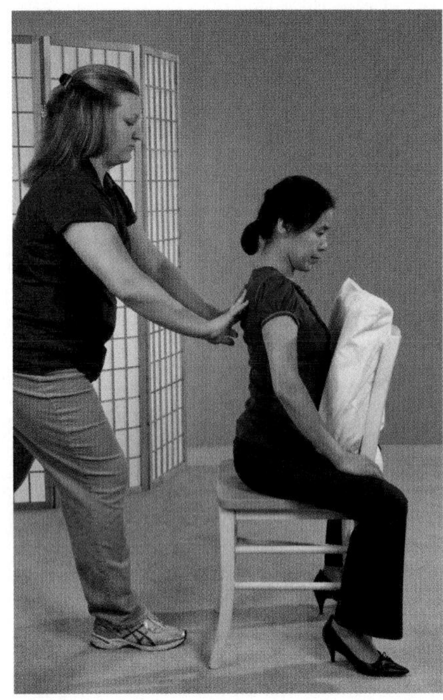

FIGURE 5-85 Performing brush strokes on the back.

client can be propped with pillows piled in the lap. Practitioners need to make sure electric wheelchairs or scooters are locked into position and all controls are turned off during the treatment.

Chair massage techniques can be adapted for clients who are in bed, whether at home, in an assisted-care facility, in hospice, or in a hospital. These clients need to be vital enough to receive massage and not have any conditions that are contraindicated for massage, and the practitioner needs to receive written clearance from the client's physician to perform any treatments. The treatment session needs to be documented properly, which includes a pretreatment (intake) form and accurate session notes for every treatment performed.

Proper propping is important, and the practitioner needs to be mindful of any medical equipment or cautionary sites on the client's body. If the client is able to sit on the side of the bed with the feet on the floor, it is possible to prop with pillows and a chair. Otherwise, if the client is able to sit up in bed it is possible to place the pillows in front that the client leans onto forward.

Performing treatments on clients in a hospital environment requires much sensitivity to the client's level of physical, emotional, and mental stamina. These environments are also likely places to encounter pathogens, so practitioners should take proper steps to maintain good health. Practitioners also need to be of the emotional impact of working in a healthcare setting.

Chair massage treatments can be provided with the client sitting in a straight-back chair. One method involves placing pillows or foam rubber bolsters on a table, then have the client sit on a stool or chair and lean forward onto the pillows or bolsters. In another method, the client sits in the chair backward, straddling the seat. A pillow is placed between the client and the back of the chair for comfort as the client leans forward into the support of the chairback. The client keeps the head upright during the treatment.

STUDY QUESTIONS

Multiple Choice

Answers to the Study Questions are on page 227.

1. Which of the following is an indication for neck stretches?
   a. Muscle tightness
   b. Arthritis
   c. Herniated disk
   d. Ankylosing spondylitis

2. In the lateral neck stretch, it is inadvisable for the practitioner to do which of the following?
   a. Have the client place her hand over her head and touch her ear.
   b. Have the client take a deep breath.
   c. Press down on the client's head.
   d. Place the forearm on the client's upper trapezius.

3. In the triceps brachii stretch, how is the point of the client's elbow facing?
   a. Down
   b. Laterally
   c. Medially
   d. Up

4. Which of the following techniques can be performed on the client's calf muscles while in the massage chair?
   a. Kneading
   b. Circular friction
   c. Thumb pressure
   d. All of the above

5. Which of the following is a consideration when working on a client who is sitting in a straight-backed chair?
   a. The client's neck may get stiff from being turned to one side.
   b. The pillow is placed in the client's lap.
   c. The lunge stance is ineffective for providing pressure.
   d. The practitioner should work against gravity when applying pressure.

Fill in the Blank

1. The posterior neck stretch should be held for approximately ____________________ seconds before being released.

2. Myofascial ____________________ is a technique that involves stabilizing a muscle attachment site then having the client move so that the muscle or muscles involved elongate.

3. For a treatment that includes both chair and table massage, communication about how the client will make the transition from the massage chair to the massage table is best done during the ____________________ ____________________.

4. While working on clients in beds, the practitioner must be conscious of the client's body mechanics as it can be easy to ignore ____________________ ____________________ while working.

5. With permission from the client, ____________________ behind him or her on the hospital bed to perform back massage.

Short Answer

1. Explain the benefits of performing techniques to the client's IT band.

____

____

____

____

____

STUDY QUESTIONS

2. Explain why the practitioner may choose to start a full-body treatment with the client on the massage chair and finish with the client on the massage table.

____

____

____

____

____

3. Explain two ways to prop a client in a wheelchair for chair massage.

____

____

____

____

____

4. Explain the various factors practitioners should consider before providing chair massage in healthcare settings.

____

____

____

____

____

5. Explain how to prop a client in a straight-backed chair for chair massage.

ACTIVITIES

1. Practice the additional techniques and adaptations presented in this chapter on at least 10 people, such as friends and family. Work on people with various body sizes and shapes.
2. Practice the protocols for clients in wheelchairs, hospital beds, and straight-backed chairs. If you do not know someone who uses a wheelchair or is in a hospital bed, stage these situations for practice.
3. Create your own treatment protocols for clients in wheelchairs, beds, and straight-backed chairs.

____

____

____

____

____

4. Design a treatment plan for a client who does not like to put his or her head in the face cradle and prefers to sit upright on the massage chair.

____

____

____

____

____

5. Design a treatment plan for a client who cannot sit comfortably on the massage chair because of a condition such as arthritis in the knees or knee replacements. What adaptations would you need to make?

____

____

____

____

____

Essentials of Business

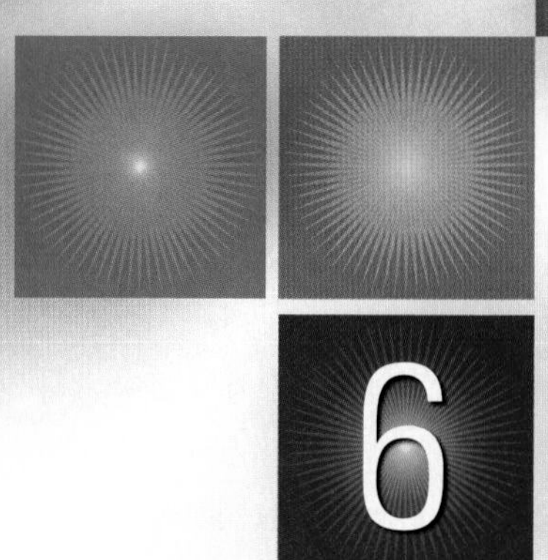

OBJECTIVES

Upon completion of this chapter, the reader will have the information necessary to do the following:

1. Explain the difference between an employee and an independent contractor.
2. Describe the factors involved in becoming a successful chair massage employee.
3. Discuss the importance and components of a business plan.
4. Delineate a target market.
5. Develop a marketing plan.
6. Discuss effective ways to approach business clients.
7. Develop and perform a chair massage presentation.
8. Create chair massage business materials including client intake forms, treatment documentation methods, client education handouts, business cards, brochures or pamphlets, and gift certificates.
9. Discuss the management of chair massage accounts, including the guidelines for organizing an efficient account.
10. Explain the components of a fair contract between a chair massage business and the companies for which chair massage services are provided.

KEY TERMS

Account	Marketing
Business plan	Marketing plan
Business relationship	Operation plan
Client base	Return on investment costs
Demographics	Sales
Indemnity agreement	Target market

ASPECTS OF A CHAIR MASSAGE BUSINESS

Providing chair massage treatments, either full-time or part-time, is a viable career choice for many practitioners. They can choose to offer chair massage solely or in conjunction with table massage. Chair massage performed at businesses is usually weekday work, which, for some practitioners, is when they are sporadically booked for table massage. Performing chair massage can be a way for practitioners to fill in empty areas of their treatment calendar.

Recall from Chapter 1 that practitioners may choose from several types of chair massage work options, such as becoming an employee or an independent contractor who provides bodywork services to the employees of a company that contracts with companies or other organizations or groups for the chair massage service. Practitioners can also choose to start their own chair massage businesses, either solely or in partnership with others. For all options, though, having knowledge of how to efficiently conduct a chair massage business adds greatly to the professionalism and career success of the practitioner.

Employee versus Independent Contractor

For practitioners who either are not in a position to start their own business or are not interested in becoming business owners, working as an employee or an independent contractor for a company that provides chair massage treatments may be the best choice. There are considerations unique to each option, which can serve as guidelines for practitioners who are undecided about which path they want to follow. Table 6-1 shows how employees and independent contractors differ.

Pay rates can vary from chair massage company to chair massage company. Some companies pay by the hour, some by a percentage of the cost of the treatment performed. Practitioners should make sure to find out the pay structure, rates, raise policy, and opportunities for career advancement in any company for which they are interested in working. In the case of gratuities, some companies do not allow their employees or independent contractors to receive gratuities, whereas other companies do. Independent contractors will receive the gratuity money directly from the client, whereas employees may receive the money directly from the client or it may be added into their paychecks.

Whether a practitioner becomes an employee of or an independent contractor for a chair massage company, it is important that a contract be signed between the

TABLE 6-1 Employee versus Independent Contractor

Features	Employee	Independent Contractor
Amount of work/benefits	Can be full-time (qualifies for benefits) or part-time (does not qualify for benefits)	Can be full-time or part-time; does not receive benefits in either case
Pay	Paid by the hour or by treatment	Pay to company either an hourly fee or percentage of cost of treatment performed
Costs of treatments	Set by company	Set by mutual agreement between company and contractor
Client payment for treatments	Clients pay company for treatments	Clients pay contractor directly
Wages	Set by company; federal and state income taxes, Social Security, and Medicare deducted from paycheck*	Responsible for paying own taxes, Social Security, Medicare[†]
Schedule	Set by company	Set by contractor
Booking of treatments	All booked by company	Booked by company or by contractor but needs to be coordinated by the company
Equipment and supplies	All provided by the company	Contractor uses own; with mutual agreement, could use company's equipment and supplies

*Employees receive the Internal Revenue Service (IRS) W-2 Wage and Tax Statement, which shows their income and deductions for Social Security and Medicare. They use this statement to file their taxes.

[†]Independent contractors need to keep track of the income they have received from their clients and follow proper Internal Revenue Service tax filing procedures. Depending on how they have contracted with the chair massage company, they may receive the IRS 1099-MISC form from the company which will show how much income they received as an independent contractor, and they can use this form to file their taxes. More information about the 1099-MISC form and other IRS forms independent contractors need can be found at www.irs.gov. Additionally, practitioners who are considering becoming independent contractors are encouraged to find a reliable accountant to assist them with their bookkeeping and tax preparation.

practitioner and the company. For employees, this contract should clearly and specifically outline the following details:

- The work schedule
- Pay rates
- Amount of sick time and vacation time
- Whether the company pays for the employee's professional liability insurance
- Any healthcare plan options

For independent contractors, the contract should include the fee or percentage of each treatment paid to the company and the days and times the independent contractor is choosing to work. Basically, contracts should include what the employee or independent contractor is responsible for and what the company is responsible for. All expectations and duties should be written in clear language. It is wise to have any contract or agreement reviewed by an attorney before signing to ensure it is legal and viable. Figure 6-1 is an example of an employee contract, and Figure 6-2 is an example of an independent contractor contract.

Chair massage companies may also have other policies and procedures of which the employee or independent contractor needs to be clearly aware and should get in writing. For example, practitioners may be required to sign a confidentiality agreement and agree not to provide treatments other than as a representative of the company or take clients with them should they no longer work for the company. The employee or independent contractor should also know what the company's leave of absence policy is. There is usually a seniority system, for both available shifts and client booking. Those who have the least amount of seniority get the last choice of shifts. Practitioners are also expected to be punctual and work with their scheduled appointments; refusing to work with a particular client is generally not acceptable. Practitioners need to set aside personal feelings and be professional.

Most massage therapy businesses have a dress code, and companies that provide chair massage are no exception. Whether an employee or an independent contractor, the practitioner will be expected to look and dress a certain way. This can include the following, for example:

- No visible tattoos or facial piercing
- Neatly groomed hair and nails
- Dressed in either a uniform (such as a company shirt and solid color pants, which the company may provide or the practitioner is expected to purchase) or clothing specified by the company, such as a polo shirt and khaki pants; the practitioner's clothing is expected to be clean and presentable (i.e., not wrinkled, not showing either breast or gluteal cleavage when the practitioner bends over, not too tight or too baggy, and so forth)
- Shoes that are clean, odor-free, and have closed toes, such as athletic shoes

Figure 6-3 shows several practitioners wearing acceptable professional dress.

STARTING A CHAIR MASSAGE BUSINESS

When a practitioner offers regular seated massage appointments at a business or organization, this is referred to as having an **account**. Maintaining the account refers to the tasks involved in making sure that the services that the practitioner is providing are meeting the needs of the clients, thus allowing the practitioner to provide massages on a regular basis. The ability to set up chair massage accounts and maintain them over a period of time is at the heart of making seated massage a viable component of a practitioner's business.

There are many factors that affect the successful establishment of chair massage accounts and then successfully maintaining them. These include choosing a name for the business, creating a business plan, approaching and communicating effectively with business contacts, having presentation skills, designing clear and appealing written marketing materials such as brochures and business cards or surveys regarding client satisfaction, and having excellent documentation skills.

CHOOSING A BUSINESS NAME

When practitioners choose a name for their chair massage business it is essential that the name reflect what their business does or what services they offer. The name must also be professional and appropriate for the massage and

Chair Massage Employment Contract
Between Stress Be Gone, Inc.
and Patricia M. Holland, LMT, MC

This contract dated, June 17, 2009, is by and between Stress Be Gone, Inc. (Employer) located at 1960 E. Pecoraro Ave. Tucson, AZ and Patricia M. Holland, LMT, MC (Employee).

Services to Be Provided by the Employee

Employee is contracted to provide seated chair massage services within the scope of licensure. Employee is responsible for maintaining appropriate certification and licensure (including all costs thereof). Employee agrees to wear professional attire at all times when representing the employer. Professional attire consists of beige/khaki long pants, a black polo shirt, and closed toes shoes. Employee will maintain client records in the manner prescribed by employer.

Employee will provide transportation to and from the onsite locations.

When Employee is not engaged in sessions while on location, Employee will contact the Human Resources Department of the location to announce that there are openings available for clients.

Services to Be Provided by the Employer

Employer shall provide the following: a professional well maintained massage chair, sanitation supplies, a music source, marketing supplies, and wellness information in the form of handouts. Employer will make all arrangements to schedule appointments; communicate with the contact person at each location to arrange logistics, coordinate the collection of fees from the location, will notify the Employee within 48 hours of an employment opportunity, and will provide 24 hours' notice of a cancellation of an event to the Employee.

Other Provisions

1. Employee has the right to provide services for other companies during the term of this contract; however, he or she cannot solicit seated chair massage business from the companies already contracted with the employer.
2. Employee has the right to provide 60-minute therapeutic table massage services to individuals of the companies contracted with Employer at the Employee's private practice.
3. Upon termination of employment the Employer retains rights to all of the onsite location accounts. The Employee shall not solicit business from these accounts.
4. All client records shall remain with the Employer.
5. Employee may not display any non-Employer marketing materials except the Employee's private practice information for table massage.

Fees and Terms of Payment

Employee shall be compensated at the base rate of $40 per hour for a minimum of 3 hours and a maximum of 6 hours. Payment will be made within 48 hours of the account being complete.

FIGURE 6-1 Example of an employee contract. (Adapted from Sohnen-Moe CM: *Business mastery: a guide for creating a fulfilling, thriving business and keeping it successful*, ed 4. Tucson, 2008, Sohnen-Moe Associates.)

Continued

Local, State, and Federal Taxes

Employer is responsible for paying all required local, state, and federal withholding, Social Security, and Medicare taxes.

Workers' Compensation and Unemployment Insurance

Employer will provide Workers' Compensation and Unemployment Insurance.

Insurance

During the term of this contract, Employee shall maintain malpractice insurance of at least $2,000,000 aggregate annual and $1,000,000 per incident. Employer shall maintain insurance for liability, fire, and theft.

Term of Agreement

Either party may terminate this agreement, given reasonable cause, as provided below, or by giving 14 days' written notice to the other party of the intention to terminate this contract.

1. Material violation of the provisions of this contract.
2. Action by either party exposing the other to liability for property damage or personal injury.
3. Violation of ethical standards as defined by local, state and/or national associations and governing bodies.
4. Loss of licensure for services provided.
5. Employee fails to maintain the standard of service deemed appropriate by Employer.
6. Employee engages in any pattern or course of conduct on a continuing basis which adversely affects Employee's ability to perform services.
7. Employee engages in any pattern or course of conduct on a continuing basis which adversely affects Employer's or other employees' ability to perform services.
8. It is agreed that any unresolved disputes will be settled by arbitration, including costs thereof.

This constitutes the entire agreement between Employee and Employer and supersedes any and all prior written or verbal agreements. Should and part of this agreement be deemed unenforceable, the remainder of the agreement continues in effect. This agreement is governed by the laws of the state of Arizona.

Employee: ______________________ Date: ____________

Employer: ______________________ Date: ____________

Witness: ______________________ Date: ____________

FIGURE 6-1, cont'd.

bodywork profession. The names should be short enough fit in one line on a business card. This makes it easier for clients and potential clients to remember the business.

Sometimes practitioners come up with business names they think are clear or witty, only to have them completely misunderstood by potential clients. For example, consider the reaction the practitioner may get who names his or her business "Complete Massage! Treating Clients Head to Toe and Everything in Between." The practitioner may think that it is clear that the name means that he or she can effectively address the head, neck, shoulders, upper, mid and low back, hips, legs, and feet. Potential clients, on the other hand, may think the name means that sexual services are available. Practitioners should consider having trusted family members, friends, and mentors evaluate names they are considering to get more objective opinions on what the names may be conveying.

CREATING A BUSINESS PLAN

Many times people have great ideas but do not necessarily know the steps necessary to put the ideas into action, or they many not have realistic expectations about implementation costs versus revenue. When considering whether to create a chair massage business either as part of an existing bodywork practice or as the entire practice, it is highly recommended that a cohesive **business plan** be developed. A business plan is an outline of definable business goals, the reasoning behind why the business goals are attainable, and a realistic plan for reaching those goals.

There are many resources for creating business plans, such as *Business and Professional Skills for Massage Therapists*, by Sandy Fritz (Elsevier, 2010), *Business Mastery*, 4th edition, by Cherie Sohnen-Moe (published by Sohnen-Moe Associates, Inc., 2008), the Small Business Administration (www.sba.gov), local chambers of commerce, and the Better Business Bureau (www.bbb.org). Additionally, business coaches and mentors can be found in many cities and towns. It is important that practitioners make informed decisions when determining what steps they need to take to successfully incorporate chair massage into their businesses.

The following information does not constitute a business plan; rather, it is intended as a template for the research needed to be done to develop a business plan. Again, it is

Chair Massage Practitioner Independent Contractor Business Contract
Between Patricia Holland, Mindful Touch Therapeutic Massage
And Corporate Chair Massage, Inc.

This document, _______________, 20____, is by and between Patricia Holland of Mindful Touch Therapeutic Massage (Contractor) with principal office located at 423 E. Hewitt Ave. Tucson, AZ and Corporate Chair Massage, Inc. (owner of corporate account), with principal office located at 360 N. Locust St. Tucson, AZ.

Independent Contractor Status

Patricia Holland is an independent contractor and not an employee of Corporate Chair Massage, Inc.
As an independent contractor, Patricia Holland and Corporate Chair Massage, Inc. (CCM, Inc.) agree to the following:

1. Ms. Holland has the authority to determine the means, manner, and method by which seated chair massages services are provided.
2. Ms. Holland will provide all necessary equipment, supplies and materials used for this service, including a massage chair, face cradle covers, sanitation materials, music source, and wellness information in the form of handouts describing the benefits of massage in the workplace.
3. Ms. Holland has the right to conduct services for others during the terms of this contract but will not solicit nor provide services to Corporate Chair Massage, Inc. clients for private practice during the terms of this contract or for 9 months after termination. Upon termination of Contract, Ms. Holland has the right to approach any contacts made while providing services for Corporate Chair Massage, Inc.
4. Ms. Holland shall indemnify and hold Corporate Chair Massage, Inc. harmless from liability or loss of property arising from services being provided under this contract.
5. Ms. Holland is responsible for maintaining appropriate certification and licensure for the regions in services are provided.

Services to Be Provided by Independent Contractor

- Patricia Holland, LMT, MC agrees to provide seated chair massage therapy, and will at all times remain within the scope of practice for massage therapy as designated by the American Massage Therapy Association, and will follow all standards of practice as designated by the National Certification Board for Therapeutic Massage and Bodyworkers (NCBTMB).
- Ms. Holland will provide a minimum of three (3) hours of chair massage or a maximum of six (6) hours of chair massage in twenty–minute (20–minute) increments to on-site businesses who have contracted with CCM, Inc.
- Ms. Holland will dress in a manner that is professional and appropriate which includes wearing long black pants, a white polo shirt and close-toed tennis shoes.
- Ms. Holland shall maintain all client records as directed by CCM, Inc.

Services to Be Provided by Corporate Chair Massage, Inc.

- CCM, Inc. shall provide corporate chair massage clientele for Patricia Holland, LMT, MC with at least 48 hours' notice. This notice will include the name of a contact person on location, travel directions to the location, and the exact time frame in which the services will be provided.
- CCM, Inc. will make all logistic and financial arrangements with corporate clients as well as manage all aspects of payment from the corporate client.

FIGURE 6-2 Example of an independent contractor contract. (Adapted from Sohnen-Moe CM: *Business mastery: a guide for creating a fulfilling, thriving business and keeping it successful*, ed 4. Tucson, 2008, Sohnen-Moe Associates.)

Continued

highly recommended that readers find additional resources to assist them in the creation of their actual business plan.

The four crucial areas that need to be considered when building or expanding a business involve determining the following:

1. The target market
2. The services and products to offer
3. How to deliver the services and products (also known as the operation plan)
4. The financial plan for investment costs and revenue

Target Markets

The term **target market** refers to the specific type of clients (customers) that a business wants to attract. Having a target market helps to narrow down the scope of people on whom the business will spend its money, time, and effort in order to be noticed. Because most businesses have a specific amount of money to spend on marketing, it is cost-efficient to find out who is most likely to have the needs the business can fill and get those people to notice the business.

The key to having a successful bodywork business is to have a dependable number of clients actively making regular appointments for services. This is referred to as a **client base**. How do practitioners attract clients to their business, and how many clients does it take to be considered a successful practice? These are two fundamental questions that practitioners must ask themselves as they venture into the world of self-employment. When just starting out or starting a new business direction, it is best that practitioners have a clear vision of the kinds of clients for whom they will provide their services. Narrowing the focus to a few specific groups of people will help save money as well as effort when it comes to marketing to these groups.

Fees, Terms of Payment

CCM, Inc. will pay Patricia Holland $50 per hour while on location as well as provide and additional sum of $20 to cover travel and meal expenses. This payment will be made within five (5) business days of the completion of the account.

Local, State, and Federal Taxes

Ms. Holland is responsible for paying and filing all applicable local, state, and federal withholding, Social Security, and Medicare taxes.

Workers' Compensation and Unemployment Insurance

CCM, Inc. is not responsible for payment of Workers' Compensation and Unemployment Insurance.

Insurance

During the term of this contract, Ms. Holland shall maintain professional liability insurance of at least $2,000,000 aggregate annual and $1,000,000 per incident.

Terms of Agreement

Either party may terminate this contract, given reasonable cause, as provided below, or by giving 30 days' written notice to CCM, Inc. of the intention to terminate this contract.

a. Material violation of the provisions of this contract.
b. Action by either party exposing the other to liability for property damage or personal injury.
c. Violation of ethical standards as defined by local, state, and or national associations and governing bodies.
d. Loss of licensure for services provided.
e. Ms. Holland engages in any pattern of behavior on a continuing basis which adversely affects Ms. Holland's ability to perform services.
f. Ms. Holland engages in any pattern of behavior on a continuing basis which adversely affects CCM, Inc. or CCM, Inc. associates' ability to perform services.
h. It is agreed that any unresolved disputes will be settled by arbitration, including costs thereof.

This contract constitutes the entire agreement between independent contractor, Patricia Holland, LMT, LC of Mindful Touch Therapeutic Massage and Corporate Chair Massage, Inc. and supersedes any and all prior written or verbal agreements. Should any part of this contract be deemed unenforceable, the remainder of the contract continues in effect. This contract is governed by the laws of the State of Arizona.

Independent Contractor: ____________________ Date: ____________

CCM, Inc., Representative: ____________________ Date: ____________

Witness: ____________________ Date: ____________

FIGURE 6-2, cont'd.

When determining the target market, practitioners need to consider **demographics**. Demographics refer to characteristics of various populations, such as age, income, profession, family size (i.e., how many children a couple has), level of education, and so forth. Based on this information, the following are some questions practitioners can ask themselves:

- What type of clients do I want to attract? For example, what is the age group I'd like to market to? What income level, professions, and recreational activities are these clients likely to have?
- Where are these clients located? Are they in one specific area of my community, or are they scattered throughout?
- What will these clients pay for treatments?
- What types of treatments do these clients need? In other words, what types of conditions and situations would these clients have that would make them interested in chair massage? Do they have professions where they sit at desks all day and so might be interested in treatments that relieve low back pain? Do they work at computers most of the day and so have sore neck muscles that can benefit from chair massage techniques? Do they stand on their feet all day and so would be interested in overall muscle tension relief? Are they of the age that many are getting married and starting families and so may have bridal or baby showers at which they might want chair massage provided as a treat?

Another way to determine a target market is to consider what industries and businesses in the community do. Do their workforces sit most of the day at a computer or phone or stand all day, such as in law offices, call centers, or security firms? In other words, the practitioner should become familiar with the local workforce to determine if there are

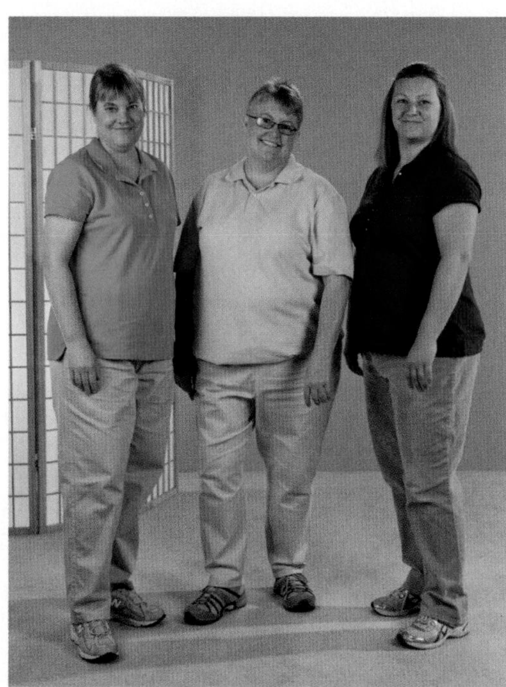

FIGURE 6-3 Practitioners wearing examples of professional dress.

companies or types of professions that would be open to having a practitioner provide services that would benefit their employees. Practitioners can also try entering "sedentary occupations" in an Internet search engine to get more ideas. Other resources involve searching the yellow pages (for associations, organizations, competing chair massage businesses, and so forth), by using local libraries, contacting local chambers of commerce, and sometimes simply driving around neighborhoods and business districts.

The Internet is also an excellent resource for demographics and trends, especially such websites as the American Massage Therapy Association (www.amtamassage.org), the Associated Bodywork and Massage Professionals (www.abmp.com), and the National Certification Board for Therapeutic Massage and Bodywork (www.ncbtmb.org). There should also be websites for professional associations to which members of the target market belong.

After identifying companies, professions, and organizations in the community that the practitioner is considering approaching, the next step is to research them. For each business, find out how many employees there are and the type of work done (e.g., computer tasks, phone calls, telemarketing, physical labor, and so forth). Then do some research about what impact the work may have on the employees' bodies and how seated massage may benefit them. For example, are the employees on the phone all day but do not use headsets? In this case, create a presentation on neck and shoulder dysfunctions and how seated massage can relieve muscle tension and pain in these areas. If a certain percentage of the workforce uses computers, the employees are at risk of repetitive stress syndrome in the wrist and finger joints. Given this information, develop a specific treatment plan to prevent the condition from happening or from getting worse in those who are showing signs of it. Because seated massage is such a flexible modality, there are really no limits to the possible target markets. The key is to narrow down interest to one or two groups, then find a way to introduce chair massage to the targeted business, profession, or organization.

Marketing

Marketing involves promoting, selling, and distributing a product or service to prospective consumers (or clients, in the case of massage and bodywork). The purpose of marketing is to generate interest in the product or service with the goal of forming business relationships with those who are interested. The **business relationship** consists of providing the product or service in a mutually agreed-upon manner in return for payment. While marketing is usually done to a wide audience, **sales**, a part of marketing, are more focused on those who have expressed at least some interest in the product or service. It occurs one on one, with the provider (or a representative of the provider) of the product or service communicating directly with a prospective client to create the business relationship. Sales are covered in more detailed in the "Sales" section of this chapter.

Marketing Plan

Once practitioners have determined their target market or markets, it is time to develop a **marketing plan**—a written document detailing the necessary actions to achieve one or more marketing objectives. In short, it is a plan on how to reach the practitioner's target markets. It needs to include the following information:

- Methods to reach the target market(s)
- Estimated costs of these methods
- A timeline for implementing the marketing methods
- A system for evaluating the effectiveness of the various marketing methods

It is essential to be clear about the vision of the business in the course of developing a marketing plan. This will make it much easier to communicate in a positive, straightforward, and professional manner, which tends to make prospective clients more receptive to what the practitioner has to say. To help with clarity, practitioners should always keep in mind the question, "How do I differentiate my business from all the other businesses offering chair massage?" It would be useful for practitioners to make a list of answers to this question, such as these:

- My level of education, experience, and professionalism differentiates my business from others offering chair massage.
- The level of education, experience, and professionalism of all the practitioners who work for me differentiates my business from others offering chair massage.

PERSPECTIVES

Kneaded Energy, Kneaded Energy School of Massage, NCBTMB CE Provider #450524-07, and National Massage Network

408 ½ State St., Greensboro, NC 27405
Telephone number: *(336) 273-1260*
Website: *www.kneadedenergy.com*
Co-owners: *Bill Norman, LMBT, and Shelley Johnson, LMBT*
In business since 1999

Bill and Shelley started their private massage practice, Kneaded Energy, in Greensboro, North Carolina, in 1999. Since then they have added several divisions to their parent company, including a massage school and CE provider program, and they have authored: **The Enviable Lifestyle: Creating a Successful Massage Therapy Business;** National Massage Network is one of those divisions. They have an extensive team of licensed contracted massage therapists across the country who perform treatments at companies and events.

The onsite business happened organically when someone they knew in a city near their office called to hire a massage therapist for seated treatments. Since the philosophy of the business is "Say yes first, then figure out the details," they were able to find a therapist for the event. Soon, another call came in from another city nearby, and they were able to get a therapist for that job. As word got out, they began getting calls from companies across the nation who wanted to hire chair massage therapists, and they figured out the details as they went along. They currently have 600 therapists nationwide to draw on at any given moment.

Chair massage treatments are delivered in 10- or 15-minute sessions. Both employees and independent contractors work through the North Carolina location. However, the chair massage therapists the co-owners hire across the country to provide treatments are independent contractors. They pay massage therapists $42 per hour, and Kneaded Energy's National Massage Network requires that there be a 3-hour minimum before sending a therapist out for the job.

The types of businesses and events to which practitioners are sent to perform chair massage include the following:

- Health screening events—Kneaded Energy National Massage Network has a nationwide contract with different wellness companies that contract with major corporations to supply nurses for insurance screenings that in return help lower the corporations' insurance cost. National Massage Network provides the chair massage as incentive for employees to receive the screening tests.
- Outside events like street fairs and festivals
- Trade shows
- Conventions
- Sports events
- Locally, the company sends its employees to a variety of settings such as schools, businesses, and so forth

To work with Kneaded Energy's National Massage Network, the practitioner must be licensed in the state where he or she is working, must be a member of a professional association that provides liability insurance, must be professionally dressed and well groomed, and must be able to arrive to the chair massage location prepared and on time. When interviewing practitioners, the co-owners look for someone who is willing to represent the massage profession first and his or her own business second. They want to be sure that the practitioner understands that it is the profession as a whole that is being hired, not just this individual's interpretation of the profession.

Norman and Johnson prefer to hire people who have a Web page and who can supply a photo (although that is not absolutely necessary). They want to get a good sense of how the person represents the profession, and the person's picture and the information on the website help them do this. To Kneaded Energy's National Massage Network, a website is a sign that practitioners are invested in their businesses. It also provides a direct way to get specific information about a potential independent contractor rather than by playing "phone tag," which can sometimes happen when trying to make contact by telephone. Websites are usually more efficient.

Another consideration for hire is the willingness, or lack of willingness, of the potential contractor to work within the parameters of the company, such as following dress codes and personal grooming requirements.

The biggest challenge is trusting that practitioners who are hired through the Internet and phone calls will represent the profession with integrity and provide excellent service to the company for which they have been contracted. For example, sometimes Norman and Johnson receive follow-up calls from a contact person who organized the event for which they provided practitioners. The contact person may report that the practitioner took all of the leftover juice boxes and energy bars before leaving, or that she or he tried to solicit business or gratuities outside of what the contract stated. For this reason, Kneaded Energy's National Massage Network demands the utmost in professionalism and skills from the practitioners the company hires.

Bill Norman and Shelley Johnson say that the biggest reward of their business is being able to make a living doing massage therapy. They enjoy having much diversity in the services they offer, which makes it unnecessary to have another job unrelated to massage therapy to supplement their living.

- I provide treatments of varying durations (i.e., 10 minutes, 15 minutes, 20 minutes).
- I can provide treatments on short notice.
- I can provide treatments in many different settings.
- My treatment fees make my business more competitive.
- My equipment and supplies are of the highest quality.

Methods to Reach Target Markets

After practitioners have identified possible target markets, they need to find ways to reach them. They can start with their personal networks: family, friends, neighbors, social and professional acquaintances, and so forth. Perhaps the practitioner has a neighbor who is a tax accountant and talks about long hours in front of the computer during tax season. This is a person the practitioner could talk to about the benefits of chair massage and who might then help set up a meeting at the person's company where the practitioner can make a presentation about chair massage. Or perhaps the practitioner attends a weekly yoga class and hears someone talking about a group that needs chair massage. This is an opportunity

PERSPECTIVES

The Right Touch Massage Therapy, Inc.

2984 E. Ft. Lowell Rd., Tucson, AZ 85716
Telephone number: *(520) 326-7675*
Website: *www.righttouchmassagetherapy.com*
Owner: *Kathy Rinn, BS, LMT, ABT, NCTMB*
In business since 1984

The Right Touch Massage Therapy, Inc. offers seated chair massage services in a variety of settings, ranging from a high-profile reality TV show that remodeled an entire home in 7 days to a management company offering an incentive for tenants to renew their lease for another year. The key to the success of Right Touch Massage Therapy, Inc. in offering chair massage services is that Kathy prefers to consult with the companies to determine what is the best way to utilize the service so that the company, as well as the practitioners, benefit.

This consultation consists of an on-location visit to get a sense of what the company's goal is for offering chair massage, such as honoring a particular department for meeting a deadline or drawing attention to the company's vendor table at a conference. Rinn also finds out if there will be such a high volume of treatments needed that more than one practitioner is necessary, what time frame will be most suitable, and whether 15-, 20-, or 30-minute sessions are needed. Knowing where the event will take place helps Rinn determine what space would be the most appropriate to comfortably accommodate the practitioners. For example, if the event is outdoors she needs to make sure there will be proper shelter to protect the practitioners from elements such as wind, rain, or hot sun.

Rinn states that this consultation allows her to collaborate with the company contact person or the event coordinator to design a program that will ensure the best benefits from the chair massage services. It also reduces the possibilities of misunderstandings between the two parties in terms of what exactly is expected from the practitioners, as well as what is expected from the company.

Rinn reports that she has contracted with chair massage brokers from other states to provide services locally. "There is a lot of trust needed in this arrangement because you often do not get paid until after the event is over. In addition, you are communicating via email or phone calls with the event coordinator, and sometimes miscommunication or misunderstandings happen, which can make a working relationship difficult." She recommends that anyone who contracts to provide services with an out-of-state company get all agreements in writing and require that payment be due the same day of the event, and if not at that time, then within 2 weeks of the date that services were provided.

The Right Touch Massage Therapy, Inc. has both employees and independent contractors who provide the chair massage services. Payment is based on the practitioner's employment status with the company. Employees receive a higher compensation for their work than do independent contractors. The Right Touch Massage Therapy, Inc. charges $80 per hour for chair massage services per practitioner, which includes the initial consultation. Employees receive 75% of the treatment fee, and independent contractors receive 65%. Rinn encourages the practitioners she hires to promote their own business while on location.

When she is interviewing applicants to provide treatments, Rinn says she looks for the "marines of chair massage." She wants to ensure that the practitioner has the physical stamina to work the account without becoming fatigued or injured as well as have a positive professional attitude throughout the event. She also wants someone who has a solid work ethic and will not be taking a lot of breaks while on duty or behave in ways that do not represent her company or the massage profession well. Finally, Rinn tries to match practitioners with the types of events or locations that reflect their personality and their interests.

"Being a connector is what makes this work rewarding and challenging for me at the same time. I like the challenge of finding the right practitioner for the right event, which in turn allows for the actual client who is receiving the massage to benefit as well. When all parties are pleased, that is a successful connection."

Words of advice that Rinn has for chair massage practitioners are "Don't give it away." Chair massage is an excellent educational tool, allowing people who are new to massage an opportunity to see that it is safe and accessible. Although it is very easy to offer free chair massage treatments as an educational or marketing tool, she cautions practitioners to limit this activity so that the public will place a value on chair massage services rather than thinking it is something to get for free, for example, at a grand opening. She states that it is not uncommon for new practitioners to offer many deals and discounts as they build their practice. Although this may bring in new clients initially, it does not ensure that the clients completely value the service enough to pay full price once the discount is used.

for practitioners to introduce themselves and describe their businesses.

Many successful contacts in business are made in ordinary day-to-day conversations, or through activities that the practitioner enjoys such as sports, shopping, buying or selling Tupperware or cosmetics, and so forth. Practitioners should keep business cards with them—it could be a chance conversation at the grocery store that gives them the perfect opportunity to talk about chair massage.

Conventions and trade shows are great marketing opportunities for practitioners who live in larger cities that host such events. The local Chamber of Commerce is an ideal place to contact to find out what events are coming to the area and who the contact person is for the event. Some Chambers of Commerce require business owners to join before they give out such information; others will provide the information for a fee. Joining the local Chamber of Commerce is a good step to take if practitioners are not sure in which direction they want to go in terms of specific target markets. As a member of a Chamber of Commerce, the practitioner has the opportunity to attend mixers and networking breakfasts and luncheons with other business owners in the community. This is a way to get the word out about a business and perhaps get some leads to follow up

PERSPECTIVES

Massage Bar, Inc.

444 NE Ravenna Blvd., Suite 201, Seattle, WA 98115
Telephone number: *(206) 985-7177*
Fax number: *(206) 985-4161*
Website: *www.massagebar.com*
President: *Cary Cruea*
In business since 1993

Massage Bar, Inc., mostly operates in permanent settings in airports across the country. The company currently has 10 locations including sites in Seattle, Washington; Sacramento, California; Nashville, Tennessee; Newark, New Jersey; Dulles, Virginia; and Columbus, Ohio. Massage Bar To Go is another aspect of Massage Bar, Inc. It provides services onsite such as for companies to reward employees who have excellent job performance or as a part of marketing at health fairs, trade shows, or special events. Massage Bar To Go can also be hired for personal events such as bridal showers, parties, or sporting events.

Services consist of 15-minute treatment (called a Single Shot) for $21 and a 30-minute treatment for $39 (called a Double Shot). The names of the treatments are in keeping with the bar theme of the business's name.

Practitioners are part-time employees. They are paid a base rate and make a commission of either $5 or $10, depending on the treatment length. Massage Bar currently employs 140 part-time licensed massage practitioners.

According to its website, "Friendly and professional therapists make our business successful by sharing their own unique experience and knowledge through their work. The working dynamic provides an opportunity for continued education from co-workers, supervisors, and is supported by corporate training. Massage Bar provides an opportunity for therapists to come together in a fun, flexible and fast-paced working environment, sharing knowledge and creativity, while providing seated massage and other services to our customer base."

Resumés of practitioners who are interested in working for Massage Bar, Inc., are accepted by fax to the location where the practitioner wants to work.

on. The practitioner might even arrange to provide seated massage treatments at one of these events as a way to draw attention to the businesses and distribute business cards.

Other common marketing methods practitioners can use are email blasts, newsletters, or introductory flyers to client lists. If practitioners already have a client base, they can use that. Otherwise, it is possible to rent or buy mailing lists. To find lists, practitioners can do online searches. Here are examples of companies that provide, for a fee, targeted mailing lists:

- American Heritage Data Corporation, www.heritagelists.com
- Marketing Comparison, www.marketingcomparison.com
- Leadsplease, www.leadsplease.com

Offering complimentary sessions in different settings can also be effective. For example, it is common for a business have an open house when a new store opens or a business opens at a new location. Offering free seated chair massage treatments to all who attend is an excellent way to draw attention to the store. It is also an excellent way for practitioners to meet a large number of people in a short amount of time. Ideally, the owner of the business would be willing pay an hourly fee for the services of a licensed massage practitioner. If this is not the case, however, it is still a good opportunity for practitioners to promote their businesses. There are plenty of other venues to consider for offering complimentary chair massage; for example, locally owned bookstores, health fairs, or almost any fundraising event such as walks to raise money for cancer research.

Practitioners should be mindful, however, that they do not do so much free chair massage that the public does not value it as a viable alternative to table massage. Although it is sometimes necessary to offer services free of charge as a way to market businesses, practitioners should be careful that they do not this so often that chair massage is seen as a "freebie" modality rather than one that is worth payment for services. Practitioners may consider setting a guideline of only offering free massage services to nonprofit organizations while charging a fee to businesses and corporations.

Regardless of how specific or wide the target market is, it is in practitioners' best interests to get themselves out in the community and let potential clients know that they have a business they believe in. They should follow up any interesting leads with a phone call, a visit to the office to offer a complimentary session, or a note of thanks to someone who made an impression and spent some time with them at a networking event. Thank-you notes are easy to write and a gracious follow-up method that makes a positive impression and helps others remember the practitioner when they want the services the practitioner provides.

Estimated Costs of Marketing Methods

Before proceeding with any marketing methods, practitioners should determine their marketing budget. Marketing budgets should be realistic and should be what the practitioner can afford. It is easy to get caught up in the idea of exciting marketing methods such as, for example, a radio or television commercial. However, if the cost is beyond the practitioner's means or if practitioners do not have the client base to support it, then the practitioners can find themselves in the predicament of having spent money they do not have for a venture that may or may not pay off in terms of increased business.

After determining their marketing budgets, practitioners can decide what marketing methods fall within them. This is best done by listing the methods practitioners find appealing and researching the costs. The costs should include every aspect of the marketing methods. For example, if the practitioner decides to send flyers promoting the practitioner's chair massage business, $75 to rent a mailing list of 1,000 names may seem to be reasonable. However, there are other costs, such as those for the following:

- Shipping the list to the practitioner
- Return address labels
- Printing the names addresses on peel-and-stick labels
- Designing the flyer
- Printing the flyer
- Envelopes to mail the flyer
- Postage

As this list shows, costs can add up quickly, and what may have seemed like a reasonably priced marketing method at first may turn out not to be so. It is better for practitioners to investigate ahead of time than to receive an unpleasant surprise when actual costs are added up.

Timeline for Implementing Marketing Methods

Once practitioners have decided on marketing methods that are within their marketing budgets, they should determine a timeline for implementing these methods. The timeline should also be realistic. Some marketing methods can be implemented immediately, such as practitioners spreading the word about their business through their personal networks. Other methods take longer, such as creating and mailing flyers. Some marketing methods can be done over and over, but because of financial considerations or to see if the marketing methods are working, or both, practitioners may choose to have gaps of time in between repetitions, such as for attending Chamber of Commerce networking breakfasts every two months or sending out flyers once every three months.

Practitioners may find it helpful to create an actual timeline as a reference tool in their marketing plan. It could be something as simple as a written list of dates when each marketing method will be implemented (Figure 6-4), or practitioners can design more elaborate timelines if that suits their needs.

System for Evaluating the Effectiveness of Marketing Methods

Because it only makes sense to continue marketing methods for which practitioners see returns, such as an increase in chair massage accounts or client base, practitioners need to have a way of evaluating how effective their marketing methods are. That way, time, effort, and money can be spent wisely on what is working, and nonuseful marketing techniques can be discarded.

The easiest and most direct system for evaluating the effectiveness of marketing methods is for practitioners to ask new clients how they found out about the practitioner's business. The clients can be asked face to face, on an intake form, or through the use of written surveys. Practitioners should keep written records of how many new clients they have, when these clients starting receiving treatments, and what marketing method(s) spurred the client to contact the practitioner. These records allow practitioners to cross-reference when they see an increase in clients with the implementation dates of specific marketing methods. Practitioners can then use this information to see how they are marketing their business most successfully, which methods are having lesser degrees of success, and which methods are not working at all.

What Services and Products to Offer

To effectively communicate about their chair massage businesses, practitioners need to decide what services and products to offer. To assist them with this process, practitioners can ask themselves the following questions:

- Do I want to offer only onsite seated massage, or do I intend to offer it as an added service within an established bodywork practice?
- Do I want to perform all the treatments myself, do I want to have employees or independent contractors, or do I want to both perform treatments as well as manage other practitioners?
- Do I want to provide chair massage treatments only at businesses, or am I open to other types of events such as health fairs and birthday parties?
- Do I want to provide only 15-minute treatments, or am I willing to do shorter and longer treatments?
- Do I want to offer only the massage treatment, or do I want to offer other services such as aromatherapy or hand and ear reflexology (possibly at an additional fee) along with the treatment?
- Do I want to sell products along with my chair massage treatments such as hand strengthening tools, large rubber bands to help clients stretch and strengthen, or aromatherapy oils?

The answers to these questions will help practitioners get as clear as possible about their range of services, which is crucial to a successful business.

How to Deliver the Services and Products

Once practitioners are clear about the services they intend to offer (as well as any products they intend to sell), determining how to deliver them is known as the **operation plan**. The operation plan will include, for example, the following aspects:

January 5	Attend Chamber of Commerce networking breakfast
January 12	
January 19	
January 26	Mail out flyers
February 2	
February 9	
February 16	
February 23	
March 2	Attend Chamber of Commerce networking breakfast
March 9	
March 16	
March 23	
March 30	Participate in Women's Wellness Health Fair
April 6	
April 13	
April 20	
April 27	
May 4	Attend Chamber of Commerce networking breakfast
May 11	
May 18	
May 25	Mail out flyers
June 1	
June 9	
June 15	
June 22	
June 29	
July 6	Attend Chamber of Commerce networking breakfast
July 13	
July 20	
July 27	
August 3	
August 10	Participate in Diabetes Research Rock-n-Roll Run
August 17	
August 31	
September 7	Attend Chamber of Commerce networking breakfast
September 14	
September 21	
September 28	Mail out flyers
October 5	
October 12	Participate in Harvest Farmer's Market
October 19	
October 26	
November 2	Attend Chamber of Commerce networking breakfast
November 9	
November 16	
November 23	
November 30	
December 7	Participate in Cancer Research Jingle Bell Run
December 14	
December 21	
December 28	

FIGURE 6-4 Marketing timeline using written dates.

- *Determining the timeline of the treatments.* Are they to be given on a one-time-only basis, such as for a special event, or is the goal to set up an account with a business? If it is an account, how often will the services be provided? Once a week? Once a month?
- *Deciding the frequency and length of the treatments.* When will the chair massage service start and end, and how long will each session be?
- *Deciding who will deliver the chair massage treatments.* How many chair massage practitioners will be performing the

treatments? If there is more than one practitioner, how will the responsibilities for equipment, scheduling, and providing treatments be dealt with?

- *Determining how potential clients will be notified of the availability of chair massage at an event or business.* How will this be done? Is it the responsibility of the event or business contact person, or is it the responsibility of the chair massage practitioner?
- *Finding out treatment space parameters.* How and where will the treatment space be created? How much setup and takedown time will practitioners have?
- *Determining how the practitioner or practitioners will be paid.* Will clients pay them directly? Will the business or event planner pay them?

From these examples, practitioners can see that a clear operation plan is also crucial to the success of a business.

The Financial Plan for Investment Costs and Revenue

As with any business, having a profitable chair massage business means that the income from the business is greater than the costs invested in it. To help determine the costs for investment and income, practitioners may find filling out the worksheets in Figure 6-5, "Investment Costs," and Figure 6-6, "Return on Investment Costs," helpful. **Return on investment costs** is the amount the practitioner needs to make from chair massage treatments to return the amount of money invested (i.e., break even) and above which is profit.

Subtract your investment costs (line A) from your total gross revenue (line B). The difference is your profit (or loss). Does this number work for you? Is this an achievable goal, in terms of money and time invested? If not, what would need to be adjusted? Do you need to charge more for your chair massage treatments? Should you offer longer treatments at a higher price? Are there less expensive ways to market your business? To improve the bottom line, you can increase your income, decrease your expenses, or do both. The challenge is to devise a plan that is ambitious enough to be fun and stimulating while also being attainable.

SALES

While marketing is about increasing awareness of the practitioner's business and services by as many people as possible, sales is about closing the deal. This is the point at which the service/product provider (or a representative of the provider) is communicating directly with a prospective client in an effort to have the client agree to pay for a product or service. This generally includes a discussion of how the product or service would benefit the client and the costs of and methods to deliver the product or service. In some types of sales, the client and provider can negotiate costs and delivery methods, and this is certainly true in chair massage businesses.

Chair massage services are not necessarily "one size fits all" but can be customized to fit clients' specific, unique situations. Therefore it is important that practitioners ask prospective clients what their needs and preferences are. Not only does this show genuine interest in the client, but it is valuable information practitioners can use to deliver their services or to determine if the client is a good fit for the practitioner's business, because not all prospective clients are a good match. Practitioners may find it helpful to ask the following questions:

- How many employees do you have?
- Does your company have an employee wellness program? Please tell me about it.
- Do you think your employees would be interested in receiving chair massage treatments? If so, how often? Weekly? Monthly?
- Can your employees be away from their desks (or work stations) for 10, 15, or 20 minutes to receive treatments? If not, can they receive treatments at their desks or in their workstations?
- What day of the week and time of day would be best for the majority of your employees to receive chair massage treatments?
- Is there a certain time each month that would be best for your employees to receive chair massage?
- How do you see your company paying for chair massage services? Would the company pay for the entire cost of treatments, would employees pay for the entire cost, or would it be split between the company and the employees?
- If the employees would need to pay for the entire cost of treatments, are they able to afford to do so?
- With whom should I speak to discuss the possibility of providing chair massage treatments to your employees? The CEO? The human resources administrator? May I make an appointment with this person to discuss my chair massage services and give him or her a complimentary treatment so he or she can experience my work?
- Would it be possible for me to offer free minichair massage treatments to your employees to see if they like them?

Something else practitioners can let prospective clients know is that an **indemnity agreement** can be included as part of the contract the practitioner would sign with the company. Indemnity agreements mean that employees cannot hold the company liable if the employee is harmed from receiving chair massage on the company's premises. Also, practitioners' professional liability insurance will provide the coverage needed should any client injuries occur as the result of the treatments performed onsite.

Approaching Business Contacts

Getting the attention of potential clients at an open house is one thing, but transforming that attention and interest soon after the event is over into paying clients is a skill that must be developed if the practitioner is to be successful.

One way to transform or build on an initial conversation with a business contact is to offer complimentary treatments in the contact's workplace and see how management receives the proposal. The key to this approach is arranging to meet and, ideally, work on the person who is in charge of making the decision about hiring a seated chair massage practitioner. Depending on the size of the business, this person may be the owner, the human resources manager, or a health and benefits manager.

The follow-up contact can be a brief phone call requesting some time to meet with one or two individuals who have the decision-making power. During the phone call, practitioners should do the following:

- Explain who they are, what their business is, and why they are calling.
- Mention the name of the initial contact person if talking with someone else.
- Offer several dates and times to come by and give a presentation and demonstration of seated chair massage, free of charge.

Investment Costs

The following is meant to give you a general idea of the typical costs of a chair massage business. Be sure to carefully research the costs of each item.

Administration $ ________

Examples:
- Payroll for staff (to schedule appointments, to perform treatments)
- Accounting services

Marketing

Examples:
- Mailing lists
- Designing and printing flyers
- Postage for mailing flyers
- Cost to join Chamber of Commerce

Equipment $ ________

Examples:
- Massage chair
- Optional sternum pad
- Carrying case
- Desktop massage support system
- Foam rubber bolster
- Pillows
- Stool
- Music player
- Clock
- Small spray bottle
- Small basket (for client keys, glasses, and so forth.)
- Mirror
- T-shirts in various sizes
- Small blanket or beach towel
- Carrying case for supplies

Supplies $ ________

Examples:
- Pillow cases for pillows
- Coverings for bolsters
- Face cradle covers (disposable paper or fiber, or rewashable cloth)
- Paper towels
- Hand sanitizer
- Nail clippers
- Hair ties
- Receipt book
- Appointment book, pen, and appointment cards
- Price list
- Client intake forms
- Aromatherapy bottles

FIGURE 6-5 Investment costs worksheet.

Tools for Client Education

Small, portable flip charts showing bones and muscles of the body, or trigger points
Handouts of stretches/exercises clients can do for themselves to continue the benefits of the chair massage

Emergency Spill Kit

Professional, commercial-grade germicidal wipes
At least 2 sets of latex, vinyl, or nitirile rubber gloves
Gallon plastic bags that can be sealed
Garbage bags that can be tied securely

Marketing Costs $__________

Examples:
- Print advertisements
- Booth rental at wellness fair
- Brochures
- Flyers
- Newsletters
- Business cards
- Website
- Other

Inventory (for product sales) $__________

Other $__________

Examples:
- Gift certificates
- Client gifts (e.g., water bottles or magnets with the practitioner's business name and business phone number on them)
- Professional memberships to bodywork associations

Total Investment Costs $__________

FIGURE 6-5, cont'd.

Return on Investment Costs

Total Investment Costs (from **Investment Costs Worksheet**) $__________(A)

To calculate the amount you need in order to make a return on your investment costs, and to make a profit, calculate the following:

Total number of chair massage sessions for a year (Column 1) multiplied by the price of each session (Column 2) for a Total (Column 3)

	1		2		3
10 minutes	________	×	$________	=	$________
15 minutes	________	×	$________	=	$________
20 minutes	________	×	$________	=	$________
Other	________	×	$________	=	$________

Total Gross Session Income $__________

Other Business Income $__________

Total Gross Revenue $__________(B)

FIGURE 6-6 Return on investment costs worksheet.

- Establish a time to call back to set the actual date and time for the presentation.
- End the conversation politely and with a thank you, whether or not the person is interested in chair massage.

Depending on the situation, follow-up contact can instead be made by sending a letter and perhaps enclosing a brochure. The letter should include the following information:

- An introductory paragraph about the practitioner, the practitioner's credentials, and what type of treatments the practitioner provides
- Why the practitioner chose to contact this company
- What services the practitioner can provide to the company or organization
- How the employees will benefit from the services
- The practitioner's contact information
- A request for an interview or to call the person who would make the decision about hiring chair massage services to arrange a meeting

Once the letter is sent, practitioners can follow up by phone to ask for a meeting to demonstrate the seated massage techniques.

PRESENTATION SKILLS

A well-prepared presentation including solid knowledge about the company can be impressive to the company's contact people, who then may be more open to how chair massage services can benefit the company's employees. The presentation should be brief, focus on the benefits of seated chair massage, and include a demonstration.

In the presentation, practitioners should be careful not to make it sound as though the business is stress filled and the employees are on the edge of becoming injured. This could insult the manager or owner of the business. Instead, the presentation should reflect the practitioner's knowledge about what the employees do during their daily job activities, followed by how seated chair massage can benefit the company by bringing more wellness to the workplace. If the practitioner can make a case for increased productivity, even better.

Some practitioners may find it difficult to make a presentation in front of people; public speaking may not be their best skill or may, in fact, be scary to them. However, one thing to keep in mind is that the presentation is an opportunity to talk about something the practitioner believes in, namely, the benefits of massage and bodywork. If performing chair massage is something the practitioner loves to do, the passion for the work will come through the presentation and may make it easier to talk about it with others.

Practicing the presentation out loud a number of times can help practitioners become comfortable with the content, and they can consider asking a friend or colleague to listen and offer feedback before meeting with the business contact. Well-rehearsed presentations tend to go much more smoothly than "winging it." A sign of professionalism is being able to articulate clearly and concisely what is important about chair massage services and to do so in a manner that is enjoyable for both the practitioner and the audience.

If the prospect of public speaking is still too daunting, consider attending speech preparation and delivery classes at a local community college or joining Toastmasters International (TI). Toastmasters is a nonprofit, educational organization dedicated to helping their members improve their public speaking, communication, and leadership skills. More information can be found on its website at www.toastmasters.org.

The Presentation

The presentation itself should include three parts:

The Introduction

Practitioners should do the following:

- Introduce themselves, and give their credentials.
- Describe when and where they received their training.
- Describe the services they provide.
- Explain why they are speaking with the group today.

The Body

Practitioners should do the following:

- Explain what seated massage is.
- List some of the benefits of seated massage.
- Describe what seated chair massage looks and feels like.
- Provide brief demonstration treatments.
- Describe what a seated massage account would consist of for the company.

The Conclusion

Practitioners should do the following:

- Summarize the benefits and value of offering seated massage to the employees.
- Invite questions.
- Express their gratitude for the opportunity to speak with the group.
- Leave their contact information.

To save time and give a more dynamic as well as efficient presentation, practitioners can talk while performing the demonstration.

After the presentation practitioners should personally thank the person who arranged for the presentation and ask when would be a good time to call for a follow-up meeting. If practitioners are not given a definite time, they can simply indicate they will check back in a week. One week is an adequate amount of time for the decision makers to meet and determine if they will hire chair massage services. Practitioners should also send a thank-you note the next day, again stating that they are looking forward to hearing from the company's representatives or that they will be contacting them in a week.

Chair Massage Intake Form

Name: ______________________________

Phone: ______________________________

Email: ______________________________

Please check any of the following that apply:

Are you under a physician's care? ________ Do you have any recent injuries? ________

Have you had a recent illness? ________ Are you taking any medications? ________

Where in your body do you have discomfort? ________ Do you have any allergies? ________

Head ________ Neck ________ Shoulders ________ Arms ________

Wrists ________ Hands ________ Back ________ Hips ________

Legs ________ Feet ________

By signing below you are stating that you do not have any contraindications for chair massage at this time.

________________________ Signature ________________________ Date

FIGURE 6-7 Brief intake form.

WRITTEN INFORMATION

Seated massage is typically a mobile business. As such, it may be inconvenient to take much paperwork from location to location. However, like any bodywork session, it is important to get as much information as possible about the client to provide a safe and appropriate treatment. Options include a brief yet concise interview to obtain the information or using an intake form. Either approach is acceptable as long as the appropriate information is gathered. Other written material to consider includes treatment documentation forms, handouts for clients, business cards, brochures, pamphlets, and gift certificates. Practitioners should note that in some municipalities, laws mandate that practitioners have their massage therapist or their massage establishment license number on all forms of advertising, which includes all written material except documentation forms. They should check with the laws governing their practice to see if this applies to them.

Intake Forms

The intake form for a chair massage session can be brief. Because treatments are usually 15 to 20 minutes in length, an in-depth medical history may not be needed. Therefore, the intake form can be a simple checklist for the client to note such things as medications, recent injuries, and focus areas for the treatment session (Figure 6-7). If need be, practitioners can clarify with the client any of the information checked on the form. These intake forms are typically about a half page in length and, for convenience, can even be printed in a tear-off page format.

Some practitioners prefer a more detailed intake form. However, it is important to keep in mind whether the client will be completing it before or within the time frame of the treatment session (Figure 6-8). Because there is usually a short amount of time for each treatment, clients will not want to spend most of it writing. Keeping in mind what information is most essential can help practitioners create an intake form that gathers that information.

Documentation Methods

Some practitioners do not write any documentation for chair massage, thinking that it is not warranted because each treatment is so brief compared to a full-body table massage. Other practitioners who have regular chair massage accounts may be concerned about possibly confusing clients with one another, and not performing the best treatments possible, or even injuring clients because of a lack of a written history about client treatment sessions. In this case, it would be best to create a personalized documentation system that is readily accessible, convenient to use, and portable.

Documenting what transpired during the chair massage treatment session includes the following:

- *Subjective information.* What the client states she is feeling or experiencing that is relevant to the treatment.

Chair Massage Intake Form

Name: ____________________

Address: ____________________

____

Phone: ____________________

Email: ____________________

DOB: ____________________

Please answer the following:

Are you under a physician's care? If so, please indicate why and if there are any contraindications for massage at this time: ____________________

____

____

Do you have any recent illnesses? If so, what are they? ____________________

____

____

Do you have any recent injuries? If so, what are they? ____________________

____

____

Are you currently taking any medications? If so, what are they? ____________________

____

____

Do you have any allergies? If so, what are they? ____________________

____

____

What would you like the focus of today's treatment to be? ____________________

____

____

What is your pressure preference? Mild Moderate Deep

Do you have any additional comments? If so, what are they? ____________________

____

____

By signing below you are stating that you do not have any contraindications for massage therapy at this time.

____________________ Signature

____________________ Date

FIGURE 6-8 Longer intake form.

FIGURE 6-9 SOAP chart.

- *Objective information.* What the practitioner observes about the client during visual and palpatory evaluations, and while performing the treatment.
- *Assessments.* The changes in the client's tissue and body that the practitioner notices as a result of the treatment.
- *A plan.* Suggestions for the client to help continue the effects of the treatment and to enhance the client's health and well-being, as well as ideas for techniques or areas of focus for the next treatment session.

All of this information can be referred to as SOAP charting: **S**ubjective, **O**bjective, **A**ssessment, and **P**lan. It is easy to design a treatment documentation form that uses these four components, which can then be completed quickly after each client. Figure 6-9 is an example of a simple SOAP chart.

Practitioners who do business with insurance carriers need to keep treatment notes, as most insurance companies require SOAP notes before reimbursing the client. In this case, remember to keep detailed notes of those client treatment sessions and submit them promptly when asked. Insurance companies are also particular about how SOAP charts are written and what abbreviations are used. More information on SOAP charting can be found in *Essential Sciences for Therapeutic Massage*, 3rd edition (2009), by Sandy Fritz and M. James Grosenback (published by Mosby Elsevier); *Fundamentals of Therapeutic Massage*, 4th edition (2009), by Sandy Fritz (Mosby Elsevier); and *Hands Heal,* 3rd edition (2005), by Diana Thompson (Lippincott Williams & Wilkins).

Documentation can also be done in a narrative form describing what the client presented with, what techniques the practitioner performed to alleviate muscular tension and pain the client was experiencing, and the results of the massage treatment. This is similar to the information in SOAP charting but in a less formal style.

Another method is to use 3-inch-by-5-inch note cards and carry them in a box. This can be a convenient and easy way to manage client data. Each client card could include contact information, notes about typical areas of muscular tension and pain, and client preferences for techniques, types of music, the face cradle, or aromatherapy. Any other information relevant to the massage treatment could be noted, as well as events that may be happening in the client's life such as a long-awaited trip or the birth of a grandchild. Referring to these life events is a great way to stay connected with the client.

For those technologically inclined, a laptop computer could be a portable and effective way of maintaining client documentation. There are various software programs available that are designed specifically for massage therapists that include SOAP charting, tracking payments, and listing client data and preferences. Practitioners can even track birthdays, sending out cards with good wishes and perhaps a discount on their next appointment. To research software programs, start with any massage supply website and search keyword "software." Sites to search include the following:

- Massage Warehouse, www.massagewarehouse.com
- Sunset Park Massage Supplies, www.massagesupplies.com
- Natural Touch Marketing for the Healing Arts, www.naturaltouchmarketing.com

Handouts

Handouts of educational material are good to give to clients because it demonstrates interest in their well-being between sessions. The handouts could be of stretches, nutritional information, or exercises that focus on a problem area the client is experiencing. However, in some municipalities, giving clients this information is considered beyond the scope of practice for massage therapists. Practitioners should check with the laws governing their practice to see what types of information they are legally allowed to disseminate.

For some clients without a lot of support or resources in their lives, the gesture of being given written information designed to enhance their health and well-being can have a big impact. Handouts also give clients something to take away from the session, and it may inspire them to call for another treatment. For this reason, practitioners should be sure to have their business name and contact information on every handout given to clients (and massage therapist or massage establishment license number, if applicable).

Some resources practitioner can explore for handouts are the following:

- Natural Touch Marketing for the Healing Arts, www.naturaltouchmarketing.com
- Stretching Inc., www.stretching.com
- WaterColorsCards, www.watercolorscards.com

Business Cards

Business cards are one of the most useful ways to market chair massage businesses. The card should be easy to read and include the pertinent information without being cluttered. The following information should be included in the design:

- Name
- Credentials (e.g., LMT [Licensed Massage Therapist], NCTMB [Nationally Certified in Therapeutic Massage and Bodywork])
- Phone number(s)
- Business address
- Website information or email address, if applicable.
- Massage therapist or massage establishment license number, if applicable

Equally important to the written information is the presentation—the colors and font type used. The practitioner should make sure the color is easy to read and that the font is simple; intricate fonts are much harder to read. There are software programs and websites that offer design help and inexpensive cards, or working with someone (a friend or a paid consultant) to create the design is another option. Remember that, generally, simple is better.

Some resources for business cards are as follows:

- Natural Touch Marketing for the Healing Arts, www.naturaltouchmarketing.com
- WaterColorsCards, www.watercolorscards.com
- American Massage Therapy Association (AMTA), www.amtamassage.org
- VistaPrint, www.vistaprint.biz

Brochures and Pamphlets

The purpose of brochures and pamphlets is to provide potential clients information about the practitioner and the practitioner's business. Brochures are typically printed on 8½-by-11-inch paper and then folded in half or thirds (twofold or threefold), depending on the amount of information. Pamphlets tend to be simpler; they are usually a two-sided sheet of paper and are less expensive to produce than brochures.

A basic brochure will have a brief description and summary of the chair massage services offered as well as contact and location information. Practitioners can consider including a personal profile that outlines their training, experience, and intentions for their work with clients. Some practitioners choose to list prices; however, this requires new brochures every time there are changes in treatment prices. Other items to include are as follows:

- Business policies, such as for clients who cancel with less than 24 hours' notice
- Guidelines for receiving chair massage treatments
- Benefits of chair massage treatments
- Testimonials from satisfied clients
- Massage therapist or massage establishment license number, if applicable

Just as with a business card, the same design considerations apply: easy-to-read colors and simple fonts generally work the best.

Brochures about the benefits of chair massage and other bodywork in general are also great to give to clients. These are brochures that are not specific to practitioners' businesses, but they can put their contact information on them. Some resources for these brochures are as follows:

- Natural Touch Marketing for the Healing Arts, www.naturaltouchmarketing.com
- WaterColorsCards, www.watercolorscards.com
- Massage Warehouse, www.massagewarehouse.com
- American Massage Therapy Association (AMTA), www.amtamassage.org
- VistaPrint, www.vistaprint.biz

Gift Certificates

Because many satisfied clients will also want their family and friends to have the opportunity to enjoy the benefits of chair massage, consider having a display of gift certificates near where treatments are performed on clients. That way, clients can buy them while they are thinking about them. If clients need to wait to purchase gift certificates (for example, until their next session when the practitioner brings some) or if they have to travel to the practitioner's office to purchase them, these are added obstacles and contribute to the likelihood that they may forget to come by or may change their minds altogether.

There are many styles of gift certificates for practitioners to choose from and many companies from which to buy them. The following are some resources for practitioners to explore:

- Natural Touch Marketing for the Healing Arts, www.naturaltouchmarketing.com
- WaterColorsCards, www.watercolorscards.com
- Massage Warehouse, www.massagewarehouse.com
- Massage Gift Certificate, www.massagegiftcertificate.com
- American Massage Therapy Association (AMTA), www.amtamassage.org
- VistaPrint, www.vistaprint.biz

Practitioners may find it useful to keep record of the sale of gift certificates. For one thing, they may notice that more are sold at certain times of year and that could be something to build on. It is also good to know just how many gift certificates are out there, waiting to be claimed. Practitioners should remember that they have already been paid for those sessions, so there could possibly be an impact on their cash flow if many gift certificates are claimed at one time long after they were purchased.

MANAGING CHAIR MASSAGE ACCOUNTS

It is important for practitioners to be specific about the services that their chair massage businesses offer. When making a pitch to a company or an organization, it is essential to have as many of the details about their businesses determined beforehand; otherwise it can be difficult to negotiate an agreement that works for the practitioners as well as the company. However, flexibility is just as important.

For example, a software company sets up a meeting with the practitioner about providing chair massage treatments. The company does not have a private room for the treatments and wants them provided to the employees at their desks. The practitioner turns down the account because she thinks she cannot provide quality treatments in such a manner. She mentions this to a colleague who meets with the company and accepts the account, performing the treatments as requested. Within a month, a private treatment space becomes available and the employees now receive treatments while sitting on the colleague's massage chair in a separate room away from their desks. Of course, if the practitioner had accepted the account in the beginning, the private space may never have materialized. But she also might have found that she could give very good treatments to employees at their desks or, at the very least, reconfirmed for herself that she cannot give effective treatments on employees at their desks and found someone else to take over the account.

Guidelines for Organizing an Efficient Account

There is much more to setting up and maintaining a chair massage account than simply performing the treatments. While that is an understandable area of focus, there are other equally important factors to consider. These include defining the services offered, determining the account's contact person, establishing the frequency of service and the length of the individual treatment sessions, creating a signup system for clients, establishing a means of communicating to prospective clients what to expect in chair massage, arranging for and setting up the treatment space, determining payment methods, having written policies and procedures available, providing client satisfaction surveys, and, finally, getting a signed contract with the company, group, organization, or event with which the practitioner will be working.

The following are guidelines to assist in organizing an efficient account:

- *Define the services being offered.* This may sound obvious, but some practitioners not only provide chair massage, but they also provide workshops on health-related topics such as nutrition, fibromyalgia, ergonomics in the workplace, and so forth. Offering aromatherapy with the sessions and selling health-related items such as large rubber bands that clients can use for stretching and strengthening (if it is within the practitioner's scope of practice) are examples of additional services that can be included. It is important to be specific and clear about the description and price of each of the services.
- *Determine the frequency of appointments at the location.* The frequency of appointments with a company, organization, or group depends on its needs as well as the number of people there who will receive treatments. For example, a large company may want a practitioner there on a weekly basis for several hours each time. A more common frequency is once or twice a month for a certain number of hours. Practitioners should know their schedules before making any commitments.
- *Determine how long the sessions will be.* The duration of each session depends on the needs of the individual client; the needs of the company, organization, or group; the length of time the practitioner has been hired to work; and who is responsible for payment. A chair massage session typically takes 15 to 20 minutes but can be lengthened or shortened depending on circumstances. If a business is hiring a practitioner to be on location for a preset amount of time, the length of each session will be determined by how many employees are expected to receive treatments in that amount of time. A large company may need more than one practitioner to provide the treatments in the preset length of time. If the individual client is responsible for payment, then the treatment may be shorter (or longer) than if the company is paying for it.
- *Find a contact person at the location.* It is helpful to have a contact person at the location to help with logistics such as sending out email blasts to employees to let them know the dates for chair massage, reserving a treatment space, getting parking tickets validated, and so forth. This contact person is essential at the beginning of a new account for a tour of the facilities, staff introductions, and advice on how to get the word out about chair massage to the employees. The contact person can also help drum up business when things are slow by letting individual employees know that the chair massage service is available with no waiting. Consider giving the contact person a free or discounted treatment as a gesture of gratitude for the help.
- *Inform clients about how to receive the service.* The contact person, in the same email that informs of the upcoming chair massage sessions, could let the employees know how to receive chair massage. For example, the email could state, "Be sure to wear clothes you don't mind getting wrinkled, or bring something you can change into for the chair massage. Please don't wear tight skirts or thick sweaters, which can interfere with receiving the best treatment possible. Also, your face will rest in a face cradle, and the treatment might include a scalp massage. Be sure to let the practitioner know if you are uncomfortable with either of these, and adjustments will be made to the treatment for you."
- *Inform employees about how to sign up for the service.* Practitioners should call the contact person at the beginning of the week they are scheduled to be there as well as the day before (or the preceding Friday if treatments are scheduled for Monday) to confirm that the company is prepared for their arrival.

First come, first served

10- or 15-minute sessions

Name	10 minutes	15 minutes
José Montoya	X	
Louise Frost		X
Mary Wilson		X
Jeff Padeem	X	
Nadia Romana		X

FIGURE 6-10 Simple signup sheet with handwritten names.

Ideally, the contact person would send out an email at the beginning of the week that the practitioner is coming and another email the day before (or the preceding Friday if treatments are scheduled for Monday) the practitioner is scheduled to arrive. The email should also inform the employees where they can sign up to receive a treatment. The options for signing up include email to the contact person, who would then add names to the signup sheet, or a paper signup sheet on which employees can handwrite their names (Figure 6-10). This signup sheet could be posted in a common area or break room of the company so all can see it. Ideally, clients will sign up ahead of time, giving practitioners an idea of what the day will be like.

The signup sheet should be simple and easy to read. Smaller businesses, however, may not require a signup sheet; instead, when one employee is finished, the next employee receives a treatment, and so on, until all employees who want treatments have been worked on.

Another type of signup sheet has treatment sections marked out in 10- to 15-minute intervals and a place for employees to include their contact phone numbers (or company phone extensions) so that if they are running late, the practitioner can call to remind them (Figure 6-11). There can also be a standby list, complete with phone numbers, to accommodate those who did not get chance to sign up before all the time slots filled (Figure 6-12). This system will ensure that the practitioners stay busy and do not waste time because of a no-show or a cancellation. If more than one practitioner will be providing treatments onsite, then the signup sheet should reflect this fact (Figure 6-13).

Signup Sheet for Chair Massage
Provided by Patricia Holland, LMT

Wednesday, February 13
10 am - 2 pm

2nd Floor Conference Room

Cost: $20.00 per session, payable at time of treatment (cash or check accepted)

Contact Felicia Torres in Human Resources for more information

Time	Name	Extension
10:00 - 10:15 am	Peggy Hanson	x723
10:20 - 10:35 am	William DeLuca	x692
10:40 - 10:55 am	Portia Martinez	x503
11:00 - 11:15 am	Eloise Blanchard	x712
11:20 - 11:35 am	Fred Abelard	x240
11:40 - 11:55 am	Radeem Azad	x337
Break		
12:20 - 12:35 pm	Florence Carpenter	x221
12:40 - 12:55 pm		
1:00 - 1:15 pm	Mary Ann Brooks	x454
1:20 - 1:35 pm	Tyler Montgomery	x109
1:40 - 1:55 pm	Keiko Shimoto	x489

FIGURE 6-11 Signup sheet with time intervals.

To allow for a day not going exactly as planned, consider not filling the last half-hour or hour of the schedule. That way, if the schedule is going as planned, that time could be filled from a standby list. And if running late, leaving on time may still be a possibility.

- *Creating a treatment space.* As has been discussed previously, the space that a practitioner is provided to work in can vary in size, accessibility, and neatness. To make the space as comfortable as possible, keep equipment and supplies neat, orderly, and out of the way. This will also make the space safer for clients. A way to make a utilitarian space feel more therapeutic is to dim the lights if possible, bring a music source, display bone and muscle flip charts, and provide educational handouts for clients (if within the scope of the practitioner's practice). Some practitioners use aromatherapy products to enhance the sense of calm and quiet. It is always good form to display business cards, brochures, and gift certificates. Many times clients see the gift certificates and are reminded that they need to purchase a last-minute gift for someone, and it lets them know they can call the practitioner for gift certificates in the future.
- *Payment methods.* There are three primary ways that chair massage treatments are usually paid for:
  - *Payment by the individual.* The client pays the entire treatment fee at the time of service. The practitioner

Signup Sheet for Chair Massage
Provided by Patricia Holland, LMT

Wednesday, February 13
10 am - 2 pm

2nd Floor Conference Room

Cost: $20.00 per session, payable at time of treatment (cash or check accepted)

Contact Felicia Torres in Human Resources for more information

Time	Name	Extension	Standby Client	Extension
10:00 - 10:15 am	Peggy Hanson	x723		
10:20 - 10:35 am	William DeLuca	x692	Connie Smith	x582
10:40 - 10:55 am	Portia Martinez	x503	Elizabeth Cho	x984
11:00 - 11:15 am	Eloise Blanchard	x712		
11:20 - 11:35 am	Fred Abelard	x240	Kelly Winthrop	x196
11:40 - 11:55 am	Radeem Azad	x337		
Break				
12:20 - 12:35 pm	Amber Carpenter	x221		
12:40 - 12:55 pm				
1:00 - 1:15 pm	Mary Ann Brooks	x454	Abby Hutchinson	x358
1:20 - 1:35 pm	Tyler Montgomery	x109		
1:40 - 1:55 pm	Keiko Shimoto	x489	Charlie Balad	x413

FIGURE 6-12 Signup sheet with standby clients.

can choose how to receive the payment (e.g., cash, check, or credit card).

- *Payment by the company.* The company pays the practitioner by the hour; the practitioner is paid regardless of whether or not there is a client for every treatment session. There is usually a high turnout with this payment method because most employees recognize a good thing when they see it and appreciate the company's contribution to their health and well-being.
- *Co-payment.* Individual clients pay for half of the treatment and the company picks up the other half. This method can also be great for office morale as it shows that the company is willing to help with part of the treatment fee.

When receiving payment from the sponsoring group or company, it is important to agree ahead of time whether the practitioner will be paid the day of service or will be billing the organization. If a billing arrangement is agreed upon, it is crucial that a contract be drawn up to spell out the terms of payment. It is also important to have an accurate and timely billing procedure to ensure getting paid.

- *Policies and procedures.* It is important to have as many guidelines and expectations written out ahead of time to prevent misunderstandings and potential difficult

Signup Sheet for Chair Massage
Provided by Mindful Touch Therapeutic Massage, LLC
3 practitioners will be available for 15-minute sessions on February 15 in the Break Room
Sign Up Today!

Time	Chair 1 Name	Ext.	Chair 2 Name	Ext.	Chair 3 Name	Ext.
9:00 - 9:15 am						
9:20 - 9:35 am						
9:40 - 9:55 am						
10:00 - 10:15 am	Break					
10:20 - 10:35 am			Break			
10:40 - 10:55 am					Break	
11:00 - 11:15 am						
11:20 - 11:35 am	Break					
11:40 - 11:55 am			Break			
12:00 - 12:15 pm					Break	

FIGURE 6-13 Signup sheet for multiple practitioners.

interactions with chair massage accounts. The policies and procedures include, for example, the procedures for booking (and canceling) an appointment, consequences for clients who are late or fail to show up for scheduled treatments, tips on how best to receive chair massage, and the payment schedule. For example, a no-show policy could be that clients prepay for their massage session and forfeit the fee if they do not show for the treatment. Practitioners must decide what policies and procedures are important to them and the success of their businesses, and they must write them accordingly.

- *Client satisfaction surveys.* One of the nice things about a regular chair massage account is the sense of connection, of community that can develop. However, it is important not to take the long-term nature of the therapeutic relationship for granted and start to slack off. One way to prevent this is by giving out surveys at random that ask the clients (anonymously, of course) to evaluate the practitioner's performance. The surveys can include questions such as "Did the practitioner arrive on time?" "Do your sessions feel therapeutic?" "Do you feel relief from muscular pain and tension?" "Do you feel more productive as a result of the chair massage sessions?" It is always important to check in regularly with those who keep the practitioner in business.

CONTRACTS

Written contracts are always a good idea, whether the practitioner is working with a large company where she or he does not know anyone or with a small group of friends. A written contract protects the interests of both the receivers of the massage treatments and the practitioner who is performing them. These interests can be very complicated or very simple, depending on the nature and size of the company, group, or organization involved. Many chair massage practitioners work without contracts because the accounts are so small or they have an understanding with the owner; they think a handshake is the only contract they need. However, human nature being what it is, it is best that all parties involved create a mutually beneficial contract to make sure everyone is protected.

Components of the Contract

The contract should include, but not necessarily be limited to, the following:

- The names, addresses, and contact information of both parties
- A description of services the practitioner agrees to provide for the company—what, where, when, how often, for how long

**Business Agreement between
Carole's Farmer's Market and
Desert Touch Massage Center**

This agreement made this 17th day of May, 2009, by and between Carole's Farmer's Market (hereinafter called CFG), an Arizona corporation located at 4400 N. Grapevine Way, Tucson, AZ , (520) 555-4259 and Desert Touch Massage Center (hereinafter called DTMC), 329 E. Saguaro Cactus Drive, Tucson, AZ (520) 555-3764.

Contact Information

The contact person for CFG is Carole Manchester, business phone (520) 555-4259, cell phone (520) 555-4583.

The contact person for DTMC is Rosalie Aguirre, business phone (520) 555-3764, cell phone (520) 555-5981.

Services to Be Provided by DTMC

DTMC will provide 2 licensed massage therapists (LMTs) to provide seated chair massage services within the scope of licensure.

DTMC practitioners are responsible for maintaining appropriate certification and licensure.

DTMC will provide all equipment and supplies deemed necessary to provide this service.

DTMC will provide educational materials to promote health and wellness to the patrons of the Farmer's Market.

DTMC will provide seated chair massage services every Friday, Saturday, and Sunday for 6 hours each day for the term of this contract.

One LMT will work a 3-hour shift from 9:00 am to Noon. The second LMT will work a 3-hour shift from Noon to 3:00 pm. Each LMT will arrive on location 20 minutes before the shift begins to provide continuity of service.

Services to Be Provided By CFM

CFM will provide a tented space with the measurements of 12 ft x 12 ft to accommodate the seated massage therapy services.

CFM will provide marketing materials to advertise the seated chair massage services to the patrons of the Farmer's Market.

CFM will provide an onsite manager, on an on-call basis, to assist the employees of DTMC if any problems arise with logistics or difficult patrons.

FIGURE 6-14 Example of chair massage contract with a company. (Adapted from Sohnen-Moe CM: *Business mastery: a guide for creating a fulfilling, thriving business and keeping it successful*, ed 4. Tucson, 2008, Sohnen-Moe Associates.)

- A description of the equipment and supplies the practitioner agrees to provide for the treatments (e.g., a massage chair in good working order, sanitation methods for cleaning the chair in between clients, and so forth)
- A list of accommodations that the company agrees to provide for the practitioner, such as a space to provide the treatments, an onsite contact person, advertisement of the service, and an explanation of how employees will sign up for the treatments
- Specific dollar amounts for how much the company, organization, or group will pay for the service
- Payment method–from the individual client, from the company, or co-pay arrangement
- Schedule of payments–the day service is provided or a billing arrangement
- Grounds for discontinuance of service by either party and how much notice is required
- Consequences for each party if any of these terms is violated.

Consider contacting a lawyer who specializes in small businesses for drafting the contracts. Figure 6-14 is an example of a contract written between a provider of chair massage and companies.

SUMMARY

Chair massage practitioners can choose to become an employee or independent contractor for companies who provide chair massage services. In contrast to employees, independent contractors set their own schedules, use their own equipment, and receive payment directly from clients. They also pay their own taxes, Social Security, and Medicare. Chair massage companies may also have other policies and procedures of which the employee or independent contractors needs to be clearly aware and should get in writing. Whether a practitioner becomes an employee of or an independent contractor for a chair massage company, it is important that a contract be signed between the practitioner and the company.

Other Provisions

DTMC is allowed to advertise all services available at the Center via brochures, business cards, and flyers.

DTMC is allowed to schedule appointments with the patrons of the Farmer's Market for treatments at DTMC's business location as requested.

DTMC shall indemnify and hold CFM harmless for any loss or liability arising from services provided under this agreement.

Fees, Terms of Payment, and Fringe Benefits

CFM shall compensate DTMC $50 per hour for a total of $900 per week.

DTMC shall receive payment from CFM by check on the 30th of each month.

DTMC employees are given a 15% discount on all merchandise at the Farmer's Market.

CFM employees are given a 15% discount on all services provided at the DTMC.

Local, State, and Federal Taxes

DTMC shall be responsible for paying all required local, state, and federal withholding, Social Security, and Medicare taxes.

Insurance

During the term of this agreement, all DTMC practitioners must have professional liability insurance of at least $2,000,000 aggregate annual and $1,000,000 per incident.

Term of Agreement

Either party may terminate this agreement, given reasonable cause, as provided below, or by giving 30 days' written notice to the other party of the intention to terminate this agreement.

1. Material violation of the provisions of this agreement.
2. Violation of ethical standards as defined by local, state, and/or national associations and governing bodies.
3. Loss of licensure for services provided.
4. DTMC fails to maintain the standard of service deemed appropriate by CFM.
5. It is agreed that any unresolved disputes will be settled by arbitration, including costs thereof.

This constitutes the entire agreement between CFM and DTMC and supersedes any and all prior written or verbal agreements. Should any part of this agreement be deemed unenforceable, the remainder of the agreement continues in effect. This agreement is governed by the laws of the state of Arizona

____________________ Representative from CFM — __________ Date

____________________ Representative from DTMC — __________ Date

____________________ Witness — __________ Date

FIGURE 6-14, cont'd.

Practitioners can also choose to start their own chair massage businesses, either solely or in partnership with others. There are many factors that affect the success of a chair massage business, and practitioners who choose to do this should create a business plan that includes the practitioner's target market, the services and products that he or she will offer, the operation plan, and the financial plan for investment costs and revenue. Target markets can be determined through the use of demographics, giving practitioners information that can help them to create a marketing plan. A marketing plan needs to include methods to reach the target market(s), estimated costs of these methods, a timeline for implementing the marketing methods, and a system for evaluating the effectiveness of the various marketing methods. Having a profitable chair massage business means that the income from the business is greater than the costs invested in it. Practitioners need to determine their investment costs and the amount of income they need to make a return on their investment.

When selling their chair massage services to potential clients, it is important that practitioners ask prospective clients what their needs and preferences are so that practitioners can determine if the client is a good fit for the practitioner's business and, if so, customize the delivery of their services. To approach prospective clients, practitioners can make contact face-to-face or on the telephone and through follow-up letters. Practitioners can deliver a presentation to the decision makers at the company, group, or organization, outlining the benefits of chair massage to their staff or members while giving a demonstration on chair massage and offering complimentary treatments.

Written information necessary to a chair massage business includes intake forms, SOAP charting or other documentation methods, educational handouts for clients, business cards, brochures and pamphlets, and gift certificates. All written information given to clients should be clear and easy to read and should include the practitioner's contact information.

Managing chair massage accounts efficiently includes defining the services offered, determining the frequency of appointments at the location, determining how long the sessions will be, finding a contact person at the location, informing clients about how to receive the service, informing employees about how to sign up for the service, creating a treatment space, determining payment methods, having written policies and procedures, and using client satisfaction surveys. It is best if there is a written contract between the company and provider of chair massage services to protect the interests of all parties involved.

STUDY QUESTIONS

Answers to the Study Questions are on page 227.

Multiple Choice

1. What is the term for the specific type of client that a business wants to attract?
   a. Customer base
   b. Target market
   c. Company account
   d. Marketing plan

2. What is the term for how much the practitioner needs to earn from chair massage treatments to make a chair massage business worthwhile?
   a. Return on investment costs
   b. Investment costs
   c. Marketing plan
   d. Gross revenue

3. Which of the following should be included in a chair massage presentation?
   a. Introduction of the practitioner and his or her credentials
   b. A brief demonstration of techniques
   c. Information on how the practitioner can be contacted
   d. All of the above

4. Which of the following helps practitioners to enhance their chair massage skills?
   a. Co-payment of services
   b. Business contracts
   c. Client surveys
   d. Gift certificates

5. Which of the following is a purpose of a chair massage business contract?
   a. Protect all parties involved
   b. Ensure the clients are satisfied with their treatments
   c. Delineate the practitioner's policies and procedures
   d. Create a signup sheet

Fill in the Blank

1. A practitioner who sets his or her own schedule and receives payment directly from clients is considered a(n) ____________________.

2. A(n) ____________________ is an outline of definable business goals, the reasoning behind why the goals are attainable, and a realistic plan for reaching those goals.

3. Handouts of educational material demonstrate to clients that the practitioner is interested in their ____________________ between sessions.

4. Brochures and pamphlets provide potential clients with ____________________ about the practitioner and the practitioner's business.

5. Announcing chair massage services to employees, explaining how to receive chair massage, and managing the treatment signup sheet can be done through the company's ____________________.

Short Answer

1. When determining a target market, what are four questions practitioners can ask themselves?

____

____

____

____

____

2. Describe six methods practitioners can use to reach their target market or markets.

____

____

____

____

____

STUDY QUESTIONS

3. Describe the appropriate topics practitioners can include in follow-up phone calls to business contacts.

4. Explain three ways practitioners can document chair massage treatments.

5. Explain why it is important that practitioners have their policies and procedures written out.

ACTIVITIES

1. Describe your ideal chair massage business. Include the name of your business, type(s) of clients you would like to work with, how many treatments in a session and the length of each treatment in a session, the type of treatments you would like to perform, your fee structure, and whether you would like to be the sole practitioner or work with other practitioners. If you envision a business in which you would employ other chair massage practitioners, describe the qualifications you would require for employment and how you would recruit the employees.

2. Choose a name for your business. Design a business card, brochure, documentation form, gift certificate, signup sheet, and client satisfaction survey for your business.

3. Research local companies, organizations, and groups by looking online, through the Yellow Pages, and contacting the Chamber of Commerce. List the companies, organizations, and groups that could benefit from chair massage, and, for each one, write down specifically why it would benefit from chair massage.

4. Choose one or two target markets from Activity 1, and design a chair massage treatment plan for conditions the members of the target market(s) could be experiencing.

STUDY QUESTIONS

5. Create a business plan for your chair massage business.

____

____

____

____

____

6. Create a marketing plan for your chair massage business.

____

____

____

____

____

Communication and Ethics

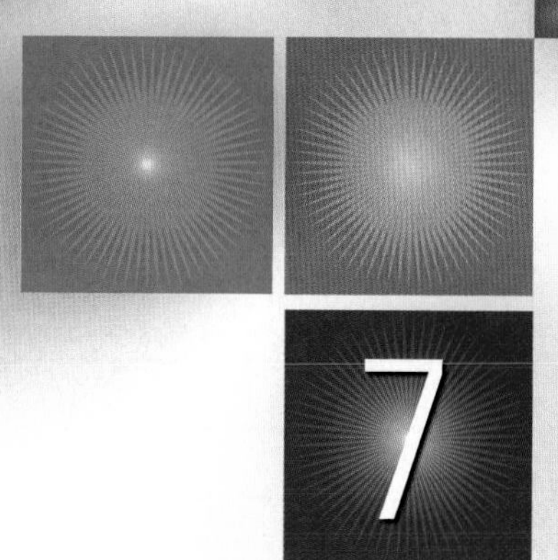

OBJECTIVES

Upon completion of this chapter, the reader will have the information necessary to do the following:

1. Explain the importance of ethics and effective communication for practitioners.
2. Define code of ethics.
3. Describe the components of professional presentation of self.
4. Define boundaries, and explain the importance of boundaries for the bodywork practitioner.
5. Communicate with new clients about chair massage procedures.
6. Define feedback, explain its importance, and conduct a posttreatment interview.
7. Describe different methods of preparing emotionally and physically to perform chair massage.
8. Communicate with special-needs clients about the best ways for them to receive chair massage.

KEY TERMS

Boundaries
Code of ethics
Ethics
Feedback
Office politics
Professional presentation
Therapeutic relationship

THE IMPORTANCE OF ETHICS AND EFFECTIVE COMMUNICATION FOR PRACTITIONERS

The mark of a practitioner's professionalism consists of much more than the level of hands-on skill. It includes such factors as level of integrity, accountability (i.e., ethics), and quality of self-presentation. Generally, the higher the level of professionalism, the greater the client satisfaction (and return business). Although ethics and communication classes are taught in most massage and bodywork programs, it is crucial for practitioners to remember that ethics are also part of everyday life. Practitioners should make sure that the personal principles that guide their professional behaviors are in alignment with the code of ethics of the massage and bodywork profession.

Codes of Ethics

An **ethic** (or **ethics**) is a set of moral principles, such as a *work ethic* or *conservation ethic*. Whether people have ever articulated the principles to themselves, they all operate under some ethic, which informs their day-to-day decisions (e.g., I found a wallet; do I keep it? I'm mad at a coworker; should I "forget" to pass on the important telephone message?). Professional massage and bodywork practitioners need to be guided by ethical standards that ensure conduct that will protect the physical and emotional well-being of the client, guide the business affairs of the practice, and hold the practitioners accountable for taking the appropriate measures to run their businesses with integrity. Practitioners do this by following the code of ethics set forth by the profession.

A **code of ethics** is a set of guidelines that a profession has determined is essential to ensure that all members of the profession have a basic understanding of what is expected of them in terms of behavior with clients, colleagues, and members of other professions. Simply put, the code outlines the principles of conduct governing the profession. Box 7-1 is the Code of Ethics for the American Massage Therapy Association; Box 7-2 is the Code of Ethics for Associated Bodywork and Massage Professionals; Box 7-3 is the Code of Ethics for the National Certification Board for Therapeutic Massage and Bodywork.

It is also important that clients are aware that the massage and bodywork profession has codes of ethics in place to protect them from practitioners who may not have their best interests in mind. For example, many clients do not know that performing spinal adjustments is beyond the scope of practice for massage therapists. Should a client request these adjustments, it is the massage therapist's responsibility to tell the client that he cannot comply with the request because he does not have the training to do them and would most likely injure the client. The practitioner should also say that a massage therapist who would do spinal adjustments is violating the profession's code of ethics. Practitioners can consider posting the code of ethics

BOX 7-1 American Massage Therapy Association Code of Ethics

This code of ethics is a summary statement of the standards by which massage therapists agree to conduct their practices and is a declaration of the general principles of acceptable, ethical, professional behavior.

Massage Therapists Shall:

1. Demonstrate commitment to provide the highest quality massage therapy/bodywork to those who seek their professional service.
2. Acknowledge the inherent worth and individuality of each person by not discriminating or behaving in any prejudicial manner with clients and/or colleagues.
3. Demonstrate professional excellence through regular self-assessment of strengths, limitations, and effectiveness by continued education and training.
4. Acknowledge the confidential nature of the professional relationship with clients and respect each client's right to privacy.
5. Conduct all business and professional activities within their scope of practice, the law of the land, and project a professional image.
6. Refrain from engaging in any sexual conduct or sexual activities involving their clients.
7. Accept responsibility to do no harm to the physical, mental, and emotional well-being of self, clients, and associates.

From the American Massage Therapy Association, 2009.

BOX 7-2 Associated Bodywork and Massage Professionals' Code of Ethics

Code of Ethics

As a member of Associated Bodywork and Massage Professionals, I hereby pledge to abide by the ABMP Code of Ethics as outlined below.

Client Relationships

- I shall endeavor to serve the best interests of my clients at all times and to provide the highest quality service possible.
- I shall maintain clear and honest communications with my clients and shall keep client communications confidential.
- I shall acknowledge the limitations of my skills and, when necessary, refer clients to the appropriate qualified health care professional.
- I shall in no way instigate or tolerate any kind of sexual advance while acting in the capacity of a massage, bodywork, somatic therapy, or esthetic practitioner.

Professionalism

- I shall maintain the highest standards of professional conduct, providing services in an ethical and professional manner in relation to my clientele, business associates, health care professionals, and the general public.
- I shall respect the rights of all ethical practitioners and will cooperate with all health care professionals in a friendly and professional manner.
- I shall refrain from the use of any mind-altering drugs, alcohol, or intoxicants prior to or during professional sessions.
- I shall always dress in a professional manner, proper dress being defined as attire suitable and consistent with accepted business and professional practice.
- I shall not be affiliated with or employed by any business that utilizes any form of sexual suggestiveness or explicit sexuality in its advertising or promotion of services, or in the actual practice of its services.

Scope of Practice/Appropriate Techniques

- I shall provide services within the scope of the ABMP definition of massage, bodywork, somatic therapies and skin care, and the limits of my training. I will not employ those massage, bodywork, or skin care techniques for which I have not had adequate training and shall represent my education, training, qualifications, and abilities honestly.
- I shall be conscious of the intent of the services that I am providing and shall be aware of and practice good judgment regarding the application of massage, bodywork, or somatic techniques utilized.
- I shall not perform manipulations or adjustments of the human skeletal structure, diagnose, prescribe, or provide any other service, procedure, or therapy which requires a license to practice chiropractic, osteopathy, physical therapy, podiatry, orthopedics, psychotherapy, acupuncture, dermatology, cosmetology, or any other profession or branch of medicine unless specifically licensed to do so.
- I shall be thoroughly educated and understand the physiological effects of the specific massage, bodywork, somatic, or skin care techniques utilized in order to determine whether such application is contraindicated and/or to determine the most beneficial techniques to apply to a given individual. I shall not apply massage, bodywork, somatic, or skin care techniques in those cases where they may be contraindicated without a written referral from the client's primary care provider.

Image/Advertising Claims

- I shall strive to project a professional image for myself, my business or place of employment, and the profession in general.
- I shall actively participate in educating the public regarding the actual benefits of massage, bodywork, somatic therapies, and skin care.
- I shall practice honesty in advertising, promote my services ethically and in good taste, and practice and/or advertise only those techniques for which I have received adequate training and/or certification. I shall not make false claims regarding the potential benefits of the techniques rendered.

From the Associated Bodywork and Massage Professionals, 2009.

BOX 7-3 National Certification Board for Therapeutic Massage and Bodywork Code of Ethics

Code of Ethics

Revised October of 2008

NCBTMB certificants and applicants for certification shall act in a manner that justifies public trust and confidence, enhances the reputation of the profession, and safeguards the interest of individual clients. Certificants and applicants for certification will:

I. Have a sincere commitment to provide the highest quality of care to those who seek their professional services.
II. Represent their qualifications honestly, including education and professional affiliations, and provide only those services that they are qualified to perform.
III. Accurately inform clients, other health care practitioners, and the public of the scope and limitations of their discipline.
IV. Acknowledge the limitations of and contraindications for massage and bodywork and refer clients to appropriate health professionals.
V. Provide treatment only where there is reasonable expectation that it will be advantageous to the client.
VI. Consistently maintain and improve professional knowledge and competence, striving for professional excellence through regular assessment of personal and professional strengths and weaknesses, and through continued education training.
VII. Conduct their business and professional activities with honesty and integrity, and respect the inherent worth of all persons.
VIII. Refuse to unjustly discriminate against clients and/or health professionals.
IX. Safeguard the confidentiality of all client information, unless disclosure is requested by the client in writing, is medically necessary, is required by law, or is necessary for the protection of the public.
X. Respect the client's right to treatment with informed and voluntary consent. The certified practitioner will obtain and record the informed consent of the client, or client's advocate, before providing treatment. This consent may be written or verbal.
XI. Respect the client's right to refuse, modify, or terminate treatment regardless of prior consent given.
XII. Provide draping and treatment in a way that ensures the safety, comfort, and privacy of the client.
XIII. Exercise the right to refuse to treat any person or part of the body for just and reasonable cause.
XIV. Refrain, under all circumstances, from initiating or engaging in any sexual conduct, sexual activities, or sexualizing behavior involving a client, even if the client attempts to sexualize the relationship unless a pre-existing relationship exists between an applicant or a practitioner and the client prior to the applicant or practitioner applying to be certified by NCBTMB.
XV. Avoid any interest, activity, or influence which might be in conflict with the practitioner's obligation to act in the best interests of the client or the profession.
XVI. Respect the client's boundaries with regard to privacy, disclosure, exposure, emotional expression, beliefs, and the client's reasonable expectations of professional behavior. Practitioners will respect the client's autonomy.
XVII. Refuse any gifts or benefits that are intended to influence a referral, decision, or treatment, or that are purely for personal gain and not for the good of the client.
XVIII. Follow the NCBTMB Standards of Practice, this Code of Ethics, and all policies, procedures, guidelines, regulations, codes, and requirements promulgated by the National Certification Board for Therapeutic Massage & Bodywork.

From the National Certification Board for Therapeutic Massage and Bodywork, 2009.

in their massage and bodywork offices, or they should take a small, portable copy with them onsite to perform chair massage.

Effective Communication

To develop an appropriate treatment plan for clients, the practitioner must be skilled in knowing what questions to ask, how best to ask them, and how to transform the answers into a bodywork session that will address the client's symptoms while taking into account the client's expressed needs and preferences. Listening to the client and then accurately reflecting back what is heard is an essential tool for success.

Communication skills are necessary not only for pre- and posttreatment interviewing. A lot of clients like to talk. Hands-on work promotes a certain level of intimacy, and sometimes clients will share fairly intimate details of their life as well as their body issues. Being able to communicate skillfully with the client during these times includes not letting the conversation get in the way of the treatment. This sometimes can be difficult, especially when performing treatments in a business setting. Many times clients want to discuss office politics or problems they are having with coworkers, people whom the practitioner could also be working on during the course of the treatment session. In this instance, communication skills meet ethics, as practitioners need to be able to maintain their professionalism, keep these communications confidential, and not pass on what employees have said about each other.

Additionally, it is important to be able to distinguish between when the client is asking for advice or when the client just needs to talk. The therapeutic connection between practitioner and client can be easily broken if the practitioner continually offers unwanted solutions. It could also be unethical or a violation of scope of practice, even if the client wants advice. In this case, the practitioner could say something like, "I am not qualified to provide you with the type of support you are asking for, but I am happy to refer you to a resource who is." If the client just wants to relax and not interact, practitioners need to be able to keep silent during a treatment as well.

Effective communication (both listening and speaking) is essential because serious misunderstandings can occur when practitioners are not mindful of the content, the tone, and the delivery of their speech (i.e., not only what they are saying, but how they are saying it). This is a major component of professionalism, something practitioners should keep in mind because onsite treatments involve working in professional settings.

PROFESSIONAL PRESENTATION OF SELF

Generally a first impression takes 4 to 20 seconds. These are crucial seconds for practitioners because first impressions can be the deciding factor in whether or not a client will choose to work with them. If clients do not feel comfortable with what they see or hear from the practitioner, chances are they will not be receptive to the bodywork session. **Professional presentation** refers to practitioners' abilities to present themselves in a poised, confident, qualified, and skilled manner. It is further demonstrated through the practitioner's ethics. There are several aspects to professional presentation. These include the following:

- Arriving early for appointments and being set up and ready to start exactly at the designated time
- Having professional attire and clean hygiene, demonstrating to clients that practitioners are conscious of their personal appearance and take care to be presentable
- Greeting clients in a friendly and respectful manner
- Using equipment that is clean and well maintained
- Setting the same fees for services for all clients

These examples may seem like common sense. However, what may be common sense to one person may not be to another. Age, life, work experience, and personal belief systems are all factors that determine how practitioners interpret their professional responsibilities and obligations.

Professional Attitudes and Behaviors

How people perceive the world is reflected in their attitudes, and attitudes reflect how people engage with the world. It is not healthy to live in a state of prolonged negativity, as it depletes the immune system, tends to drive people away, and impairs the practitioner's ability to build a thriving practice, as clients can detect the negativity through the practitioner's touch. A professional attitude is generally one that is positive and open to new ideas, with an inherent flexibility (useful for when things do not go as planned and some creative problem-solving is needed). A more negative and less professional attitude tends to amplify any faults seen in others and generally expresses dissatisfaction without any inclination to try to change. Which of these attitudes will project to the client an image that invokes trust and compassion? Everyone has bad days. Responsible and ethical practitioners who experience prolonged periods of less than positive outlooks, though, are willing to be honest and acknowledge it, seek help in understanding what it is about, and work to change it.

A professional attitude flows into professional behavior (i.e., how practitioners conduct themselves in a professional setting). Showing up on time for appointments is a professional behavior displaying an attitude of respect for self and client. Dealing effectively with a client who makes demands that are outside the practitioner's established policies and guidelines for the account demonstrates clarity of purpose and fairness.

Being professional means that practitioners put the client's appropriate needs (needs that fall within the scope of practice of chair massage) first and do not use the practitioner/client relationship as a means to get their own needs met. The relationship or connection that is created between the practitioner and the client in which the beneficial effects of treatment are able to take place is referred to as a **therapeutic relationship**. The connection must be appropriate, safe, and client centered. It is mandatory that practitioners recognize that it is always their responsibility to safeguard the therapeutic relationship.

Talking during the Treatment

In general, the therapeutic relationship is compromised when the practitioner's needs take precedence over the client's. For example, when a client asks how a practitioner's week went, some practitioners may talk endlessly about themselves rather than allowing clients to speak. A professional practitioner is able to respond politely and keep the focus on the client. The following statements are examples of how the practitioner can be brief in answering a personal question and then bring the attention back to the client:

- "Thank you for asking. My week was fine. Now, take a deep breath and exhale. Take another deep breath and exhale."
- "I had a good week. Thank you for asking. How is this shoulder feeling today?"

In other words, always thank the client for the interest, and then redirect the focus back to the client. Some practitioners are afraid of sounding rude or impersonal if they do not engage in conversation with a client. This does not have to be the case, especially as the seated massage sessions are brief. As long as the practitioner acknowledges the question and provides a brief response, he or she does not have to offer long and involved answers.

For some clients, talking is means of relaxing; for others, it is a sign of nervousness. Sometimes clients just need to talk, and practitioners should let them. Continuing to tell the client to take a deep breath and relax in an effort to help the client "get out of her head and into her body" may not work or, worse, may annoy the client.

Even if the practitioner is very knowledgeable about a given subject matter, the treatment is not the time or the setting to offer opinions. Although boundaries are discussed later in this chapter, this is an example of practitioners setting a boundary on how much they will disclose about themselves. Boundaries are essential, because without them practitioners could potentially find themselves embroiled in deep, introspective conversations or heated arguments with clients, neither of which is conducive to providing therapeutic, client-centered treatments.

Balancing Practitioner/Client Relationships

This is not to say that practitioners will never have heartfelt conversations with clients, particularly if they perform treatments in the same office with the same employees over an extended period of time. A sense of familiarity and connection on a personal level does tend to develop because of continuity over time, the quality of the practitioner's work, and the success of the therapeutic relationship. The job, then, of practitioners is to know how to balance the relationship so that they are always mindful that they are not working on friends, that they are in a professional setting, and that they are being paid to provide a service. The ability to balance these factors comes with practice and experience, but it must start with a professional understanding of what the practitioner's role is and an acknowledgment that the client comes first.

If practitioners find that they are talking a lot about themselves during sessions with clients, it is important for them to ask themselves why that is. Doing this in the professional setting generally means they lack an outlet for personal sharing elsewhere in their lives. Perhaps they are new to the area and have not yet made friends, or perhaps they have gotten isolated from friends and family for whatever reason, and clients are the only people they see on a regular basis that they feel close to. There could be as many reasons as there are practitioners. However, this behavior indicates a need to seek supervision from trusted mentors, peers, or colleagues or to work with a professional counselor to explore what this issue means and how to manage it personally so it does not interfere professionally.

Other Unprofessional Behaviors

It cannot be stressed enough that practitioners need to make sure they behave professionally at all times and do not, for whatever reason, slide into unprofessional behavior, no matter how comfortable they feel with clients or how long they have been working with them. Examples of other unprofessional behaviors that practitioners need to guard against include the following:

- Telling childish or off-color jokes, even if the client tells these types of jokes
- Making comments that denigrate the massage profession
- Engaging in gossip or mean-spirited conversation
- Being disrespectful of other professions, especially in an attempt to make massage therapy appear superior (e.g., "I'd never get a chiropractic adjustment! They just crack your back and then you have to keep going back. Massage is much better for you.")
- Making a habit of last-minute cancellations (e.g., because a better offer came up, such as a higher-paying client, or because the practitioner just does not feel like working that day)
- Taking a chair massage account for granted and getting sloppy (e.g., frequently running late, being less conscientious about the hands-on work, sharing gossip with the clients, and so forth)
- Arguing with a client (for whatever reason) rather than speaking calmly, getting a mediator within the office, or choosing to walk away

Practitioners who conduct themselves with a high regard for professional integrity and behavior project strong and confident images to their clients. This image is what will initially attract clients to want to experience their work. Consistency, effective techniques, and client-centered treatments should keep clients coming back.

Professional Appearance

As discussed previously, first impressions are made quickly and are predominantly visual (unless, of course, the person has a striking odor). What practitioners wear, its condition and fit, how their hair is styled, and their level of hygiene convey an enormous amount of information to which people have an immediate response. For example, it has been the authors' experience that at community service events such as walks and runs to raise money for various organizations, people will often wait in longer lines just to be sure they get worked on by a particular practitioner, even if other practitioners are available. Generally, the popular practitioners are wearing clean pressed pants or shorts in good condition, a clean polo shirt, a neat hairstyle (pulled back in a hair tie if the hair is long), clean athletic shoes, and have warm smiles as they greet and work with each new client. In contrast, practitioners at the same event wearing wrinkled pants or shorts with frays around the hems, wrinkled or ill-fitting polo shirts (or tank tops or other unprofessional shirts), soiled shoes, and who have unkempt hair and a dour look on their faces are usually not nearly as busy. Even if directed to these available practitioners, clients often politely decline, point to the first type of practitioner, and say, "I've been watching him. Can I wait until he is free?"

This scenario exemplifies how much power image has on how people make choices. This is not true for everyone, of course, but humans commonly respond more positively to what they find appealing. To be successful, practitioners need to pay attention to this tendency, and dress and act accordingly. If practitioners have made the commitment to invest time and money into successfully completing an educational bodywork program, the next step is to invest in their businesses. In addition to equipment and supplies, a professional wardrobe is necessary (recall the professional dress described in Chapter 6). This does not mean the clothing needs to be expensive; inexpensive clothing that is neat and well kept sends the same message of professionalism.

The setting in which the practitioner is working will inform what the appropriate attire should be. All bodywork professionals must note that there have been many pioneers in the profession who have worked very hard over the past 50 years to move bodywork, especially massage therapy, out of the shadows of adult entertainment and into the healthcare field. Therefore, it is essential that practitioners' attire reflect the position and respect the profession has gained in the eyes of the public and other healthcare providers.

BOUNDARIES

Boundaries, at the simplest, are limits. Boundaries are about a person's actions. They are determined by what people choose to reveal about themselves and what behavior and information they will accept from others. When people set a boundary for themselves, they are making the statement, "This is where I draw the line." Some examples of types of boundaries include the following:

- *Physical.* People determine for themselves how their bodies will be touched and by whom.
- *Mental and emotional.* People determine how much they think and feel about various topics, choose how much they disclose about what they think and feel, and decide how much to mentally and emotionally engage with others.

There are personal as well as professional boundaries. Personal boundaries are those that, through their life experiences, upbringing, and education, people have chosen to govern their words and actions. Some personal boundaries are consciously chosen, and some are not, but all depend on one's personal ethics. Another factor about personal boundaries is that they create safety and provide structure. When people feel safe in their environments and know what is expected of them, and of others, they can then connect more deeply with others. They are also conscious of the fact that they can *choose* to change their boundaries at any time, depending on the situation.

Professional boundaries govern a person's conduct at work. Professional boundaries are an integral part of professional ethics. A code of ethics is, in fact, a way to take ethical concepts and present them as appropriate behaviors defined by appropriate boundaries. When practitioners are clear about their scope of practice, for instance, they have the information they need to set boundaries around what techniques they will and will not perform.

Professional boundaries differ from personal boundaries in the nature of their intent. In the bodywork profession, the intention is to provide professional and quality treatments. In a professional setting, practitioners must be conscious of that fact that the clients are not there just to share personal stories with, or ask advice from, the practitioner. Well-defined professional boundaries on the part of the practitioner assures clients that they do not have to be concerned about the practitioner wanting or needing anything from them. This then allows the therapeutic relationship to form.

As discussed previously, boundaries can be physical. In the bodywork profession, this is shown when clients tell practitioners exactly how much pressure they want to experience and inform practitioners when the limit is passed. Emotional boundaries in the bodywork profession can be shown through the example of a client who is having a difficult day at work and then is short-tempered with the practitioner. The practitioner can set a boundary by choosing not to take the client's bad mood personally and, therefore, not engage with it, in order to give the client an effective treatment.

Boundaries can also be set around money. Money is a part of the therapeutic relationship with clients when practitioners' intentions are to be paid for their chair massage services. The more clear practitioners are about the importance of being paid, the more successful their practices will be. Why? Because they are being clear about the value of their work and their own sense of self-worth, and they are willing and able to share this with clients. Although many practitioners are happy to donate their time and energy doing bodywork for charitable causes, practitioners should not undermine the value of their training and their work by always giving it away for free.

The purpose of boundaries in the bodywork field is to create safety for all parties involved and to promote transparency so that the client and the practitioner are clear about each other's expectations and requests within the therapeutic relationship. In the onsite setting where the practitioner has developed an ongoing relationship with clients, it can be easy to get personal about each other's lives as well as hear comments about other employees the practitioner eventually will be working on. The goal is to be able to find the balance between being open to all clients and yet not set boundaries so firmly that the practitioner is viewed as detached. If practitioners are clear about their professional boundaries, it is easier to develop the ability to remain warm and friendly with clients while tactfully deflecting or redirecting as needed.

If practitioners are having difficulty recognizing, understanding, setting, or maintaining personal and professional boundaries, it is highly recommended they seek assistance. This can be through discussion with trusted mentors and colleagues, participating in boundaries and ethics workshops or online courses, and reading texts devoted to ethics for massage therapists and bodyworkers. The website www.thebodyworker.com is also a good resource for information.

Office Politics

Companies, organizations, and groups are like small communities with their own sets of rules and guidelines. Some rules are clearly defined and adhered to. What can trip up a newcomer to a group, however, are the unspoken rules and any longstanding alliances or feuds. In this context, **office politics** refers to the total complex of relationships in the organization and any competing interests for power or leadership. The bigger the group, the more likely the chance that not everyone will get along. Practitioners will sometimes massage someone who will be telling them horrible things about a coworker and then that very coworker is the next person on the schedule. The professional practitioner will be able to navigate the waters of office politics and not get involved or choose sides. This aspect of professionalism means the practitioner is the same person with all clients, does not treat some better than others, and does not engage in gossip with clients. Maintaining clear boundaries, which includes being specific about the policies and procedures for receiving services, makes it easier for the practitioner to connect with all the clients in each setting as they come in for treatments, without any notion that the practitioner might be playing favorites (and thus adding themselves to the swirl of office politics).

The following are some examples of typical situations that may occur in the office setting that could challenge the practitioner's ability or willingness to provide quality services.

Relationship between the Supervisor and a Co-Worker

One example of office politics that requires poise and calmness from the practitioner is the scenario involving a supervisor who has a personal (intimate) relationship with one of the employees. As a result, the boss's significant other may get special treatment in the office, which could extend to the practitioner (for example, the boss may tell the practitioner to provide this particular employee with an extra 15 minutes of chair massage beyond what other employees receive). This could cause resentment among the other employees and the expectation that the practitioner should be the one keeping all treatments equitable.

In this case, practitioners need to maintain professionalism and set clear boundaries about the work they are contracted to provide to all clients. To those who comment on favorable treatment for the boss's significant other, practitioners could say something like "I'm not responsible for setting the treatment schedule. But since this is your treatment time, I'm happy to keep the focus on your needs."

Watching the Clock and Demanding a Specific Time Slot

Each chair massage account will have standards of practice in terms of how long each treatment will last and how each client will be notified of his or her appointment time. These standards are to ensure an organized flow to the account and allow practitioners to estimate how long they will be at a particular location.

There are instances in which one or more employees might complain that they are not getting the same amount of time as another employee. There are two methods to handle this situation. One way is to have a clock in a visible place in the room. When the client arrives for the appointment, the practitioner can say, "Hi, Raphael. Welcome to your 3 o'clock appointment," while pointing to the clock. "We will be doing a 15-minute session, so let's get started." These cues let the client know what time the treatment is starting as well as verbally clarifying how long the session will last. It is especially helpful to state how long the session is if the practitioner offers a variety of treatment lengths that clients can sign up for.

Another way to ensure that all treatments are same length of time is to use a timer. It can be placed in view of the client and set for the treatment time. However, the ringer or buzzer that goes off at the end of the session can be unsettling, so be sure to alert the client to that eventuality. This method of assuring clients that they are receiving their allotted treatment time is not usually recommended except in situations where clients have expressed doubts about the fairness or equality of treatment length.

It is also important to make the distinction to the client between the treatment length and the amount of time the practitioner is actually doing hands-on work. For example, a 20-minute session may include a 2-minute pretreatment interview and a 1-minute posttreatment interview, making the actual hands-on time 17 minutes. A statement in the practitioner's policy and procedure guidelines should clarify this. It is an important distinction to make to the clients so that they do not think they are being shortchanged. It may also prevent them from talking so much that they delay, and shorten, their treatment time, allowing the treatment to begin as quickly as possible.

Sometimes clients become territorial about the time slot in which they get their treatment. For example, a practitioner has a standing appointment with a company every other Thursday at 1 p.m., and there is an employee that always insists on getting that first appointment. This is not necessarily a problem until that employee is running late and expects the practitioner to hold the appointment for him, thus throwing off the entire treatment schedule. It could also become a problem if it prevents flexibility in scheduling, such as another employee needing that time because she is leaving early, but the first client still insisting on having the first treatment slot. If the practitioner is being paid per individual client, the practitioner then loses potential income if the second employee's schedule cannot be accommodated.

Depending on the tone and the accessibility of the office, it may be possible to speak to the contact person about the situation. The practitioner could say, for example, "Jean told me that she would love to get a treatment but she cannot stay into the afternoon. Is it possible to schedule her first or fit her in earlier?" That way, the contact person can make the decision. If practitioners have some flexibility in their schedule that day, they can let the contact person know that as well by saying something like "In fact, I can start 30 minutes earlier if that would help to accommodate employees who are not able to stay later in the afternoon." It would be wise of practitioners to not make this suggestion unless they are certain that a definite client will fill the early spot. Otherwise, practitioners may come in early and then not be busy.

Sometimes not everyone at a company, organization, or group who wants a massage can get one. If this becomes a concern for either the company or the practitioner, it might be worthwhile to formally survey the employees and assess whether the amount of time the practitioner is at the location is sufficient. If not, consider talking with the office manager to negotiate an increase in treatment hours.

Venting about the Supervisor

Comparisons have been made between bodywork practitioners and counselors in the sense that many are easy to talk to and people tend to feel safe and free about disclosing intimate details about their lives. In the work setting, this happens frequently when there is unrest about the supervisor among the employees. One of the reasons the practitioner is at the office is to promote health and well-being. The employee might reason that one way to feel better is to let off some steam about the supervisor. If this happens, it is imperative that the practitioner listen respectfully and not engage in the conversation. Not only would this be unprofessional and crossing an ethical boundary, it would be violating the trust that the supervisor placed in the practitioner to offer wellness care to the employees.

If it seems like clients are trying to engage the practitioner in their displeasure with the supervisor, the practitioner can tactfully say something like "I can hear how frustrated you are about your supervisor, and I can feel how tense you are in your shoulders. I hope this massage will help work out some of that tension, and you won't feel so frustrated when you go back to your desk." This response does not involve the practitioner's opinion of the supervisor. However, it does acknowledge to the client that the practitioner hears her frustration, while bringing attention back to the client and the reason for the treatment. Whether or not the practitioner likes the supervisor or the employee at a location, it is neither appropriate nor professional to share those feelings or opinions.

COMMUNICATING WITH CLIENTS WHO ARE NEW TO SEATED MASSAGE

Chapter 3 covered what to say to first-time chair massage clients and how to show them the proper way to sit in the massage chair. Sometimes, however, before the practitioner can stop him, a client new to seated massage approaches the massage chair and promptly sits in it with his back against the sternum pad. To prevent this from happening and to minimize any embarrassment to the client, practitioners should always greet new clients with a handshake, introduce themselves, and ask, "Have you ever had a chair massage?" If the answer is no, then the practitioner can model how to sit while explaining the adjusting mechanisms of the chair.

If clients get ahead of practitioners and sit on the chair backward before practitioners can stop them, it is important that practitioners tactfully educate the clients and not embarrass them. After all, it is possible to receive a seated massage treatment in this position; it is just not common. The following is an example of how the practitioner could redirect the client:

"Would you mind standing for a moment? I'd like to show you the different features of the massage chair. You can actually sit in either of two directions. Facing this way (pointing), this pad supports your chest, and your knees go on these pads. This is a face cradle that supports your face, and this is where your arms would go. Sometimes clients prefer to sit with their backs to the chest pad, and that can work as well, although sitting the other way allows better access to the neck, shoulder, and back muscles. How would you like to sit today?" This brief conversation will give clients a choice as well as the opportunity to recognize that practitioners are willing to accommodate client needs.

Also, it is important to ask clients if they have any physical conditions or limitations that would make it difficult for them to sit on the chair frontward. Practitioners should keep in mind, though, that clients do not always know if they will be comfortable on the chair until they are actually sitting on it, so they should not assume that clients will speak up. For example, if the client is has had knee surgery recently, the practitioner can quickly demonstrate how to bring the legs forward or to the side of knee pads for support, so that the client will not have to kneel, or perhaps the client would be more comfortable sitting backward on the chair.

With new clients, the primary need is to set them at ease, to give them permission to ask questions about their comfort level on the chair, and to tell the practitioner if that comfort level changes once the massage has started.

Feedback

Another brief conversation to have with new clients, and returning clients, is the importance of providing feedback on how the session is proceeding. **Feedback** is the term used in the bodywork profession for the sharing of information between client and practitioner regarding the effectiveness of the treatment. Speaking about this before the treatment starts will give the client permission to speak up about, for example, needing less or more pressure in an area or that she would rather not have any massage on the neck. Clients should not have to suffer through a treatment session because they did not know they could make a request for change; they might assume that all seated massage sessions would be like this and therefore may not ever receive another one. Or a client could keep coming back but risk being injured from not telling the practitioner if pressure is too deep, or a stretch is not comfortable, and so forth.

From the practitioner's perspective, it can be disheartening to hear, after the fact, that a client was not satisfied with a treatment but did not say anything until it was over. Or, in the worst case scenario, a coworker tells the practitioner that a particular client has stopped coming because he did not like something that the practitioner did in a treatment. Timely feedback is essential for the practitioner to understand, in the moment, what is working and what is not working; it also gives clients a voice in their treatments. When the practitioner invites the client to give feedback, the client knows that it is okay to speak up, make requests, and state preferences.

An example of how to communicate to the client the importance of giving feedback is to say something like "I invite you to give me feedback at any time during the treatment, especially if you are not comfortable, if the pressure is too much or not enough, if a stretch is uncomfortable, or if a technique is not working for you. Do not hesitate to let me know so that I can do my best to meet your needs."

This brief statement not only gives the client permission to give feedback, it also gives examples of possible types of feedback, and it assures the client that the practitioner is a professional and will not be offended by the feedback. The practitioner is demonstrating concern about the client's experience. It is also appropriate to check in with a client (e.g., 'Is this enough pressure?') at points throughout the session, as long as it is not disruptive to the relaxing flow of a session.

Because the client is usually not facing the practitioner during a chair massage treatment, different signals could be offered for alerting the practitioner when the client needs to communicate something. For example, the client could lift the head out of the face cradle when needing to speak, or maybe raise the right hand if the pressure is too much and the left hand if the pressure is not enough. Whatever the system is, the client and the practitioner should agree on it ahead of time, it should be easy to follow, and it should not interfere with the client relaxing into the treatment. Some clients may just speak loudly from the face cradle whenever they need to say something. This is another reason why practitioners should limit conversations about themselves. If practitioners are not focusing on the client, they may miss some crucial feedback cues.

Every bit as important as inviting feedback is the way in which practitioners hear the feedback. It is critical that practitioners not take feedback personally. If a client says that the pressure performed during techniques is too much, that information is about the client and not about the practitioner's skills. This is a matter of temperament and experience. If the practitioner is the kind of person who tends to take things personally, something to keep in mind is that with more experience comes the ability to receive feedback easier.

Posttreatment Interview

After the session is over, it is appropriate for the practitioner to ask the client how the session felt. This can be a brief posttreatment interview, or feedback session, that focuses on the results of the treatment. The questions should be brief and concise, and they should seek to clarify for the practitioner if the goals of the session were met and if the client was satisfied with the session. It should also be conducted after the client gets off the chair. The practitioner could say something like "How are you feeling? Do you feel less tension in your right shoulder? Is there anything that I should do differently or be sure to do again next time I come in? Thank you so much. Be sure and drink lots of water this afternoon."

This posttreatment feedback session keeps the practitioner focused on one client at a time, and allows the client to say something that she may have forgotten to say during the treatment or wanted to say while facing the practitioner instead of while her face was in the face cradle.

Sometimes no matter how clear about feedback the practitioner is or no matter how much the practitioner encourages it, clients may still choose not to provide it. There really is nothing the practitioner can do about this fact. Some people are reluctant to mention if they did not like something no matter the circumstances. This is just a fact of human nature.

For this reason, the practitioner should always be alert for nonverbal cues from clients. For example, the client's body tightening could indicate that the practitioner's pressure may be too deep, or a stretch may not be comfortable if the client braces the arm rather than relaxes it. If the client avoids eye contact at the end of a session, it may mean there was something he didn't like about the treatment but does not want to talk about it. When picking up on such cues, err on the side of caution and, for example, lighten up on the pressure, relax the stretch, and be gracious with a client who seems distant. Collaboration between client and practitioner is important for a successful therapeutic relationship. The more that practitioner can guide and model this collaboration, the more likely it will be that the client will follow.

Feedback Forms

To assess client satisfaction, an option is to offer written feedback forms that clients can fill out anonymously. This is particularly useful for long-term accounts where practitioners may have become complacent and perhaps not realize that they are letting some of their professional skills slide.

To make it easy and efficient for an office to provide feedback, mail the feedback forms to the contact person, and enclose them in a self-addressed stamped envelope large enough to hold all of the forms. Or the practitioner could just leave the feedback forms, along with instructions on how to complete them, with the designated contact person. The contact person could distribute them and then collect them for the practitioner. Both ways encourage more honest feedback by taking the practitioner out of the equation because the contact person distributes and collects the forms. The written forms also allow clients who are not comfortable giving feedback in person the opportunity to write down their comments.

PREPARATION TO WORK

As discussed previously, one sign of professionalism is arriving early enough to be fully set up and ready for your first appointment. Being early indicates that the practitioner is eager to work with the company, is prepared to start right on time, and can be counted on to be there on a consistent basis. As stated in Chapter 2, one of the ways to make sure practitioners arrive in a timely fashion on their first visit to an office suite or business is to get as much information as possible from the contact person on how to find the location. Another way is to scout out the location at least a day before the first appointment. This will alleviate the stress that can happen if practitioners get lost, run behind schedule, or miscalculate travel time. Nothing makes a poor first impression more than being late for a new account or arriving with minutes to spare, out of breath, and looking frazzled.

Upon arrival, practitioners should plan on at least 20 to 30 minutes to set up. This setup time is used not only to prepare the treatment space; it can be used for the practitioner to prepare both emotionally and physically. All practitioners have their own methods that prepare them for being present (i.e., physically warmed up and mentally focused for their clients). These methods will differ according to personality type, business setting, and amount of preparation needed to get the treatments started at the location. When practitioners are on time and prepared, they are able to be flexible when the unexpected occurs.

Emotional Preparation

Whereas some practitioners are able to arrive at a location, set up, and start treatments immediately, others need to take a few moments to center and ground themselves. This centering and grounding is an essential component to feeling calm, relaxed, ready to perform treatments, and being open and able to make the therapeutic connection with clients.

Emotional preparation through centering and grounding can be done a number of different ways. Every practitioner has his or her own methods. Some examples are deep breathing, stretching, or sitting in quiet meditation or prayer. This quiet time allows the practitioner to put aside the drive to the location and any stresses that may have occurred with it: the work, errands, or other tasks or encounters (anticipated or dreaded) that may be waiting for the practitioner when the treatment session is over as well as the day-to-day task of making to-do lists.

Physical Preparation

Physical preparation refers to preparing both the setting and the practitioner's body. This includes such things as checking in with the contact person to get the signup sheet for the day's appointments, setting up the massage chair, organizing all the supplies (face cradle covers, spritzer, clock, business cards, brochures, gift certificates, educational handouts, music source, change bag, and so forth) for a safe and efficient treatment room, doing some warm-up stretches and exercises (as discussed in Chapter 3), and, finally, washing the hands.

SPECIAL-NEEDS CLIENTS

Some clients are not able to participate in the seated massage session in the standard format. For example, a client may feel claustrophobic and not feel comfortable with the face in the face cradle, or a client may be over the weight limit for the structure of the chair. Because it would be unprofessional, and discriminatory, to tell these client that they cannot receive a seated massage treatment, it is good to be prepared with ideas for ways to accommodate special needs. Whatever the need, keep detailed notes about the condition and the accommodation in the event that there is a long time between appointments or there is another practitioner also working on the account. The clients themselves will be the best source of information about what they need in order to receive a seated massage treatment comfortably. Do not hesitate to ask the clients what they need, and be flexible and creative in finding ways that allow an effective treatment session.

Claustrophobic Clients and Clients with Respiratory Issues

Some clients tend to prefer not to lean forward on the sternum pad with their face in the cradle. These clients might prefer to sit on the massage chair with their back to the sternum pad and the seat in the lowest position. In this case, remove the face cradle and put the armrest in its downward position, which will allow closer access to the client. The majority of the treatment will be focused on the client's upper trapezius, neck, pectoral muscles, arms, and hands. If the client does not feel comfortable sitting in the massage chair at all, try having the client sit in a straight-backed chair and perform the treatment that way. Do not use any kind of wheeled chair, however, because the pressure of performing techniques will inevitably cause the chair to move, possibly injuring the client and the practitioner.

Clients with Larger Body Sizes

Massage chairs can typically support up to 300 pounds of weight. However, this does not mean that the client with a larger body size will be comfortable, or safe, sitting in the massage chair. Therefore, the practitioner can offer the option of sitting in a standard chair, as described earlier, or straddling the chair backward to allow the practitioner access to the client's back.

An example of how the practitioner can tactfully suggest this to the client is by saying, "Do you think that you will be comfortable sitting in the chair this way (demonstrate by sitting in the chair), or would you like to try sitting in this straight-back chair for the treatment? It would allow me just as much access to your shoulders, neck, arms, and hands. If you would also like work on your low back, you could sit in the chair in this fashion." At this point the practitioner would demonstrate straddling the straight-back chair and leaning on the back of it, and ask, "What do you think?"

If the client does not agree with these ideas, then it is up to the practitioner to state clearly but gently that she is concerned that the chair might not structurally support the client, putting him at risk for injury. This comment is about the chair not being safe, not about the client. The client will, of course, interpret the practitioner's words however he wishes. However, the practitioner's primary goal is the safety of the client. If practitioners suspect that clients will not be safe, then they have a responsibility to act accordingly. Practitioners should also encourage feedback from clients and conduct a brief posttreatment interview so that they can get information about how the treatment needs to be adjusted.

SUMMARY

As with any bodywork practice, ethics and communication are important in chair massage practices because they are integral to the practitioner's professionalism. The higher the level of professionalism, the more successful the practitioner. Practitioners should make sure that their professional behaviors are in alignment with the code of ethics of the massage and bodywork profession. Effective communication skills by the practitioner are necessary for pre- and posttreatment client interviewing as well as during the treatment, especially in business settings.

Practitioners need to be mindful of their professional presentation, which includes their dress, hygiene and grooming, poise, confidence, punctuality, ways of greeting and talking with clients, and the state of the equipment they use.

The purpose of boundaries in the bodywork field is to create safety for all parties involved and to promote transparency so that the client and the practitioner are clear about each other's expectations and requests within the therapeutic relationship. By maintaining professional boundaries, practitioners will be able to successfully navigate office politics.

When communicating with clients new to massage, practitioners need to be polite should a client sit on the chair backward and be flexible about performing the treatment should the client prefer to sit that way.

Before performing any treatments, practitioners should prepare themselves emotionally and physically so that they are ready to greet clients and perform treatments in a professional manner. Also important is for practitioners to be able to communicate with special-needs clients in an effective manner and to accommodate their needs for chair massage treatments.

STUDY QUESTIONS

Answers to these questions are found on page 227.

Multiple Choice

1. What is the term for a set of guidelines that a profession has determined is essential in order for its members to understand what behavior is expected of them with clients, colleagues, and members of other professions?
   a. Boundaries
   b. Feedback
   c. Code of ethics
   d. Professional presentation

2. If, during a treatment, the client keeps asking the practitioner personal questions, what would be the best thing for the practitioner to do?
   a. Answer all of the client's questions.
   b. Keep gently bringing the focus back to the client.
   c. Say that the best therapeutic effect can be felt if the client is quiet.
   d. Remain silent in response to the client's questions.

3. What are people setting when they determine limits about what they find acceptable and in what they choose to engage?
   a. Feedback
   b. Therapeutic relationships
   c. Boundaries
   d. Codes of ethics

4. Which of the following can the practitioner do if clients are reluctant to give her feedback?
   a. State that she is open to receiving feedback that will make her treatments better.
   b. Watch for nonverbal cues during the treatment.
   c. Have the location's contact person distribute anonymous feedback forms.
   d. All of the above.

5. The practitioner taking a few moments to center himself before beginning treatments is what kind of preparation?
   a. Emotional
   b. Physical
   c. Timely
   d. Professional

Fill in the Blank

1. The practitioner's ability to present herself to the public in a poised, confident, qualified, and skilled manner is called ____________________.

2. The connection that exists between the practitioner and the client in which the beneficial effects of the treatment are able to take place is called the ____________________.

3. Clean, pressed clothing, clean undergarments, and shoes are examples of ____________________ for the practitioner.

4. The term used in the bodywork profession that denotes the shared information between client and the practitioner regarding the effectiveness of the treatment is ____________________.

5. The client who is ____________________ may not feel comfortable with her face in the face cradle.

Short Answer

1. Explain why effective communication skills are essential to the success of the bodywork practitioner.

____

____

____

____

____

STUDY QUESTIONS

2. Describe the impact professional attitudes and behavior have on the bodywork practitioner's success.

3. Give at least five examples of unprofessional behavior in which the practitioner should not engage.

4. Explain three methods practitioners can use to negotiate office politics.

5. Why is it important that practitioners arrive early at the location in which they will be providing chair massage? Give at least six reasons.

ACTIVITIES

1. Write a code of ethics for your personal life. Write a code of ethics for yourself as a bodywork practitioner. What areas overlap between the two? Are there any areas in the two codes that seem to be in opposition to each other? If so, why do you think they are opposite? Would you want to bring these areas closer together? If so, how would you do that?

2. Do you think you have professional attitudes and behaviors as a bodywork practitioner? If so, describe what they are. If there are areas where you think you have challenges, what are they? What can you do to make changes?

3. Other than the examples given in the text, think of at least three examples of office politics you think you might encounter while performing treatments on location. How would you handle each one?

4. Interview a professional chair massage practitioner. Ask about the they were challenges faced while performing treatments on location and how handled.

STUDY QUESTIONS

5. Design a feedback form that clients can fill out anonymously. Include the areas in which you would like feedback and how the clients would give the feedback. Would they give you scores in each area? Would they circle answers? Would they write out their feedback?

____

____

____

____

____

6. List three ways you center or ground yourself before you begin performing treatments. If you do not practice any centering or grounding techniques, why not? Research at least three methods and see if any of them appeal to you.

____

____

____

____

____

Appendix A

TRADITIONAL CHINESE MEDICINE CHANNEL REVIEW*

One of the foundational principles of traditional Chinese medicine (TCM) is the concept of yin and yang. Yin and yang are represented by a classic symbol (Figure A-1). To truly understand yin and yang, two apparently opposing thoughts must be held at the same time: in lightness there is dark, and in darkness there is light. In the yin/yang symbol, the dark area has a seed of light, and the light area has a seed of dark. The light and dark areas are not static; one flows into the other. Yin and yang are not fixed; they are in constant movement, always transforming each other. Yin can only go so far before it becomes yang; yang can only go so far before it becomes yin. The coldness and darkness of winter (yin) only last for so long until the warmth and light of spring (yang).

The relationship between yin and yang can be used to realize the relationship among any structures, functions, and processes. The yin characteristics of any of these are structure and substance; the yang characteristics are activity and energy. Table A-1 shows examples of yin and yang phenomena. The human body also has yin and yang aspects (Table A-2), and the qi channels are separated into yin and yang as well.

In traditional Chinese medicine, natural phenomena were systemized into Five Elements: metal, water, earth, wood, and fire. Seasons, foods, flavors, colors, and sounds were categorized into each of the elements. Ancient medicine expanded Five Element theory to include aspects of the body: organs, sense organs, tissues, emotions, and behavioral attributes. Everything categorized under the Five Elements is referred to as *correspondences*; these correspondences were used as a reference for traditional Chinese medicine physicians in their practice of diagnosis and treatment. Table A-3 shows the Five Element correspondences, including what channels are categorized under which element.

*This information is also found in *The Practice of Shiatsu* by S. K. Anderson (St. Louis, 2008, Mosby).

THE CHANNELS

Lung Channel (Figure A-2)

Yin Organ

Function: Intake of qi

Related to: Nose, sinuses, throat, bronchii, lungs, skin, breathing

Symbolism: Structure and vitality, boundaries

TCM: Governs qi and respiration, disperses fluids (mists fluids) and Wei qi, descends qi (prevents scattering and exhaustion of qi), regulates water passages, houses corporeal soul

Location: Lung channel begins at LU-1, which is approximately 1 inch inferior to the hollow under the lateral end of the clavicle. From there it travels through the most anterior portion of the deltoid, biceps brachii, and over the brachioradialis. It then runs down the lateral aspect of the anterior (yin) arm, where the skin is fairer and thinner. It proceeds along the tendon of brachioradialis, over the wrist onto the pad of muscle on the thumb side of the palm to finish at LU-11, on the tip of the radial side of the edge of the thumbnail.

Large Intestine Channel (Figure A-3)

Yang Organ

Function: Elimination

Related to: Large intestine, mouth, throat, nose, mucous secretions, bowel movements, secretions

Symbolism: Ability to release

TCM: Descends its qi, allows passage of waste

TABLE A-1 Examples of Yin and Yang Phenomena

Yin Phenomena	Yang Phenomena
Cold	Heat
Rest	Movement
Passivity	Activity
Darkness	Light
Interior	Exterior
Contraction	Expansion
Decrease	Increase
Tranquil	Noisy
Static	Dynamic
Autumn and winter	Spring and summer
Night	Day
Female	Male

From Anderson SK: *The practice of shiatsu.* St. Louis, 2008, Mosby.

TABLE A-2 Yin and Yang Aspects of Body Structure

Yin Aspects	Yang Aspects
Feet	Head
Lower body	Upper body
Anterior surface of the trunk	Posterior surface of the trunk
Medial surfaces of the extremities	Lateral surfaces of the extremities
Bones	Skin
Internal organs	Muscles
Body fluids (e.g., blood, lymph, mucus, cerebrospinal fluid, saliva)	Energy (e.g., qi, metabolism [formation of ATP, digestion, etc.], nerve impulses, the flow of blood, lymph)

ATP, Adenosine triphosphate.
From Anderson SK: *The practice of shiatsu.* St. Louis, 2008, Mosby.

TABLE A-3 Five Element Correspondences

	Metal	Water	Earth	Wood	Fire
Season	Autumn	Winter	Late summer	Spring	Summer
Direction	West	North	Center	East	South
Color	White	Black, blue	Yellow, brown	Green	Red
Taste	Pungent	Salty	Sweet	Sour	Bitter
Odor	Rotten	Putrid	Fragrant	Rancid	Burnt
Climate	Dryness	Cold	Dampness	Wind	Heat
Development stage	Harvest	Storage	Transformation	Birth	Growth
State	Quieting	Slumber	Transition	Awakening	Wakefulness
Spiritual quality	Po (Corporeal soul; body; material)	Zhu (Ambition; will)	Thought and ideas	Hun (Ethereal soul; immaterial)	Shen (Spirit; awareness)
Yin organ/time of day	Lungs 3-5 am	Kidneys 5-7 pm	Spleen 9-11 am	Liver 1-3 am	Heart 11 am-1 pm
Yang organ/time of day	Large intestine 5-7 am	Urinary bladder 3-5 pm	Stomach 7-9 am	Gallbladder 11 pm-1 am	Small intestine 1-3 pm
Sense organ	Nose	Ears	Mouth	Eyes	Tongue
Tissue	Skin and body hair	Bones	Muscles	Sinews	Vessels
Emotion	Sadness; grief	Fear	Pensiveness	Anger	Joy
Sound	Crying	Groaning	Singing	Shouting	Laughing

From Anderson SK: *The practice of shiatsu.* St. Louis, 2008, Mosby.

Location: LI starts at LI-1, located on the radial side of the nail of the index finger. It travels on the posterior (yang) arm along the extensor digitorum and extensor carpi radialis, then along the anterior edge of brachioradialis. It runs up between the two heads of the biceps brachii, through the anterior deltoid to LI-15 on the acromioclavicular joint.

From the acromioclavicular joint, LI travels over the top of the shoulder, then diagonally along the anterior neck, through the center of the sternocleidomastoid. It approaches the face at the jaw, just anterior to the ramus of the mandible.

LI follows the "smile line" to the lateral border, ending at LI-27, outside the nostril on either side of the nose.

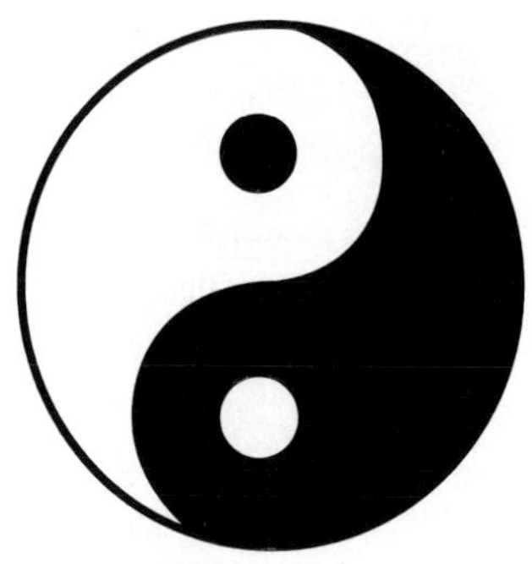

FIGURE A-1 Yin and yang symbol. (From Anderson SK: *The practice of shiatsu*. St. Louis, 2008, Mosby.)

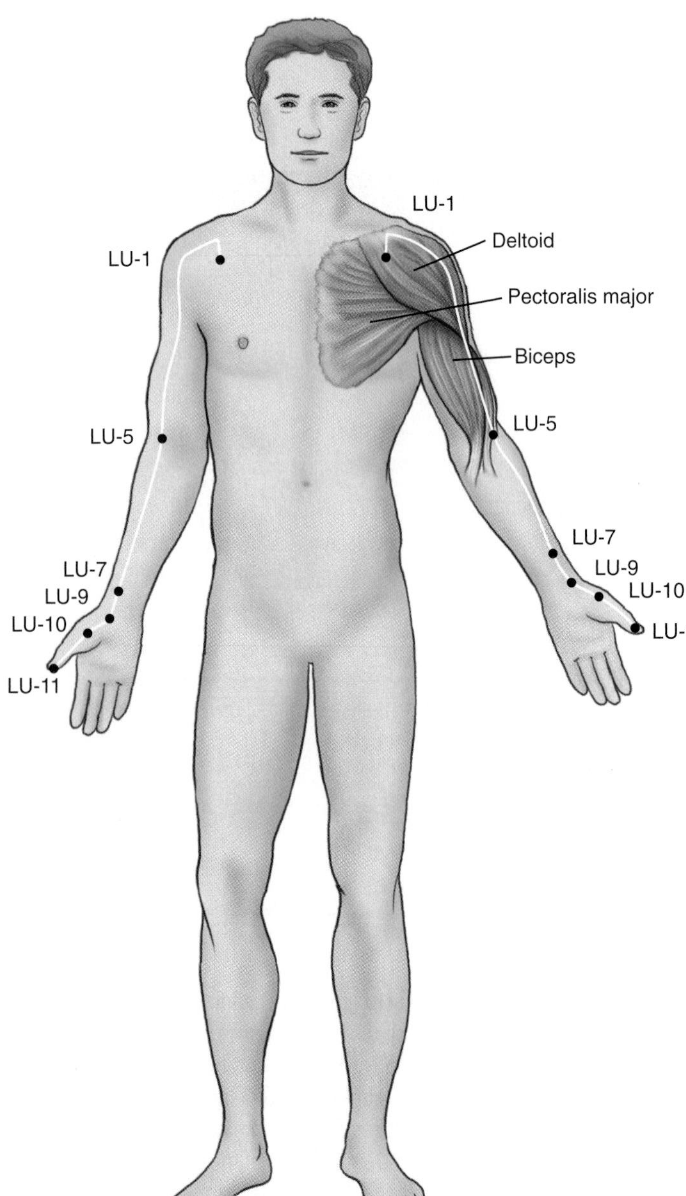

FIGURE A-2 Lung channel. (Modified from Anderson SK: *The practice of shiatsu*. St. Louis, 2008, Mosby.)

Kidney (Figure A-4)

Yin Organ

Function: Water metabolism, controls all fluid secretions, and governs endocrine system, impetus

Related to: Kidneys, pituitary gland, adrenals, stress response, fear and phobias, sexual hormones, desire for reproduction, ears, bones, and lower back

Symbolism: Impetus, flexibility, ability to respond to stimulus, ability to summon up energy when needed

TCM: Houses the essence, stores fundamental yin and yang of the body, governs water, grasps or anchors lung qi, produces marrow: brain and the central nervous system, houses willpower and ambition

Location: Kidney begins at KI-1 on the plantar surface of the foot, where the ball of the foot meets the instep, between metatarsals I and II.

KI then ascends the medial side of the foot, angling posteriorly and proximally to KI-3 on the superior surface of the medial malleolus, just anterior to the Achilles tendon. KI circles posteriorly around the medial malleolus to KI-6 on the inferior surface of the medial malleolus. From there, KI ascends the lower leg by moving proximally up the medial head of gastrocnemius to the medial side of the popliteal fossa, where the tendons of the semimembranosus and semitendinosus meet. KI continues along the medial surface of the upper leg, just posterior to the adductors, to where the inguinal region joins the perineum. At this point, KI travels internally.

KI emerges on the abdomen immediately superior to the pubic crest and approximately ½ inch from the midline of the body. KI runs superiorly on the thorax, widening to follow the lateral edges of the sternum. It terminates at KI-27, in the hollow inferior to the medial end of the clavicle.

Urinary Bladder (Figure A-5)

Yang Organ

Function: Governs autonomic nervous system, energy supply of all organ functions, transformation of fluids and purification of qi

Related to: Will, determination, intensity, fatigue, fear, uterus, urinary bladder, spine, bones, fluid balance, reproduction

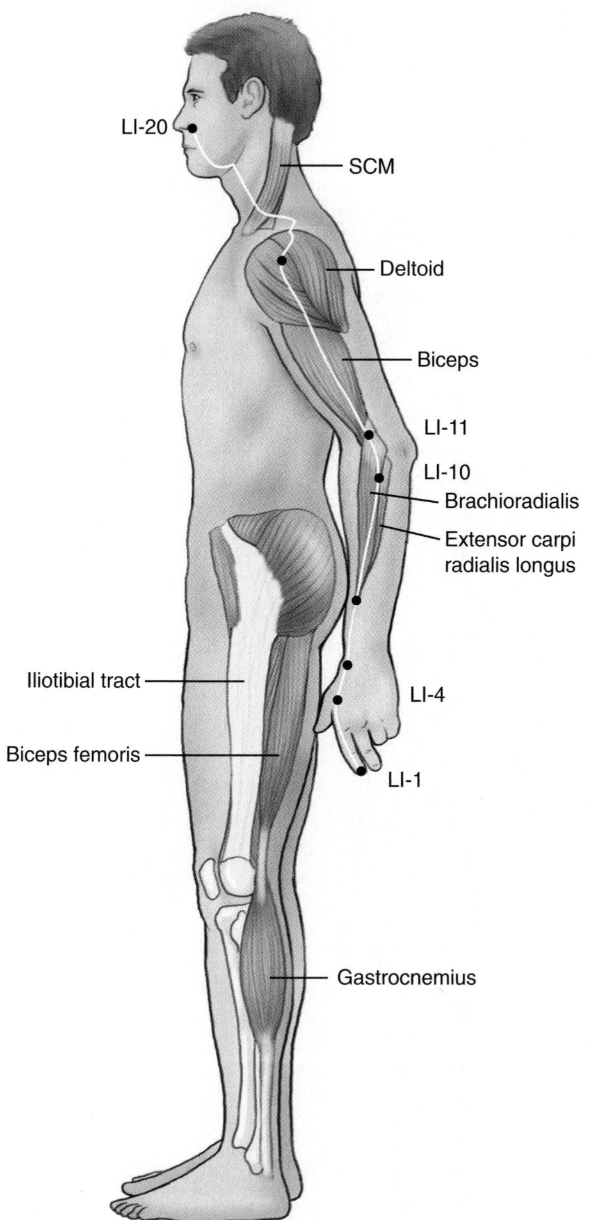

FIGURE A-3 Large intestine channel. *SCM,* Sternocleidomastoid. (Modified from Anderson SK: *The practice of shiatsu.* St. Louis, 2008, Mosby.)

Symbolism: Impetus, ability to respond, purification, fluidity

TCM: Tonifies all the organ functions, receives impure fluids from kidneys and transforms them into urine, stores and excretes urine, influences uterine function, influences posture by giving strength and support to the back

Location: UB starts at UB-1 in the hollow superior to the inner canthus of the eye and, bilaterally, travels superiorly to the forehead. It widens slightly at the superior portion of the frontal bone then travels over the top of the head, then down the posterior head to the occipital ridge. It travels down the posterior cervical region approximately 1 inch lateral to the vertebral column.

UB continues from the neck down the back in two lines. One branch travels laterally and inferiorly along the medial border of the scapula and then approximately 2 inches lateral to the vertebral column to the level of the fourth sacral foramina. The other connects continues in a straight vertical line through the erector spinae muscles in a vertical line to the lowest sacral foramina. The other branch continues in a straight vertical line through the erector spinae muscles to the lowest sacral foramina. It then ascends to the top of the sacrum to descend again more medially and diagonally over the sacral foramina to the end of the coccyx.

The two branches of UB continue through the posterior leg and meet in the center of the popliteal fossa at UB-40. The medial branch travels laterally through the gluteals to the center of the transverse gluteal fold. It descends through the center of the posterior thigh. It veers laterally for the last third of the posterior thigh to the lateral side of the popliteal fossa, then it goes to the center of the popliteal fossa to UB-40. The lateral back branch continues from the lowest sacral foramina along the lateral curve of the gluteal muscles. It angles slightly medially and crosses the other posterior thigh branch of UB approximately a hand's width superior to the popliteal fossa. It descends inferiorly to UB-40. UB then descends distally down the middle of the gastrocnemius and travels laterally to pass between the Achilles tendon and the lateral malleolus. It curves around the lateral malleolus, then travels along the lateral edge of the foot to end at UB-67, on the lateral side of the little toe's toenail.

Spleen (Figure A-6)

Yin Organ

Function: Digestive secretions, hormones

Related to: Thinking, pancreatic enzymes, saliva, stomach juices, insulin, glucagon, small intestine juices, bile

Symbolism: Nurturing, fertility, intellect, digestion of food and ideas, ability to think and learn, nourishment

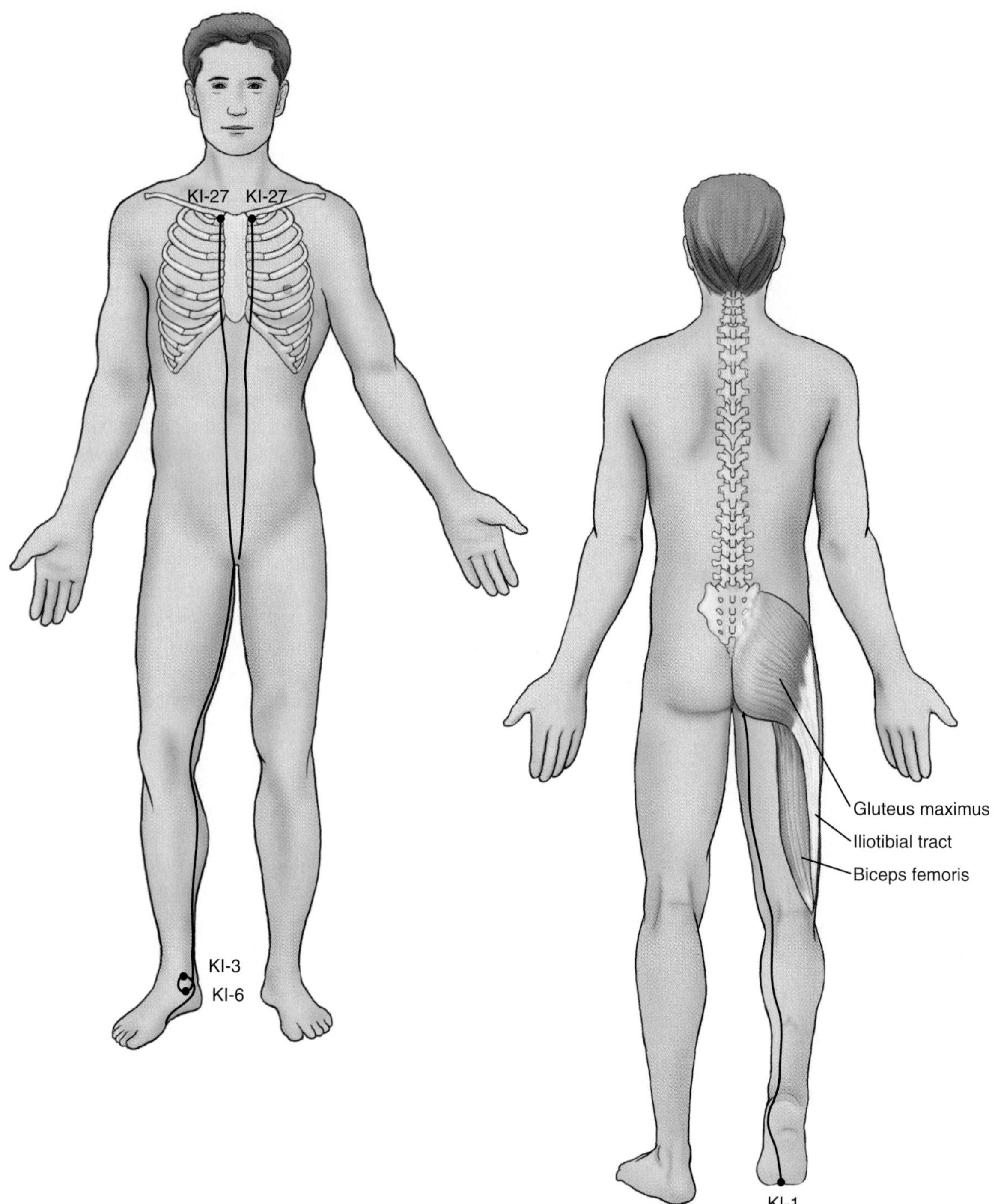

FIGURE A-4 Kidney channel. (Modified from Anderson SK: *The practice of shiatsu*. St. Louis, 2008, Mosby.)

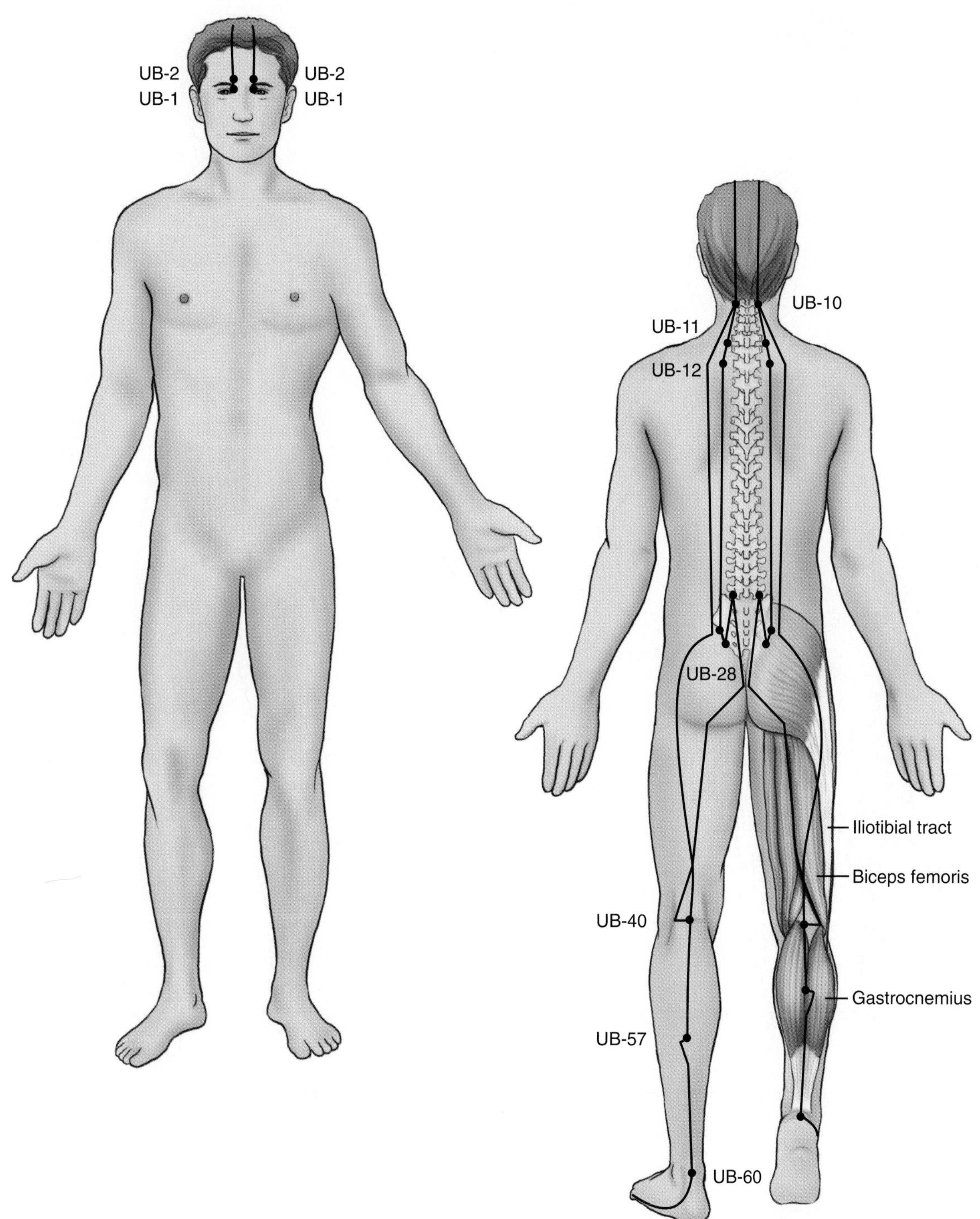

FIGURE A-5 Urinary bladder channel. (Modified from Anderson SK: *The practice of shiatsu.* St. Louis, 2008, Mosby.)

TCM: Transforms and transports food and water (root of postnatal qi), contains the blood, controls the muscles and the four limbs, lifts or raises the qi, houses thought (thinking, studying, memorizing, analyzing)

Location: SP starts on SP-1 on the medial aspect of the big toe, approximately $\frac{1}{16}$ inch from the corner of the nail. It travels medially on the foot to SP-4 at the highest point of the longitudinal arch, then runs through the ankle, anterior to the medial malleolus. It travels proximally along the calf just anterior to the gastrocnemius, past the medial border of the patella, then through the conjunction of the vastus medialis and rectus femoris into the

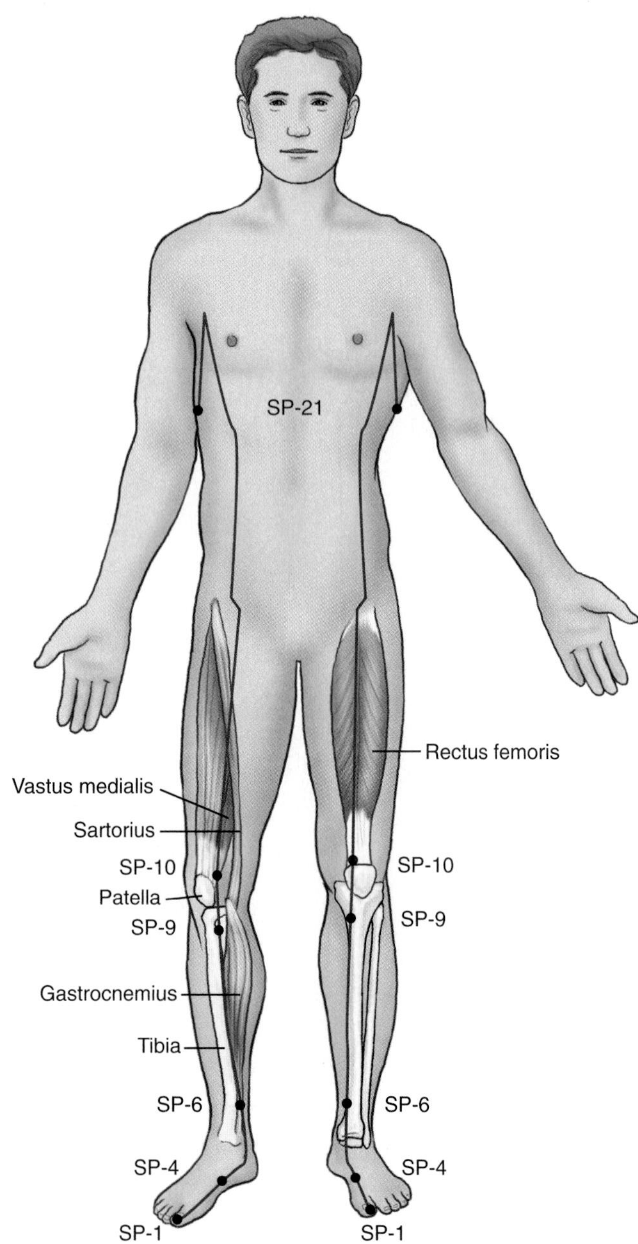

FIGURE A-6 Spleen channel. (Modified from Anderson SK: *The practice of shiatsu.* St. Louis, 2008, Mosby.)

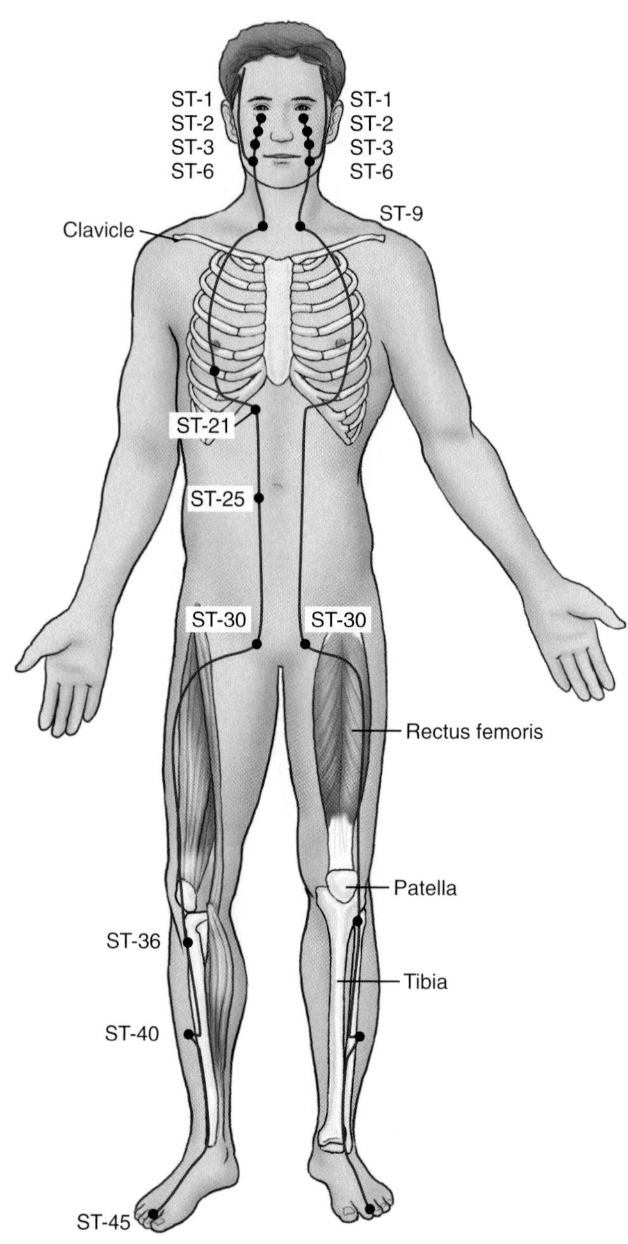

FIGURE A-7 Stomach channel. (Modified from Anderson SK: *The practice of shiatsu.* St. Louis, 2008, Mosby.)

inguinal region. SP then runs superiorly through the abdomen 1 inch lateral to the lateral border of the rectus abdominis.

Just inferior to the rib cage, SP gently angles laterally to line up with the nipple, then travels through the nipple and pectoralis major to SP-20, which is approximately 1 inch inferior and slightly medial to LU-1. It then descends inferiorly and laterally to end at SP-21, which is located at the center of the axillary line and the level of the seventh rib space (approximately one hand width inferior to the axilla).

Stomach (Figure A-7)

Yang Organ

Function: Intake of food, transportation of nutrients, digestive tubes, governs overall appetites

Related to: Esophagus, stomach, duodenum, appetite, lactation, ovaries, uterus, menstrual cycle

Symbolism: Nurturing, fertility, groundedness (heartiness)

TCM: Controls "rotting and ripening" of food ("bubbling caldron"), descends its qi

Location: ST begins under the center of the eye at ST-1 and travels down the cheek just past the corner of the mouth. It angles laterally to the jawline, then travels posteriorly along the mandible to ST-6 in the center of the masseter. From there a branch ascends directly up to the superior edge of the temporalis. ST continues inferiorly along either side of the esophagus to ST-9, then descends toward the head of the clavicle where it runs horizontally along the superior edge of the clavicle.

At the midpoint of the clavicle, ST descends to the nipple along the mammary line. At the level of the fifth rib, it angles gently toward the lateral edge of the rectus abdominis.

ST travels inferiorly along the rectus abdominis to just superior to the pubic bone, then angles diagonally across the inguinal line to the anterior, lateral edge of the rectus femoris, the lateral border of the patella, and the tibialis anterior.

At the ankle, ST travels along the lateral edge of the tendon of the second toe and follows it distally to end at ST-45, on the lateral end of the toenail.

Liver (Figure A-8)

Yin Organ

Function: Stores nutrients, controls the free flow of qi throughout the body, governs detoxification and controls the blood

Related to: Ease of flow, control, detoxification, vision, eyes, tendons, nails, excessive behavior/overindulgence, energetic and emotional ups and downs, major decision making

Symbolism: Choice and execution of one's life plan, vision, planning, action

TCM: Gives capacity for being goal-oriented, resolute, for having drive and energy, ensures the smooth flow of qi, stores the blood

Location: LV starts at LV-1, on the medial side of the big toe, $\frac{1}{16}$ inch from the corner of the toenail, and travels along the lateral aspect of the of the big toe's tendon to the anterior ankle. From there it runs along the medial edge of the tibia to approximately two-thirds up the calf, then it arcs gently up through the posterior-medial calf to approximately 1 inch inferior to the medial knee. LV then angles anteriorly for approximately 1 inch, then travels just under the gracilis in the medial thigh to the pubis.

From the pubis, LV angles laterally and superiorly to LV-13 just inferior to the tip of the eleventh rib (floating rib). It continues to angle superiorly and medially to end on LV-14, which is on the mammary line between the sixth and seventh ribs.

Gallbladder (Figure A-9)

Yang Organ

Function: Controls digestive secretions, distributes emotional and physical qi

Related to: Sides of the body, control of digestive secretions, eyes, tendons, flexibility, clarity in everyday decision making, discrimination and impartiality, ability to take risks versus timidity

Symbolism: Accomplishment, courage/spirit/gall

TCM: Stores and excretes bile, controls judgment and decision making

Location: From GB-1 at the lateral corner of the eye, GB descends posteriorly to the junction of the mandible and the earlobe. It then ascends anteriorly and superiorly to the middle of the temporalis, descends straight down approximately 1 inch, then descends posteriorly to where the top of the ear attaches to the skull at TH-21. GB then ascends straight up approximately $1\frac{1}{2}$ inches, then descends the head, moving around the ear, and down to the mastoid process. GB then curves upward and anteriorly along the superior edge of the temporalis to GB-14 in the forehead, which is approximately $\frac{1}{2}$ inch above the eyebrow, in line with the pupil of the eye. GB then curves posteriorly back over the head approximately 1 inch more medial than where it curved up onto the head, then it runs down to the occipital ridge, posterior to the mastoid process and attachment of the upper trapezius. It descends the upper border of the trapezius to the midpoint of the shoulder at GB-21, where it goes internally.

GB re-emerges below the axilla and angles inferiorly and medially to GB-24 on the eighth rib. It then travels almost straight posteriorly to GB-24 on the tip of the twelfth rib. From GB-25, GB again travels anteriorly along the anterior iliac crest to the anterior superior iliac spine.

From the anterior superior iliac spine, GB travels posteriorly to GB-30, located one third of the way between the greater trochanter and the sacrum. GB then angles anteriorly to descend the upper

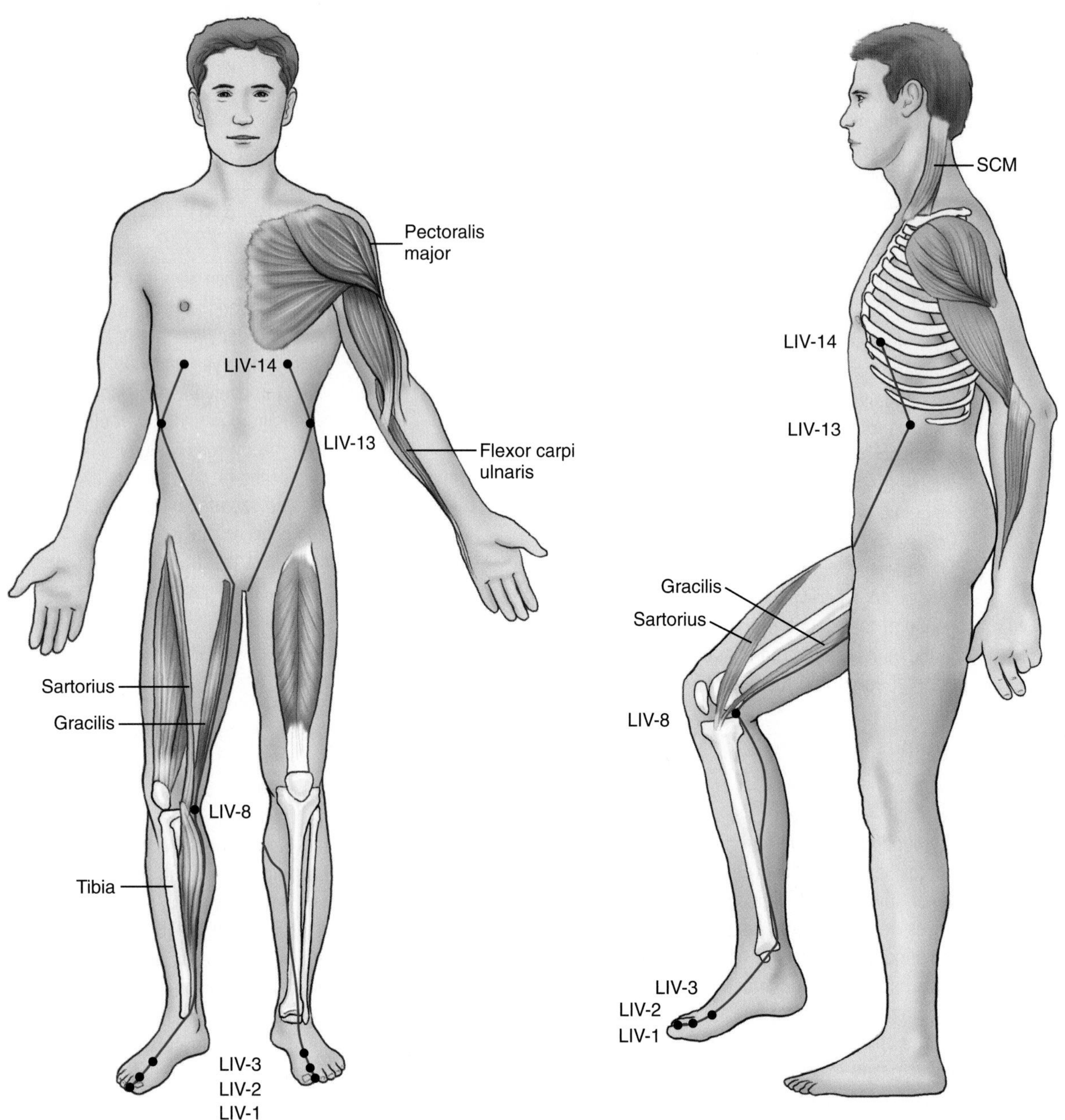

FIGURE A-8 Liver channel. *SCM,* Sternocleidomastoid. (Modified from Anderson SK: *The practice of shiatsu.* St. Louis, 2008, Mosby.)

lateral leg along the iliotibial band, and the fibula in the lower lateral leg. Approximately one third of the way down the fibula, GB travels anteriorly in a straight line approximately 1 inch to GB-36, then it angles inferiorly back to the fibula to catch the lateral tendon of the fourth toe. GB ends at GB-44, on the lateral side of the fourth toe, $\frac{1}{16}$ inch from the corner of the toenail.

Heart (Figure A-10)

Yin Organ

Function: Adaptation, emotional interpretation of experience

Related to: Heart, tongue, speech, sweat, complexion, central nervous system (brain), thymus

Symbolism: Emotional adaptation, emotional stability, spirit

TCM: Governs and propels the blood, controls the blood vessels, houses the Shen, controls sweat

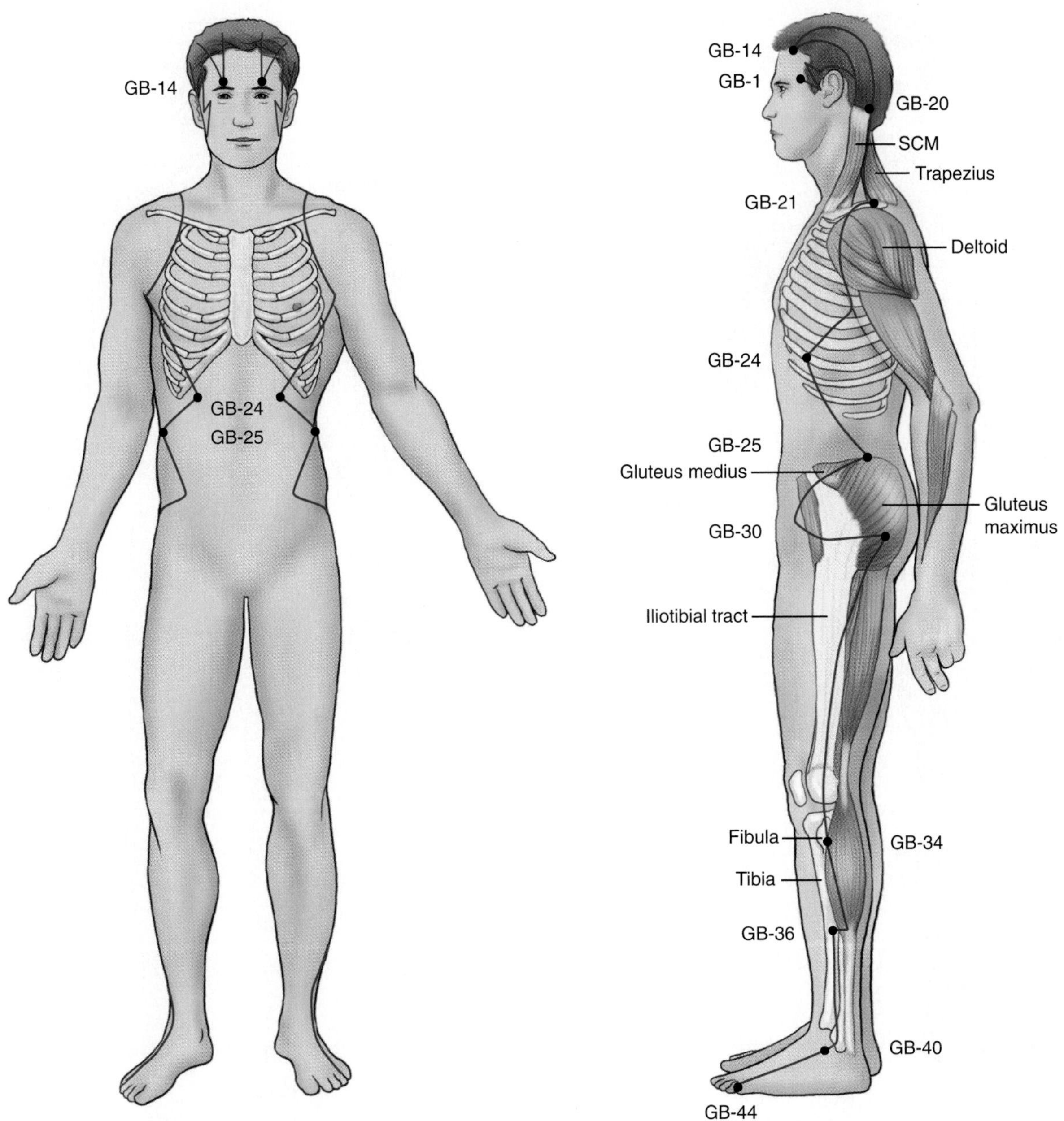

FIGURE A-9 Gallbladder channel. *SCM,* Sternocleidomastoid. (Modified from Anderson SK: *The practice of shiatsu.* St. Louis, 2008, Mosby.)

Location: HT extends from HT-1, in the center of the axilla, out along the anterior (yin) arm between the biceps brachii and triceps brachii. It travels along the medial aspect of the ulna to end on HT-9, on the radial side of the little finger, 1⁄16 inch from the corner of the nail.

Small Intestine (Figure A-11)

Yang Organ

Function: Assimilation and absorption of food and experiences of all kinds

Related to: Small intestine, the spine, cerebrospinal fluid, shock mechanism

Symbolism: Assimilation (to convert another substance into ourselves), receiving, being filled, transforming

TCM: Separates the pure from the impure (digestive function)

Location: SI starts at SI-1, on the ulnar side of the little finger, 1⁄16 inch from the corner of the nail. It travels through the medial wrist, then along the posterior (yang) side of the arm along the edge of the ulna. It crosses through the elbow between the

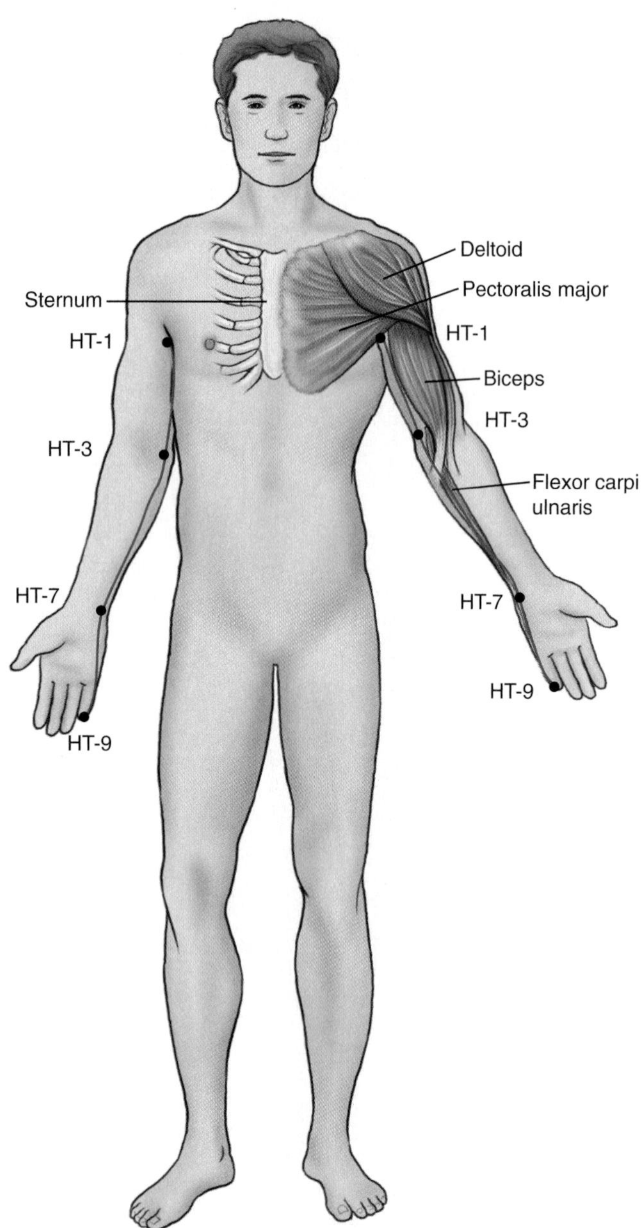

FIGURE A-10 Heart channel. (Modified from Anderson SK: *The practice of shiatsu.* St. Louis, 2008, Mosby.)

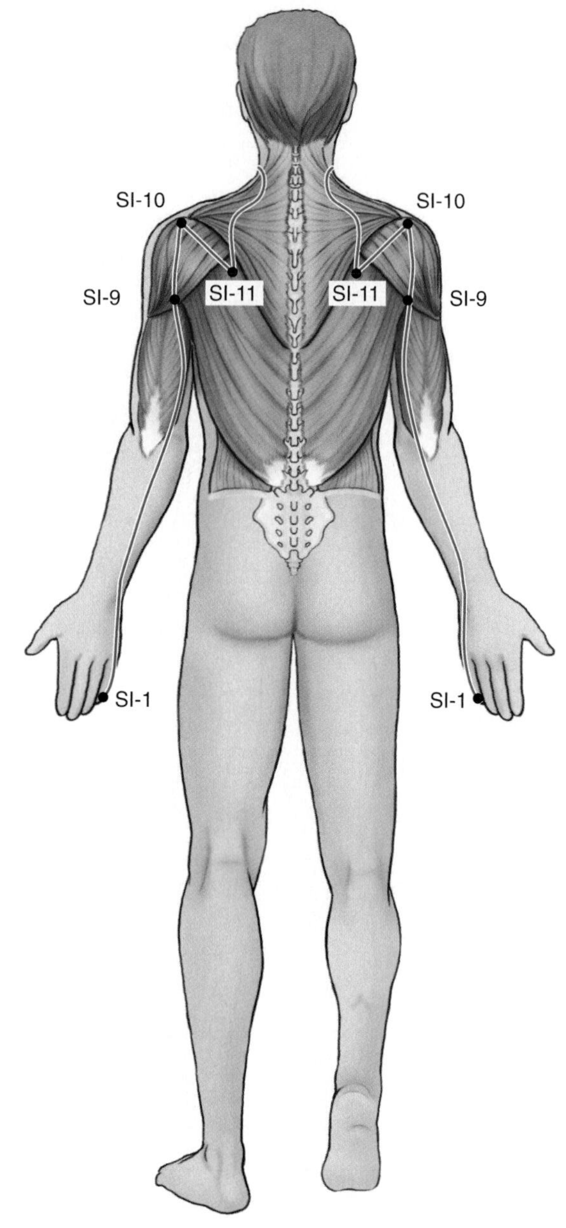

FIGURE A-11 Small intestine channel. (Modified from Anderson SK: *The practice of shiatsu.* St. Louis, 2008, Mosby.)

olecranon process and the medial epicondyle of the humerus. It travels up the arm through the center of the triceps brachii to the axillary crease to SI-10 in an indentation just posterior to the acromion process.

From SI-10, SI travels inferiorly and medially to SI-11 in the center of the scapula. It then ascends directly superior to SI-12 in the middle of the supraspinatus. SI travels medially (and slightly inferiorly) to SI-13.

From there it runs superiorly to the level of C7.

From C7, SI ascends diagonally across the neck and sternocleidomastoid to SI-17, just inferior to the earlobe. It then travels anteriorly and superiorly onto the jaw, just behind the ramus of the mandible, and up and under the cheek. It travels laterally and posteriorly back along the zygomatic arch to end at SI-19, in an indentation in front of the tragus of the ear.

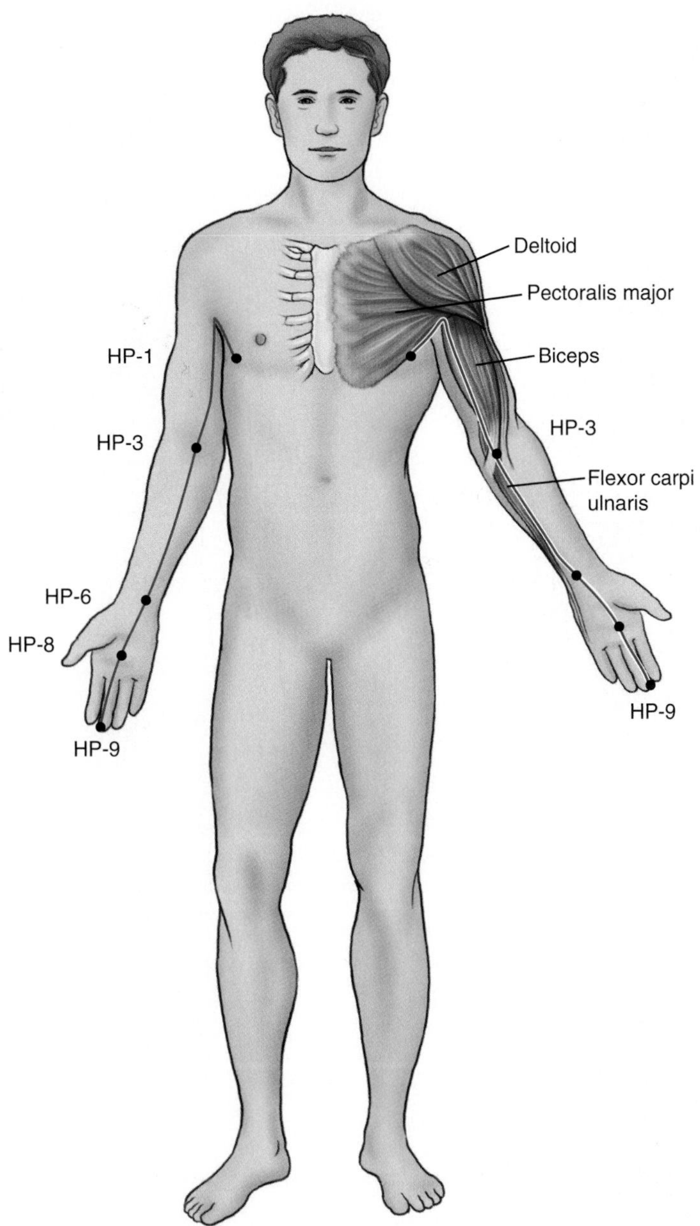

FIGURE A-12 Heart protector channel. (Modified from Anderson SK: *The practice of shiatsu.* St. Louis, 2008, Mosby.)

Heart Protector (Pericardium, Heart Constrictor) (Figure A-12)

Yin Organ

Function: "Minister of the Heart," protects the Shen, provides circulation for the inner core, governs the vascular system

Related to: Heart organ, deep/central circulation, functions of the great blood vessels, veins and arteries, blood pressure, vulnerability, inside/anterior surfaces

Symbolism: Emotional stability, messenger of the spirit/Shen by way of dreams, mother of blood/protector of blood, defends the emotional core, energetic buffer zone around the heart

TCM: Mediates with source qi on the level of consciousness by connection with the heart and Shen, energetic buffer zone around the heart, protecting it from pernicious influences, shock, emotional trauma; protects the blood of the heart and related to circulation of blood in the great vessels; ensures stability of Shen; spreads influence of Shen

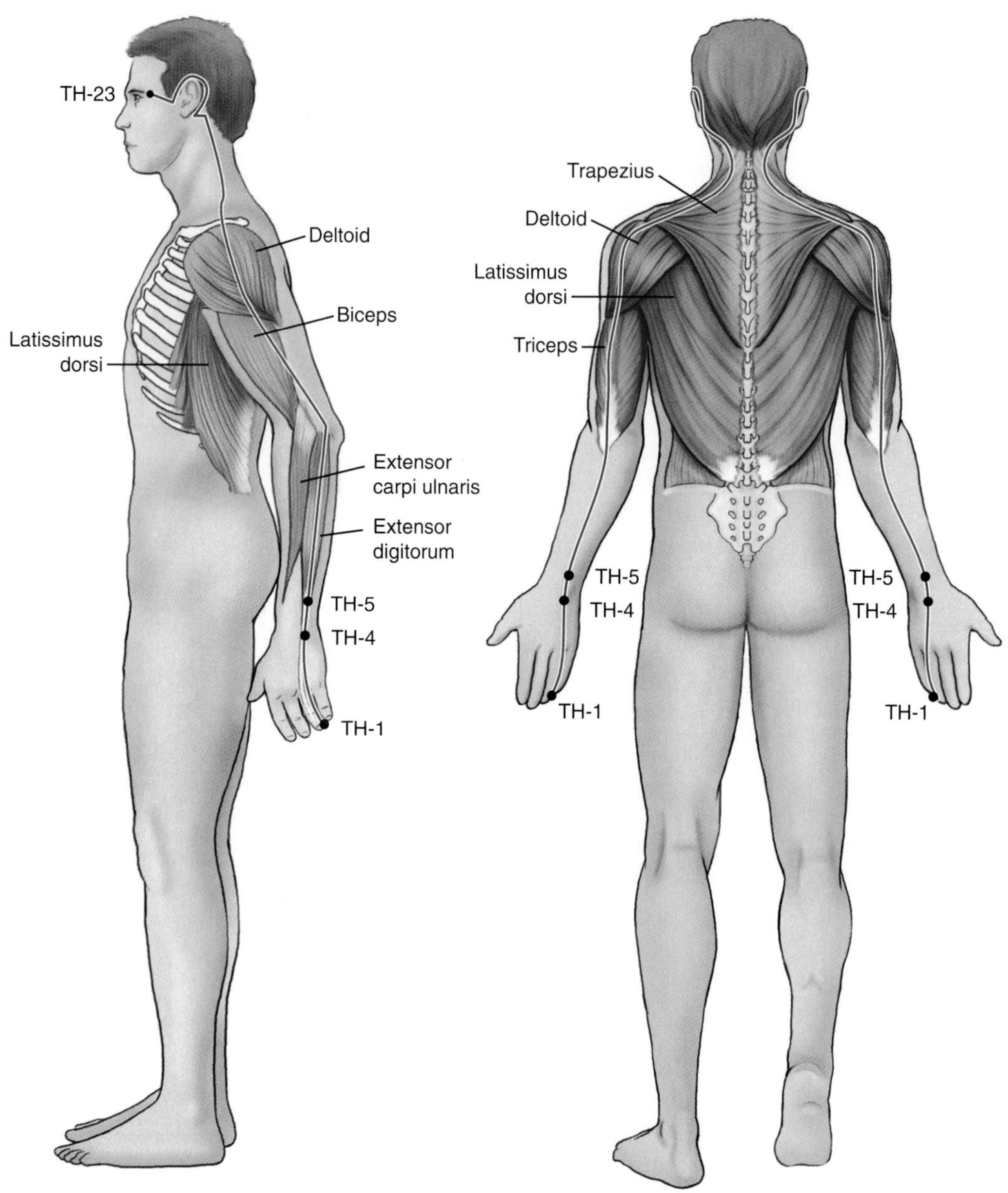

FIGURE A-13 Triple heater channel. (Modified from Anderson SK: *The practice of shiatsu.* St. Louis, 2008, Mosby.)

throughout the body-mind, works with heart to ensure a smooth flow of qi and blood in the chest and throughout the body

Location: HP starts at HP-1, which is found in the fourth intercostal space, just lateral and slightly superior to the nipple. It travels superiorly to the axilla.

Coming through the anterior axilla, HP travels along the anterior (yin) arm between the heads of the biceps brachii, then through the center of the elbow. From there it travels in between the flexor carpi radialis and palmaris longus, and through the center of the palm to end at HP-9, on the radial side of the tip of the middle finger.

Triple Heater (Triple Warmer, Triple Burner) (Figure A-13)

Triple heater is named for the three "heaters" (burners or warmers) of the body.

Yang Organ

Function: Psychological protection, peripheral circulation of blood and lymph, distributor of source qi and information between all organ systems, a warming force or feed system of kidney fire

Related to: Superficial and abdominal fascia/mesentery, blood circulation, lymphatic system, metabolism, immunity, infections, allergic reactions, thermoregulation, ears, deafness, swollen glands, tonsillitis, migraines, stiff neck and shoulders, skin, mucous membranes

Symbolism: Protection versus openness, emotional response to the process of creating physical and nonphysical boundaries, governs body surface, defends against pathogens or emotional insult

TCM: Facilitates free passage of or is an avenue for source qi; three spaces in the body that need to be warm and allow for transformation:

- Upper heater: Lungs and heart, combines air with food qi ("like a mist")
- Middle heater: Stomach, spleen, processes food into food qi ("like a bubbling caldron")
- Lower heater: Kidney, urinary bladder, small intestine, large intestine; serves to separate the pure from the impure and eliminate waste ("like a drainage ditch," involved in removing waste)

Location: TH starts at TH-1 on the tip of the ulnar side of the fourth finger, $\frac{1}{16}$ inch from the corner of the nail. It travels along the fourth finger's tendon and up the posterior forearm just to the medial side of the. midline. TH then runs over the olecranon process, up through the center of the lateral head of the triceps brachii, and through the posterior deltoid to TH-14 at the acromion process. TH then travels medially along the supraspinatus.

TH then runs up the lateral border of the trapezius to the occiput. From the most lateral edge of the occiput, TH branches anteriorly toward the face to under the earlobe. It circles laterally around the earlobe to where the earlobe attaches to the head, then rises superiorly to TH-22 on the most lateral aspect of the zygomatic arch. TH crosses in a straight line to end at TH-23, on the lateral end of the eyebrow.

Appendix B

ANATOMY AND KINESIOLOGY REVIEW*

UPPER REGION OF THE POSTERIOR BODY

Trapezius

Attachments: Occiput, nuchal ligament, and the spinous processes of C7 through T12 to the lateral third of the clavicle, acromion process, and spine of the scapula

Actions:

- Upper trapezius–elevates, retracts, and upwardly rotates the scapula; extends, laterally flexes, and contralaterally rotates the head and neck
- Middle trapezius–retracts the scapula
- Lower trapezius–depresses, retracts, and upwardly rotates the scapula

Supraspinatus (Rotator Cuff Muscle)

Attachments: Supraspinous fossa of the scapula to the greater tubercle of the humerus

Actions: Abducts and flexes the arm at the shoulder joint

Infraspinatus (Rotator Cuff Muscle)

Attachments: Infraspinous fossa of the scapula to the greater tubercle of the humerus

Actions: Laterally rotates the arm at the shoulder joint

Teres Minor (Rotator Cuff Muscle)

Attachments: Superior two thirds of the lateral border of the scapula to the greater tubercle of the humerus

Actions: Laterally rotates and adducts the arm at the shoulder joint

Subscapularis (Rotator Cuff Muscle)

Attachments: Subscapular fossa of the scapula to the lesser tubercle of the humerus

Actions: Medially rotates the arm at the shoulder joint

Teres Major

Attachments: Inferior angle and inferior third of the lateral border of the scapula to the medial lip of the bicipital groove of the humerus

Actions: Medially rotates, adducts, and extends the arm at the shoulder joint; upwardly rotates the scapula

Rhomboids

Attachments: Spinous processes of C7-T5 to the medial border of the scapula from the root of the spine to the inferior angle

Actions: Retracts, elevates, and downwardly rotates the scapula

MID AND LOW BACK REGION OF THE POSTERIOR BODY

Latissimus Dorsi

Attachments: Spinous processes of T7-L5, posterior sacrum, and the posterior iliac crest (all via the thoracolumbar fascia) to the lowest three to four ribs and the inferior angle of the scapula to the medial lip of the bicipital grooves of the humerus

Actions: Extends, adducts, and medially rotates the arm at the shoulder joint; anteriorly tilts the pelvis via its attachment to the scapula; depresses the scapula

Erector Spinae Group

Attachments: Onto the pelvis, spine, rib cage, and head

Actions: Extends, laterally flexes, and ipsilaterally rotates the trunk, neck, and head; anteriorly tilts and elevates the pelvis

Quadratus Lumborum

Attachments: Twelfth rib and the transverse processes of L1-L4 to the posteriomedial iliac crest

Actions: Elevates and anteriorly tilts the pelvis; extends and laterally flexes the trunk; depresses the twelfth rib

Gluteus Maximus

Attachments: Posterior iliac crest, posteriolateral sacrum, and the coccyx to the gluteal tuberosity of the femur and the iliotibial band

Actions:

- Entire muscle–extends and laterally rotates the thigh at the hip joint, posteriorly tilts the pelvis at the hip joint
- Upper fibers–abduct the thigh at the hip joint
- Lower fibers–adduct the thigh at the hip joint

Gluteus Medius

Attachments: External surface of the ilium to the lateral surface of the greater trochanter of the femur

*The information in this appendix is from *The Muscle and Bone Palpation Manual, with Trigger Points, Referral Patterns, and Stretching* by Joseph E. Muscolino (St. Louis, 2009, Mosby).

Actions:
- Posterior fibers–abduct, extend, and laterally rotate the thigh at the hip joint; posteriorly tilt and depress the same side of the pelvis at the hip joint
- Middle fibers–abduct the thigh at the hip joint, depress the same side of the pelvis at the hip joint
- Anterior fibers–abduct, flex, and medially rotate the thigh at the hip joint; anteriorly tilt and depress the same side of the pelvis at the hip joint

NECK AND HEAD

Trapezius

Attachments: Occiput, nuchal ligament, and the spinous processes of C7 through T12 to the lateral third of the clavicle, acromion process, and spine of the scapula

Actions:
- Upper trapezius–elevates, retracts, and upwardly rotates the scapula; extends, laterally flexes, and contralaterally rotates the head and neck
- Middle trapezius–retracts the scapula
- Lower trapezius–depresses, retracts, and upwardly rotates the scapula

Sternocleidomastoid (SCM)

Attachments: Manubrium of the sternum and the medial third of the clavicle to the mastoid process of the skull and the lateral half of the occiput

Actions: Flexes the lower neck and extends the head and upper neck, laterally flexes and contralaterally rotates the head and neck, elevates the sternum and clavicle

Splenius Capitis

Attachments: Nuchal ligament from the level of C3-C6 and the spinous processes of C7-T4 to the mastoid process of the skull and the lateral third of the superior nuchal line of the occiput

Actions: Extends, laterally flexes, and ipsilaterally rotates the head and neck

Splenius Cervicis

Attachments: Spinous processes of C3-C6 to the posterior tubercles of the transverse processes of the C1-3

Actions: Extends, laterally flexes, and ipsilaterally rotates the head and neck

Semispinalis Capitis

Attachments: Transverse processes of C7-T6 and articular processes of C4-6 to the medial half of the occipital bones between the superior and inferior nuchal lines

Actions: Extends and laterally flexes the head and neck

Scalenes

Attachments: First and second ribs to the transverse processes of C2-C7

Actions: Flex, laterally flex, and contralaterally rotate the neck; elevate the first and second ribs

Suboccipital Group

Rectus capitis posterior major (RCPMaj)
Rectus capitis posterior minor (RCPMin)
Obliquus capitis inferior (OCI)
Obliquus capitis superior (OCS)

Attachments:
- RCPMaj–spinous processes of C2 to the lateral half of the inferior nuchal line of the occiput
- RCPMin–posterior tubercle of C1 to the medial half of the inferior nuchal line of the occiput
- OCI–spinous processes of C2 to the transverse process of C1
- OCS–transverse process of C1 to the lateral occiput between the superior and inferior nuchal lines

Actions: Extend and anteriorly translate the head at the atlanto-occipital joint; OCI ispsilaterally rotates the atlas at the atlantoaxial joint

Levator Scapula

Attachments: Transverse processes of C1-C4 to the medial border of the scapula from the root of the spine to the superior angle

Actions: Elevates and downwardly rotates the scapula; extends, laterally flexes, and ipsilaterally rotates the neck

ARMS AND HANDS

Deltoid

Attachments: Lateral third of the clavicle, acromion process, and spine of the scapula to the deltoid tuberosity of the humerus

Actions:
- Entire muscle–abducts the arm at the shoulder joint, downwardly rotates the scapula
- Anterior deltoid–flexes, medially rotates, and horizontally flexes (horizontally abducts) the arm at the shoulder joint
- Posterior deltoid–extends, laterally rotates, and horizontally extends (horizontally adducts) the arm at the shoulder joint

Triceps Brachii

Attachments:
- Long head–infraglenoid tubercle of the scapula, lateral and medial heads–posterior shaft of the humerus to the olecranon process of the ulna

Actions:
- Entire muscle–extends the forearm at the elbow joint
- Long head–adducts and extends the arm at the shoulder joint

Biceps Brachii

Attachments:
- Long head–supraglenoid tubercle of the scapula, short head–coracoid process of the scapula to the radial

tuberosity and the deep fascia overlying the common flexor tendon

Actions:

- Entire muscle—flexes the forearm at the elbow joint, supinates the forearm, flexes the arm at the shoulder joint
- Long head—abducts the arm at the shoulder joint
- Short head—adducts the arm at the shoulder joint

Brachialis

Attachments: Distal half of the anterior shaft of the humerus to the tuberosity and coronoid process of the ulna

Actions: Flexes the forearm at the elbow joint

Brachioradialis

Attachments: Proximal two thirds of the lateral supracondylar ridge of the humerus to the styloid process of the radius

Actions: Flexes the forearm at the elbow joint

Pronator Teres

Attachments: Medial epicondyles of the humerus (via the common flexor tendon), the medial supracondylar ridge of the humerus, and the coronoid process of the ulna to the middle third of the lateral radius

Actions: Pronates the forearm and flexes the forearm at the elbow joint

Pronator Quadratus

Attachments: Anteriomedial surface of the distal fourth of the ulna to the anteriolateral surface of the distal fourth of the radius

Actions: Pronation of the forearm

Supinator

Attachments: Lateral epicondyle of the humerus and supinator crest of the ulna to the proximal third of the radius

Actions: Supinates the forearm

Wrist Flexor Group (Anterior Forearm)

Flexor carpi radialis, palmaris longus, flexor carpi ulnaris

Attachments:

- Proximal attachments—all three wrist flexors attach to the medial epicondyle of the humerus via the common flexor tendon; flexor carpi ulnaris also attaches to the proximal two thirds of the ulna
- Distal attachments—flexor carpi radialis attaches to the radial side of the anterior hand at the bases of the second and third metacarpals; palmaris longus attaches into the palmar aponeurosis of the palm of the hand; flexor carpi ulnaris attaches to the ulnar side of the base of the hand at the fifth metacarpal, the pisiform, and the hook of the hamate

Actions:

- All three wrist flexors—flex the wrist joint; flexor carpi radialis—radial deviation of the hand; flexor carpi ulnaris—ulnar deviation of the hand

Flexor Digitorum Superficialis

Attachments: Medial epicondyle of the humerus (via the common flexor tendon), coronoid process of the ulna and the proximal half of the anterior shaft of the radius to the anterior surfaces of the middle phalanges of fingers 2-5

Actions: Flexes fingers 2-5 at the metacarpophalangeal and proximal interphalangeal joints, flexes the wrist, and flexes the forearm at the elbow joint

Flexor Digitorum Profundus

Attachments: Proximal half of the anterior surface of the ulna and the interosseus membrane to the anterior surfaces of the distal phalanges of fingers 2-5

Actions: Flexes fingers 2-5 at the metacarpophalangeal and distal interphalangeal joints, flexes the wrist

Flexor Pollicis Longus

Attachments: Anterior surface of the distal radius and the interosseus membrane, the coronoid process of the ulna, and the medial epicondyle of the humerus to the anterior surface of the base of the distal phalanx of the thumb

Actions: Flexes the thumb at the carpometacarpal, metacarpophalangeal, and the interphalangeal joints; flexes the wrist; flexes the forearm at the elbow joint

Forearm Extensor Group (Posterior Forearm)

Extensor carpi radialis longus, extensor carpi radialis brevis, extensor carpi ulnaris, extensor digitorum, extensor digiti minimi

Attachments:

- Proximal attachments—extensor carpi radialis longus attaches to the distal third of the lateral supracondylar ridge of the humerus; the other four wrist extenders attach to the lateral epicondyle of the humerus via the common extensor tendon
- Distal attachments—extensor carpi radialis longus attaches to the radial side of the posterior hand at the base of the second metacarpal; extensor carpi radialis brevis attaches to the posterior hand at the base of the third metacarpal; extensor carpi ulnaris attaches to the ulnar side of the posterior hand at the base of the fifth metacarpal; extensor digitorum attaches to the posterior surface of the middle and distal phalanges of digits 2-5; extensor digiti minimi attaches to the posterior surface of the middle and distal phalanges of the fifth finger

Actions: All five wrist extensors extend the wrist joint

- Extensor carpi radialis longus and brevis—radial deviation of the hand and flex the forearm at the elbow joint
- Extensor carpi ulnaris—ulnar deviation of the hand and extends the forearm at the elbow joint
- Extensor digitorum—extends fingers 2-5 at the metacarpophalangeal and interphalangeal joints and extends the forearm at the elbow joint
- Extensor digiti minimi—extends finger 5 at the metacarpophalangeal and interphalangeal joints and extends the forearm at the elbow joint

Answers to Study Questions

CHAPTER 1

Multiple Choice

1. b
2. c
3. a
4. d
5. d

Fill in the Blank

1. 10, 30
2. 5,000
3. emotional, psychological
4. channels or meridians
5. time, money, modesty

CHAPTER 2

Multiple Choice

1. d
2. b
3. c
4. a
5. b

Fill in the Blank

1. return on investment costs
2. 15, 22
3. Body mechanics
4. hygiene, sanitation
5. calm

CHAPTER 3

Multiple Choice

1. b
2. c
3. a
4. d
5. b

Fill in the Blank

1. straight, larger, breathe
2. straight through, angle
3. 90-degree
4. circular, deep specific
5. cautionary sites or endangerment sites

CHAPTER 4

Multiple Choice

1. c
2. a
3. d
4. a
5. b

Fill in the Blank

1. tsubo
2. quadratus lumborum
3. noodling
4. scalenes, pectoralis minor
5. GB-21, LI-4

CHAPTER 5

Multiple Choice

1. a
2. c
3. d
4. d
5. a

Fill in the Blank

1. 7 to 10
2. pin-and-stretch
3. pretreatment interview
4. self-posture
5. kneel

CHAPTER 6

Multiple Choice

1. b
2. a
3. d
4. c
5. a

Fill in the Blank

1. independent contractor
2. business plan
3. well-being or health
4. information
5. contact person

CHAPTER 7

Multiple Choice

1. c
2. b
3. c
4. d
5. a

Fill in the Blank

1. professional presentation
2. therapeutic relationship
3. professional attire
4. feedback
5. claustrophobic

References

Abercromby P, Thomson D: *Seated Acupressure Massage,* Chichester, England, 2001, Corpus Publishing.

Adler RB, Rodman G: *Understanding Human Communication,* ed 10, New York, 2009, Oxford University Press.

American Massage Therapy Association: *2008 Massage Therapy Industry Fact Sheet.* Retrieved October 7, 2008, from http://amtamassage.org/news/MTIndustryFactSheet.html#2.

Anderson SK: *The Practice of Shiatsu,* St. Louis, MO, 2008, Mosby Elsevier.

Barker LL, Gaut DR: *Communication,* ed 8, Boston, 2002, Allyn & Bacon.

Benjamin BE, Sohnen-Moe C: *The Ethics of Touch,* Tucson, AZ, 2005, Sohnen-Moe Associates.

Benjamin PJ: *A Look Back. High Plinth, Low Plinth: Some Bodywork Tables from The Past,* 2001. Retrieved December 1, 2008, from www.amtamassage.org/journal/sp_01_journal/alookback.htm.

Benjamin PJ: *A look back: Seated massage in history,* Massage Therapy Journal, Spring 2003. Retrieved December 1, 2008, from www.amtamassage.org/journal/spring03_journal/LookBack.pdf.

Benjamin PR: *Seated massage in history,* Massage Therapy Journal, Spring 2003. Retrieved November 24, 2008, from www.amtamassage.org/journal/spring03_journal/LookBack.pdf.

Benjamin PJ, Tappan FM: *Tappan's Handbook of Healing Massage Techniques,* ed 4, Upper Saddle River, NJ, 2005, Pearson Prentice Hall.

Beresford-Cooke C: *Shiatsu Theory and Practice: A Comprehensive Text for the Student and Professional,* ed 2, Philadelphia, 2003, Churchill Livingstone.

Bilz FE: *The Natural Method of Healing,* Leipzeig, 1898, FE Bilz.

Bureau of Labor Statistics, U.S. Department of Labor, *Survey of Occupational Injuries and Illnesses in Cooperation with Participating State Agencies.* Retrieved May 12, 2009, from http://www.bls.gov/iif/oshwc/osh/case/osnr0031.pdf.

Bureau of Labor Statistics, U.S. Department of Labor, *Survey of Occupational Injuries and Illnesses in Cooperation with Participating State Agencies.* Retrieved May 12, 2009, from http://www.bls.gov/iif/oshwc/osh/case/ostb1973.pdf.

Bureau of Labor Statistics, U.S. Department of Labor, *Survey of Occupational Injuries and Illnesses in Cooperation with Participating State Agencies.* Retrieved May 12, 2009, from http://www.bls.gov/iif/oshwc/osh/case/ostb1954.txt.

Calvert RN: *The History of Massage,* Rochester, VT, 2002, Healing Arts Press.

Calvert RN: *Pages from History: The Massage Chair,* 2002. Retrieved December 26, 2008, from www.massagemag.com/Magazine/2002/issue97/history97.php.

Clay JH, Pounds DM: *Basic Clinical Massage Therapy: Integrating Anatomy and Treatment,* ed 2, Baltimore, MD, 2006, Lippincott, Williams & Wilkins.

Corey G, Corey MS, Callanan P: *Issues and Ethics in the Helping Professions,* ed 7, Belmont, CA, 2007, Brooks/Cole.

Dixon MW: *Body Mechanics and Self-Care Manual,* Upper Saddle River, NJ, 2001, Prentice-Hall.

Fritz S: *Essential Sciences for Therapeutic Massage,* ed 3, St. Louis, MO, 2009, Mosby Elsevier.

Fritz S: *Fundamentals of Therapeutic Massage,* ed 4, St. Louis, MO, 2009, Mosby Elsevier.

Frye B: *Body Mechanics for Manual Therapists,* ed 3, Baltimore, MD, 2010, Lippincott, Williams & Wilkins.

Gold R: *Thai Massage,* ed 2, St. Louis, MO, 2007, Mosby Elsevier.

Greene L, Goggins RW: *Save Your Hands!* ed 2, Coconut Creek, FL, 2008, Body of Work Books.

Lowe WW: *Orthopedic Massage: Theory & Technique,* St. Louis, MO, 2003, Elsevier Health Sciences.

McIntosh N: *The Educated Heart,* ed 2, Baltimore, MD, 2005, Lippincott, Williams & Wilkins.

Mihina AL, Anderson SK: *Natural Spa and Hydrotherapy,* Upper Saddle River, NJ, 2010, Pearson Education.

Muscolino JE: *The Muscle and Bone Palpation Manual with Trigger Points, Referral Patterns, and Stretching,* St. Louis, MO, 2009, Mosby, Elsevier.

Muscolino JE: *The Muscular System Manual,* ed 2, St. Louis, MO, 2005, Mosby, Elsevier.

Neumann DA, Wong DL: *Kinesiology of the Musculoskeletal System: Foundations for Physical Rehabilitation,* St. Louis, MO, 2002, Elsevier Science.

Oatis CA: *Kinesiology: The Mechanics and Pathomechanics of Human Movement,* ed 2, Baltimore, MD, 2008, Lippincott, Williams & Wilkins.

Palmer D: *Chair Massage History,* 2001-2004. Retrieved June 27, 2008, from www.TouchPro Institute.org: www.touchpro.org/about_touchpro/chair_massage_history.html.

Parfitt A: *Seated Acupressure Bodywork,* Berkeley, CA, 2006, North Atlantic Books.

Roth M: *The Prevention and Cure of Many Chronic Diseases by Movements,* London, England, 1851, John Churchill.

Salguero CP: *Encylopedia of Thai Massage,* Scotland, 2004, Findhorn Press.

Sohnen-Moe CM: *Business Mastery,* ed 4, Tucson, AZ, 2008, Sohnen-Moe Associates.

Stephens RR: *Therapeutic Chair Massage,* Baltimore, MD, 2006, Lippincott, Williams &. Wilkins.

Thompson DL: *Hands Heal,* ed 3, Baltimore, MD, 2005, Lippincott, Williams & Wilkins.

Tortora GJ, Derrickson B: *Principles of Anatomy and Physiology,* ed 12, Hoboken, NJ, 2008, John Wiley & Sons.

TouchPro Institute: *Founder: David Palmer,* 2008. Retrieved June 27, 2008, from www.touchpro.org: www.touchpro.org/about_touchpro/david_palmer.html.

Werner R: *A Massage Therapist's Guide to Pathology,* ed 4, Baltimore, MD, 2008, Lippincott, Williams & Wilkins.

Resources

MASSAGE CHAIR AND DESKTOP MASSAGE SUPPORT MANUFACTURERS AND DISTRIBUTORS

Earthlite
3210 Executive Ridge Drive
Vista, CA 92081
Phone: (800) 872-0560 (toll-free), (760) 599-1112
Fax: (760) 599-7374
Email: info@earthlite.com
www.earthlite.com

Living Earth Crafts
3210 Executive Ridge Drive
Vista, CA 92081
Phone: (800) 358-8292 (toll-free), (760) 597-2155
Email: sales@livingearthcrafts.com
www.livingearthcrafts.com

Oakworks
Mailing address: P.O. Box 238
Shrewsbury, PA 17361
Location address: 923 E. Wellspring Road
New Freedom, PA 17349
Phone: (800) 558-8850 (toll-free)
Fax: (717) 235-6798
Email: skrout@oakworks.com
www.oakworks.com

Pisces Production
380 A Morris Street
Sebastopol, CA 95472
Phone: (800) 822-5333 (toll-free)
International phone: (707) 829-1496
Fax: (707) 829-3491
Email: info@piscespro.com
www.piscespro.com

Stronglite, Inc.
369 S. Orange Street, #7
Salt Lake City, UT 84104
Phone: (800) 289-5487 (toll-free)
Fax: (801) 886-1411
Email: sales@stronglite.com
www.stronglite.com

Touch America
P.O. Box 1304
437 Dimmocks Mill Road
Hillsborough, NC 27278
Phone: (800) 678-6824 (toll-free)
International phone: (919) 732-6968
Fax: (919) 732-1173
Email: info@touchamerica.com
www.touchamerica.com

NRG ENERGY MASSAGE TABLES

Massage King
3827 W. Pinhook Road
Broussard, LA 70518
Phone: (800) 290-3932 (toll-free)
Email: sales@massageking.com
www.massageking.com

Massage Warehouse
360 Veterans Parkway, Suite 115
Bolingbrook, IL 60440-4607
Phone: (800) 910-9955 (toll-free), (630) 771-7400
Fax: (888) 674-4380 (toll-free)
Email: support@massagewarehouse.com
www.massagewarehouse.com

Midas Massage
22 Stewart Avenue
Beverly, MA 01915
Phone: (978) 921-2822
Email: sales@midasmassage.com
www.midasmassage.com

MEMBERSHIP WAREHOUSE CLUBS

Costco
999 Lake Drive
Issaquah, WA 98027
Phone: (800) 955-2292 (toll-free)
Email: customerservice@costco.com
www.costco.com

Sam's Club
Member Services
608 S.W. Eighth Street
Bentonville, AR 72716
Phone: (888) 746-7726 (toll-free)
www.samsclub.com

MASSAGE SUPPLIES

Antibacterial/Germicidal Wipes

Keysan
5100 North Ocean Blvd, #1114
Fort Lauderdale, FL 33308
Phone: (800) 969-5397 (toll-free)
Fax: (888) 834-9090 (toll-free)
Email: sales@keysan.com
www.keysan.com

MedRep Express
1289 Manzanita Hill Road
Prescott, AZ 86303
Phone: (877) 740-9133 (toll-free), (928) 445-2623
Fax: (800) 710-1559 (toll-free)
Email: sales@medrepexpress.com
www.medrepexpress.com

NextTag, Inc.
1300 South El Camino Real, Suite 600
San Mateo, CA 94402
Phone: (650) 645-4700
Fax: (650) 341-3779
Email: buyersupport@nextag.com
www.nextag.com

GENERAL MASSAGE SUPPLIES

Massage Depot
1736 Whitewood Lane
Herndon, VA 20170
Phone: (800) 466-1448 (toll-free)
Fax: (703) 991-8011
Email: service@massagedepot.com
www.massagedepot.com

Massage King
3827 W. Pinhook Road
Broussard, LA 70518
Phone: (800) 290-3932 (toll-free)
Email: sales@massageking.com
www.massageking.com

Massage-Tools
200 Valley Drive, #36
Brisbane, CA 94005
Phone: (866) 928-9955 (toll-free)
Email: info@massage-tools.com
www.massage-tools.com

Massage Warehouse
360 Veterans Parkway, Suite 115
Bolingbrook, IL 60440-4607
Phone: (800) 910-9955 (toll-free), (630) 771-7400
Fax: (888) 674-4380 (toll-free)
Email: support@massagewarehouse.com
www.massagewarehouse.com

Sunset Park Massage Supplies
4344 S. Manhattan Avenue
Tampa, FL 33611
Phone: (800) 344-7677 (toll-free), (813) 835-7900
Fax: (813) 835-7990
Email: sales@massagesupplies.com
www.massagesupplies.com

BUSINESS AND MARKETING

Brochures, Business Cards, Gift Certificates

American Massage Therapy Association (AMTA)
500 Davis Street, Suite 900
Evanston, IL 60201-4695
Phone: (877) 905-2700 (toll-free), (847) 864-0123
Fax: (847) 864-5196
Email: info@amtamassage.org
www.amtamassage.org

Massage King
3827 W. Pinhook Road
Broussard, LA 70518
Phone: (800) 290-3932 (toll-free)
Email: sales@massageking.com
www.massageking.com

Massage Warehouse
360 Veterans Parkway, Suite 115
Bolingbrook, IL 60440-4607
Phone: (800) 910-9955 (toll-free), (630) 771-7400
Fax: (888) 674-4380 (toll-free)
Email: support@massagewarehouse.com
www.massagewarehouse.com

Natural Touch Marketing for the Healing Arts
P.O. Box 1038
Olympia, WA 98507-1038
Phone: (800) 754-9790 (toll-free), (360) 754-9799
Fax: (360) 705-3864
Email: info@naturaltouchmarketing.com
www.naturaltouchmarketing.com

Sharper
110 Pacific Avenue, Suite 850
San Francisco, CA 94111-1900
Phone: (800) 561-6677 (toll-free)
Fax: (888) 251-4454 (toll-free)
Email: info@e-sharper.com
www.e-sharper.com

Sunset Park Massage Supplies
4344 S. Manhattan Avenue
Tampa, FL 33611
Phone: (800) 344-7677 (toll-free), (813) 835-7900
Fax: (813) 835-7990
Email: sales@massagesupplies.com
www.massagesupplies.com

VistaPrint
www.vistaprint.biz

WaterColorsCards
P.O. Box 1186
Biloxi, MS 39533-1186
Phone: (866) 541-5067 (toll-free)
www.watercolorscards.com

Demographics and Trends

American Massage Therapy Association (AMTA)
500 Davis Street, Suite 900
Evanston, IL 60201-4695
Phone: (877) 905-2700 (toll-free), (847) 864-0123
Fax: (847) 864-5196
Email: info@amtamassage.org
www.amtamassage.org

Associated Bodywork and Massage Professionals (ABMP)
25188 Genesee Trail Road, Suite 200
Golden, CO 80401
Phone: (800) 458-2267 (toll-free), (303) 674-8478
Fax: (800) 667-8260 (toll-free)
Email: expectmore@abmp.com
www.abmp.com

National Certification Board for Therapeutic Massage and Bodywork (NCBTMB)
1901 S. Meyers Road, Suite 240
Oakbrook Terrace, IL 60181
Phone: (800) 296-0664 (toll-free), (630) 627-8000
Email: info@ncbtmb.org
www.ncbtmb.org

EDUCATIONAL CHARTS AND HANDOUTS

Elsevier
Customer Service Department
3251 Riverport Lane
Maryland Heights, MO 63043
Phone: (800) 325-4177 (toll-free), (314) 447-8000
Fax: (314) 447-8033
International phone: +1 001-314-447-8000
International fax: +1 001-314-447-8033
Email: usbkinfo@elsevier.com
www.elsevier.com

Kent Health Systems
840 Deltona Boulevard, Suite L
Deltona, FL 32725
Phone: (888) 574-5600 (toll-free)
Email: info@kenthealth.com
www.kenthealth.com

Massage King
3827 W. Pinhook Road
Broussard, LA 70518
Phone: (800) 290-3932 (toll-free)
Email: sales@massageking.com
www.massageking.com

Natural Touch Marketing for the Healing Arts
P.O. Box 1038
Olympia, WA 98507-1038
Phone: (800) 754-9790 (toll-free)
(360) 754-9799
Fax: (360) 705-3864
Email: info@naturaltouchmarketing.com
www.naturaltouchmarketing.com

Stretching Inc.
P.O. Box 767
Palmer Lake, CO 80133
Phone: (800) 333-1307 (toll-free)
Fax: (719) 481-9058
Email: office@stretching.com
www.stretching.com

Sunset Park Massage Supplies
4344 S. Manhattan Avenue
Tampa, FL 33611
Phone: (800) 344-7677 (toll-free), (813) 835-7900
Fax: (813) 835-7990
Email: sales@massagesupplies.com
www.massagesupplies.com

WaterColorsCards
P.O. Box 1186
Biloxi, MS 39533-1186
Phone: (866) 541-5067 (toll-free)
www.watercolorscards.com

ORGANIZATIONS

Better Business Bureau
The Council of Better Business Bureaus
4200 Wilson Blvd, Suite 800
Arlington, VA 22203-1838
www.bbb.org

Small Business Administration
409 3rd Street, SW
Washington, DC 20416
Phone: (800) 827-5722 (toll-free)
Email: answerdesk@sba.gov
www.sba.gov

The Canadian Council of Better Business Bureaus
2 St. Clair Ave. East
Toronto, ON M4T 2T5
Phone: (703) 276-0100
Fax: (703) 525-8277
www.bbb.org

Toastmasters International
23182 Arroyo Vista
Rancho Santa Margarita, CA 92688
Phone: (949) 858-8255
Fax: (949) 858-1207
www.toastmasters.org.

U.S. Bureau of Labor Statistics, U.S. Department of Labor
2 Massachusetts Avenue, NE
Washington, DC 20212-0001
Phone: (202) 691-5200
www.bls.gov

SOFTWARE PROGRAMS

Massage King
3827 W. Pinhook Road
Broussard, LA 70518
Phone: (800) 290-3932 (toll-free)
Email: sales@massageking.com
www.massageking.com

Massage Warehouse
360 Veterans Parkway, Suite 115
Bolingbrook, IL 60440-4607
Phone: (800) 910-9955 (toll-free)
Fax: (630) 771-7400
Email: support@massagewarehouse.com
www.massagewarehouse.com

Natural Touch Marketing for the Healing Arts
P.O. Box 1038
Olympia, WA 98507-1038
Phone: (800) 754-9790 (toll-free), (360) 754-9799
Fax: (360) 705-3864
Email: info@naturaltouchmarketing.com
www.naturaltouchmarketing.com

Sunset Park Massage Supplies
4344 S. Manhattan Avenue
Tampa, FL 33611
Phone: (800) 344-7677 (toll-free), (813) 835-7900
Fax: (813) 835-7990
Email: sales@massagesupplies.com
www.massagesupplies.com

TARGETED MAILING LISTS

American Heritage Data Corporation
Phone: (888) 916-3282 (toll-free)
www.heritagelists.com

Leadsplease
Phone: (866) 306 8674 (toll-free)
www.leadsplease.com

Marketing Comparison
Phone: (866) 461-0519 (toll-free)
www.marketingcomparison.com

MODALITIES ADJUNCT TO CHAIR MASSAGE

Healing Touch
Healing Touch International, Inc.
445 Union Blvd, Suite 105
Lakewood, CO 80228
Phone: (303) 989-7982
Fax: (303) 980-8683 fax
Email: director@healingtouchinternational.org
www.healingtouchinternational.org

Jin Shin Jyutsu, Inc.
8719 E. San Alberto Drive
Scottsdale, AZ 85258
Phone: (480) 998-9331
Fax: (480) 998-9335
Email: info@jsjinc.com
www.jsjinc.net

Polarity
American Polarity Therapy Association
122 N. Elm Street, Suite 512
Greensboro, NC 27401
Phone: (336) 574-1121
Fax: (336) 574-1151
Email: APTAoffices@polaritytherapy.org
www.polaritytherapy.org

Reiki
The International Center for Reiki Training
21421 Hilltop Street, Unit #28
Southfield, MI 48033
Phone: (800) 332-8112 (toll-free), (248) 948-8112
Fax: (248) 948-9534
Email: center@reiki.org
www.reiki.org

Shiatsu
American Organization for Bodywork Therapies of Asia
1010 Haddonfield-Berlin Road, Suite 408
Voorhees, NJ 08043-3514
Phone: (856) 782-1616
Fax: (856) 782-1653
Email: office@aobta.org
www.aobta.org

Thai Massage (Yoga Massage, Thai Yoga, Ancient Massage)
The Ancient Massage Foundation
Located in Kathmandu
Email: mailserver@ancientmassage.com
www.ancientmassage.com

Tuina (Tui-Na)
The World Tui-Na Association
3409 W. Burbank Boulevard
Burbank, CA 91505
Phone: (818) 848-1111
Email: WorldTuiNa@aol.com
www.tui-na.com

HEALTH ORGANIZATIONS

American Red Cross National Headquarters
2025 E Street, NW
Washington, DC 20006
Phone: (202) 303-5000
www.redcross.org

Centers for Disease Control and Prevention (CDC)
1600 Clifton Rd, Atlanta, GA 30333
Phone: (800) CDC-INFO (800-232-4636) (toll-free)
Email: cdcinfo@cdc.gov
www.cdc.gov

ASSOCIATIONS

American Massage Therapy Association (AMTA)
500 Davis Street, Suite 900
Evanston, IL 60201-4695
Phone: (877) 905-2700 (toll-free), (847) 864-0123
Fax: (847) 864-5196
Email: info@amtamassage.org
www.amtamassage.org

Associated Bodywork and Massage Professionals (ABMP)
25188 Genesee Trail Road, Suite 200
Golden, CO 80401
Phone (800) 458-2267 (toll-free), (303) 674-8478
Fax: (800) 667-8260 (toll-free)
Email: expectmore@abmp.com
www.abmp.com

National Certification Board for Therapeutic Massage and Bodywork (NCBTMB)
1901 S. Meyers Road, Suite 240
Oakbrook Terrace, IL 60181
Phone: (800) 296-0664 (toll-free), (630) 627-8000
Email: info@ncbtmb.org
www.ncbtmb.org

ONLINE INFORMATION SITES

Massage School Notes
www.thebodyworker.com

MassageResource.com
www.massageresource.com

U

V

W

Y

Index

N

O

P

Q